# The Research and Biology of Cancer II

The Research and Biology of Cancer II

Publisher: iConcept Press Ltd.
Cover design: Pineapple Design Ltd.
Interior design: iConcept Press Ltd.
Typesetting and copy editing: iConcept Press Ltd. and Pineapple Design Ltd.

ISBN: 9781922227423

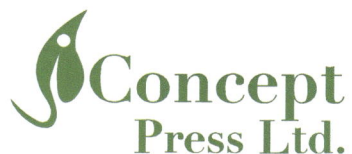

iConcept
Press Ltd.

www.iconceptpress.com

# Contents

# Preface

Cancer is a broad group of diseases involving unregulated cell growth, in which cells divide and grow uncontrollably, forming malignant tumors, and invade nearby parts of the body. Cancer may also spread to different parts of the body through the lymphatic system or the bloodstream. *The Research and Biology of Cancer* discusses some recent advances in cancer research. There are totally two volumes: Volume I mainly discusses the role of some important enzymes and proteins in cancer, whereas Volume II discusses different types of cancers, including head and neck cancer, oral cancer, kidney cancer, colon cancer, and thyroid cancer.

There are totally 11 chapters in this book. Chapter 1 discusses personalised combination therapy targeting PI3K/Akt, STAT3, ERK, and EGFR signalling pathways which may provide clinical benefits for patients with HNSCC. Such therapy is useful because molecular cross-talk between the EGFR and other RTK signalling pathways through PI3K/ Akt, STAT3, and ERK in HNSCCs, EGFR inhibitors alone may be unable to suppress EGFR downstream. Chapter 2 describes tissue based LCM, which is a powerful technique that combines morphology, histopathology, and molecular biological analysis. The ability of LCM to retrieve specific populations of interested cells, combined with the analysis of gene sequencing and gene expression in these sub-population of cells, has made LCM an critical device in clinical and investigative oral oncology. Chapter 3 discussed several aspects about the use of the Micronucleus Test to identify genetic damage in individuals at higher risk of developing oral squamous cell carcinoma and evaluated the malignant transformation potential of precancerous lesions. Chapter 4 aims to picture the landscape of metastatic renal cancer starting from its pathogenesis, molecular markers, prognostic factors, metastatic potential, with emphasis on the recent evolution in the treatment of metastatic renal cancer cases.

Chapter 5 discusses skin-level jejunostomy (SLJ) tube placement technique using the G-tube, which is a safe procedure in patients with esophageal cancer. It allows the creation of a long-term feeding jejunostomy. About 50Chapter introduces polyethylene glycols (PEGs) role as a potential therapeutic agent in decreasing bacteria induced proinvasiveness commonly seen in the event of Inflammatory Bowel Disease (IBD) and/or colon cancer, as well as its role in reestablishing extra cellular matrix (ECM) integrity in an *in-vitro* model of colon cancer. Chapter 7 offers a comprehensive review of the small bowel neoplasms, as well as its varied clinical manifestations, diagnostic challenges and management principles. Chapter 8 reviews the current research efforts to identify biomarkers suitable for non-invasive colon cancer screening.

Chapter 9 conducted a pilot study to determine the safety and feasibility of an early start of chemotherapy after the resection of colorectal cancer with distant metastases. Chemotherapy usually starts after 4 weeks of surgical resection of colorectal cancer. Unfortunately, there is no study on the optimal length of this delay. A patient may die because postoperative chemotherapy was not started soon enough and so a metastatic tumor was able to develop rapidly. This chapter gives a good review of this problem. Chapter 10 focuses on the putative role of intestinal microbiota in the development of colorectal cancer, describing his metabolic functions and relation with diet, and his interaction with host's immunity and with molecular and morpho-functional activity of gastrointestinal tract. Chapter 11 describes an approach used for identification of a novel PPI. It shows that an uncharacterized protein, two-transmembrane protein 88 (TMEM88), is a binding partner of Dishevelled (Dvl/Dsh) by using a combination of techniques, including bioinformatic, biophysical, and biochemical methods.

Editing and publishing a book is never an easy task. Each chapter in this book has gone through a peer review, a selection and an editing process so as to guarantee its quality. Without the supports and contributions of the authors and reviewers, this book can never be able to complete. We would like to thank all of the authors in this book and all of the reviewers who participated in the reviewing process: Akinyele O Adisa, T. Alcindor, Huseyin Alkim, Amedeo Amedei, Toshinori Bito, G Bobe, H. Boyle, Ronald M Bukowski, Ishveen Chopra, Cevdet Duran, Almudena Fernández-Briera, Minoru Fukuchi, Yacine Graba, Jian Gu, Masahiko Inamori, Kiran Jadhav, Anastasios K. Markopoulos, Abdul-Wahed N. Meshikhes, Eva B Ostenfeld, Santosh Kumar Patnaik, Camillo Porta, Takuji Tanaka, Satoshi Tanida, Arianne L. Theiss, Vaneja Velenik, Marco Aurelio Vinolo, J.B. Wallach, Tin Wui Wong, Juanjuan Xiang and N. Zouain. We hope that you, the reader, will find this book interesting and useful. Any advices please feel free and are always welcome to tell us.

iConcept Press Ltd
February 2014

# Overcoming Resistance to EGFR inhibitor in Head and Neck Squamous Cell Carcinoma (HNSCC)

Yuh Baba
*Department of Otolaryngology*
*Nasu Red Cross Hospital, Japan*

Masato Fujii
*National Institute of Sensory Organs*
*National Tokyo Medical Center, Japan*

Yutaka Tokumaru
*National Institute of Sensory Organs*
*National Tokyo Medical Center, Japan*

Yasumasa Kato
*Department of Oral Function & Molecular Biology*
*Ohu University School of Density, Japan*

# 1   Introduction

HNSCC (head and neck squamous cell carcinoma) is the sixth most common neoplasm worldwide, with approximately 600,000 patients newly diagnosed each year (Cripps *et al.*, 2010). Over the past 30 years, patients with recurrent and/or metastatic HNSCC have had a poor prognosis (Forastiere *et al.*, 2001; Khuri *et al.*, 2000). More than 50% of newly diagnosed patients do not achieve complete remission, and approximately 10% relapse with metastasis to distant organs (van Houten *et al.*, 2000). Therefore, research focused on gaining a better understanding of this disease and on the development of novel treatment strategies is required.

Epidermal growth factor receptor (EGFR), a ubiquitously expressed transmembrane glycoprotein belonging to the ErbB/HER family of receptor tyrosine kinases (TK), is composed of an extracellular ligand-binding domain, a hydrophobic transmembrane segment and an intracellular TK domain. Upon ligand binding to EGFR, the latter undergoes a conformational change that promotes homo- or heterodimerization with other members of the ErbB/HER family of receptors, followed by autophosphorylation and activation of the TK domain (Ciardiello & Tortora, 2003). Activation of EGFR leads to activation of intracellular signaling pathways that regulate cell proliferation, invasion, angiogenesis and metastasis.

EGFR is expressed at high levels in the majority of epithelial malignancies including HNSCC (Saranath *et al.*, 1992). Elevated expression of EGFR in HNSCC correlates with poor prognosis, and EGFR has been a target of anticancer treatments due to its critical roles in cell survival and proliferation (Burtness, 2005). Among the tyrosine kinase inhibitors targeting EGFR that have been approved by the U.S. FDA are gefitinib, erlotinib and lapatinib (Carter *et al.*, 2009). These molecules are reversible competitors, competing with adenosine triphosphate (ATP) for the tyrosine kinase binding domain of EGFR. Inhibition of receptor activation inhibits downstream signaling pathways, resulting in decreased cell proliferation and survival. The pathways mediating EGFR downstream effects have been well studied and three major signaling pathways have been identified, with the first involving the RAS-RAF-MAPK pathway. Upon ligation, ErbB receptors are activated. The activated receptor kinase phosphorylates tyrosine residues at the C-terminal end of ErbB receptors, allowing the binding of proteins containing the Src Homology 2 (SH2) domain, including intracellular docking and adaptor proteins, such as Grb2 and Shc. Upon binding to ErbB receptors, these proteins associate with other proteins, leading to the activation of serine-threonine kinases that phosphorylate serine and threonine residues on other protein kinases and/or transcription factors. This kinase cascade leads to the amplification of a network of signaling pathways, resulting in changes in protein function and activation of gene transcription. Mitogen activated protein kinases (MAPKs) are a superfamily of protein serine-threonine kinases, including Erk1/2. ErbB receptors activate Erks by binding to the adaptor protein Grb2, recruiting son of sevenless (SOS) protein to the receptor. SOS is a guanyl nucleotide-release protein (GNRP), which upon recruitment to the plasma membrane by activated cell surface receptors, causes the small G protein RAS to release GDP and bind GTP, resulting in Ras activation. Activation of Ras leads to the activation of the MKKK Raf-1, which, in turn, phosphorylates and activates the MKK Mek1/2. Activated Mek1/2 then phosphorylates and activates Erk1/2. This cascade results in the phosphorylation of a variety of substrates including 90 kDa ribosomal S6 protein kinase (Rsk), Msk1, cytosolic phospholipase A2, and the transcription factors c-Myc, NF-IL6, Tal-1, Ets-2, and Elk. This results in enhanced gene transcription and increased cellproliferation.

The second major signaling pathway mediating EGFR downstream effects is the PI3K/AKT pathway, which activates the major cellular survival and anti-apoptosis signals via activating nuclear transcription factors such as nuclear factor-kappa B (NF-kB), whereas the third major signaling pathway is the JAK/STAT pathway, which has also been implicated in activating the transcription of genes associated with cell survival.

## 2 Rare EGFR Mutations in HNSCC

Somatic mutations in the TK domain of the EGFR gene, including in-frame deletions in exon 19 and the point mutations L858, G719X and L861Q, have been associated with increased sensitivity to EGFR TK inhibitors (TKIs) and are present in 10~30% of patients with non-small cell lung carcinoma (NSCLC), depending on ethnic origin. These mutant EGFRs selectively activate the signal transduction and activator of transcription (STAT) and Akt signaling pathways, which promote cell survival. However, they have no effect on extracellular signal-regulated kinase (ERK) signaling, which induces cell proliferation. Furthermore, mutant EGFRs selectively transduce survival signals, and inhibition of these signals may contribute to the efficacy of TKIs used to treat NSCLC (Sordella *et al.*, 2004). However, molecular analysis of HNSCC tumor samples has not revealed the same spectrum of mutations (Loeffler-Ragg *et al.*, 2006; Ozawa *et al.*, 2009; Taguchi *et al.*, 2008).

One important resistance mutation in EGFR is the T790M missense mutation in the kinase domain, which may contribute to TKI resistance in NSCLCs possessing the L858R point mutation (Wong, 2008). Using the cycleave PCR method, however, we failed to detect the T790M mutation in 86 HNSCC tumor samples (Baba *et al.*, 2012).

## 3 Resistance to EGFR TKIs

EGFR TKIs have had limited results in patients with HNSCC. For example, a phase II trial of gefitinib in patients with recurrent or metastatic HNSCC showed an overall response rate of 11% (Cohen *et al.*, 2003). Similarly, a study of erlotinib in patients with recurrent and/or metastatic HNSCC showed a response rate of 4% (Soulieres *et al.*, 2004). Four mechanisms have been proposed to explain tumor resistance to EGFR TKIs.

1. ***Ras* mutations** K-*ras* mutations may cause tumor insensitivity to EGFR TKIs. Activating K-*ras* mutations may activate the Ras/mitogen activated protein kinase (MAPK) pathway independent of EGFR, thus inducing resistance to EGFR TKIs (Eberhard *et al.*, 2005). H-*ras* mutations are more common than K-*ras* mutations in HNSCC and may play an important role in tumor resistance to EGFR-targeted therapies (Anderson *et al.*, 1994).

2. **Epithelial-mesenchymal transition (EMT)** EMT results in changes in cell morphology and motility and is indicated by increased expression of vimentin and claudins 4 and 7 and by decreased expression of E-cadherin. EMT has been associated with gefitinib resistance in HNSCC (Frederick *et al.*, 2007).

3. **Upregulation of cyclin D1** Upregulation of cyclin D1 in HNSCC cell lines has been specifically associated with resistance to gefitinib. Upregulation of cyclin D1 results in the activation of cyclin D1-cyclin dependent kinase 4 (CDK4), which hyperphosphorylates retinoblastoma protein (pRb)(Kalish *et al.*, 2004).

4. **PI3K/Akt signaling as a dominant pathway** Increased expression of cortactin, a protein that increases the formation of actin networks critical to cell motility and receptor-mediated endocytosis, has been associated with gefitinib resistance and increased metastasis in HNSCC (Timpson *et al.*, 2007).

Akt has been implicated in EMT by integrin-linked kinase (ILK). The PI3K/Akt pathway not only regulates the transcriptional activity of cyclin D1, but increases its accumulation by inactivating glycogen synthase kinase-3 (GSK3), an enzyme that targets cyclin D1 for proteasomal degradation. Cortactin is thought to promote cancer cell proliferation by activating Akt (Timpson *et al.*, 2007), suggesting that factors related to resistance to EGFR TKIs are associated with the PI3K/Akt pathway.

# 4    PI3K/Akt Pathway

In this section, we will explain the activation of the PI3K/AKT pathway, its downstream effectors, and the rationale for targeting this pathway in HNSCC.

## 4.1    Activation of the PI3K/Akt Pathway

Signaling through the PI3K/Akt pathway can be initiated by several mechanisms. Once activated, this pathway can be propagated to various substrates, including mTOR, a master regulator of protein translation. The PI3K/Akt pathway is initially activated at the cell membrane, where the signal for activation is propagated through class IA PI3K. Activation of PI3K can occur through tyrosine kinase growth factor receptors such as EGFR and insulin-like growth factor-1 receptor (IGF-1R), cell adhesion molecules such as integrins, G-protein-coupled receptors (GPCRS) and oncogenes such as Ras. PI3K catalyzes the phosphorylation of the D3 position on phosphoinositides, generating the biologically active moieties phosphatidylinositol-3,4,5-triphosphate (PI(3,4,5)P3) and phosphatidylinositol-3,4-bisphosphate (PI(3,4)P2).

PI(3,4,5)P3 binds to the pleckstrin homology (PH) domains of 3'-phosphoinositide-dependent kinase 1 (PDK-1) and Akt, resulting in the translocation of these proteins to the cell membrane, where they are subsequently activated. The tumor suppressor phosphatase and tensin homolog deleted on chromosome ten (PTEN) antagonizes PI3kinase by dephosphorylating PI (3,4,5)P3 and (PI(3,4)P2), thereby preventing the activation of Akt and PDK-1. Akt exists as three structurally similar isoforms, Akt1, Akt2 and Akt3, which are expressed in most tissues. Activation of Akt1 occurs through two crucial phosphorylation events. The first, catalyzed by PDK-1, occurs at T308 in the catalytic domain of Akt1. Full activation requires a subsequent phosphorylation at S473 in the hydrophobic motif of Akt1, a reaction mediated by several kinases, including PDK-1, ILK, Akt itself, DNA-dependent protein kinase and mTOR; phosphorylation of homologous residues in Akt2 and Akt3 occurs by the same mechanism. Phosphorylation of Akt at S473 is controlled by a recently described phosphatase, PH domain leucine-rich repeat protein phosphatase (PHLPP), which has two isoforms that preferentially decrease the activation of specific Akt isoforms (Brognard *et al.*, 2007). Amplification of Akt1 has been described in human gastric adenocarcinomas, and amplification of Akt2 has been described in ovarian, breast and pancreatic carcinomas (Bellacosa *et al.*, 1995; Cheng *et al.*, 1996). Akt mutations are rare, but somatic mutations in the PH domain of Akt1 have been detected in small percentages of human breast, ovarian and colorectal cancers (Carpten *et al.*, 2007).

## 4.2  Downstream Substrates of Activated Akt

Akt recognizes and phosphorylates the consensus sequence RXRXX (S/T) when it is surrounded by hydrophobic residues. Since this sequence is present in many proteins, Akt has many substrates, many of which control key cellular processes such as apoptosis, cell cycle progression, transcription and translation. For example, Akt phosphorylates proteins in the FoxO subfamily of forkhead family transcription factors, inhibiting the transcription of several pro-apoptotic genes, including Fas-L, IGF binding protein1 (IGFBP1) and Bim. In addition, Akt can directly regulate apoptosis by phosphorylating and inactivating pro-apoptotic proteins such as BAD, which controls the release of cytochrome c from mitochondria, and apoptosis signal-regulating kinase-1 (ASK1), a mitogen-activated protein kinase involved in stress- and cytokine-induced cell death. In contrast, Akt can phosphorylate IKK, which indirectly increases the activity of nuclear factor kappa B (NF-κB) and stimulates the transcription of pro-survival genes. Cell cycle progression can also be affected by Akt; inhibitory phosphorylation of the cyclin-dependent kinase inhibitors p21 and p27 and of GSK3βby Akt has been found to stimulate cell cycle progression by stabilizing cyclin D1 expression. Akt phosphorylation of a recently described, novel pro-survival Akt substrate, proline-rich Akt substrate of 40 kDa (PRAS40), has been shown to attenuate the ability of the latter to inhibit mTORC1 kinase activity (Vander Haar et al., 2007). PRAS40 may be a specific substrate of Akt3 (Madhunapantula et al., 2007). These findings therefore indicate that Akt inhibition may have pleiotropic effects on cancer cells that contribute to an anti-tumor response. The most-studied downstream substrate of Akt is the serine/threonine kinase mammalian target of rapamycin (mTOR). Akt can directly phosphorylate and activate mTOR, as well as indirectly activating it by phosphorylating and inactivating tuberous sclerosis complex 2 (TSC2), also called tuberin, which normally inhibits mTOR through the GTP binding protein Ras homolog enriched in brain (Rheb) (Inoki et al., 2003). When TSC2 is inactivated by phosphorylation, the GTPase Rheb is maintained in its GTP-bound state, allowing increased activation of mTOR (Inoki et al., 2005). mTOR exists in two complexes: the TORC1 complex, in which mTOR is bound to Raptor; and the TORC2 complex, in which mTOR is bound to Rictor. In the TORC1 complex, mTOR signals its downstream effectors, S6 kinase/ribosomal protein and 4EBP-1/eIF-4E, to control protein translation (Inoki et al., 2005). mTOR is generally considered a downstream substrate of Akt, but it can phosphorylate Akt when bound to Rictor in TORC2 complexes (Sarbassov et al., 2005), resulting in positive feedback in the pathway. In addition, the downstream mTOR effector S6 kinase-1 (S6K1) can regulate this pathway by catalyzing the inhibitory phosphorylation of insulin receptor substrate (IRS) proteins, preventing IRS proteins from activating PI3kinase and thereby inhibiting the activation of Akt (Harrington et al., 2004).

## 4.3  Rational for Targeting the PI3K/Akt Pathway

In addition to preclinical studies, clinical observations support the targeting of the PI3K/Akt/mTOR pathway in human cancers(Vogt et al., 2009). Immunohistochemical studies using antibodies that recognize Akt phosphorylated at S473 have demonstrated that activated Akt is detectable in cancers, including head and neck cancers (Gupta et al., 2002). Moreover, antibodies against S473 and T308, two sites of Akt phosphorylation, showed that Akt was selectively activated in NSCLC compared with normal lung tissue, and that phosphorylation of Akt at both sites was a better predictor of poor prognosis in NSCLC than phosphorylation at S473 alone (Tsurutani et al., 2006). In addition, amplification of Akt isoforms has been observed in some cancers, albeit at a lower frequency. Another frequent genetic event occurring in human cancer is loss of function of the tumor suppressor PTEN, which normally suppresses activation of the PI3K/Akt/mTOR pathway by functioning as a lipid phosphatase. Loss of PTEN function in cancer can occur through mutation, deletion or epigenetic silencing, with the latter occurring in tumor types, such as lung cancer, in which PTEN mutations are rare (Forgacs *et al.*, 1998). Mutation, deletion or epigenetic silencing of PTEN has been shown to correlate with poor prognosis and reduced survival in patients with various types of cancer (Bertram *et al.*, 2006), with loss of PTEN being a common mechanism for activation of the PI3K/Akt/mTOR pathway and poor prognosis. PI3K activation in human tumors may result from the amplification, over-expression, or mutation of either its p110 catalytic or its p85 regulatory subunit. Amplification of the 3q26 chromosomal region, which contains the *PI3KCA* gene that encodes the p110α catalytic subunit of PI3K, has been observed in 40% of ovarian and 50% of cervical carcinomas (Ma *et al.*, 2000; Shayesteh *et al.*, 1999). Somatic mutations of this gene have been detected in several cancer types, with kinase activity being greater in mutant than in wild-type PI3K (Samuels & Ericson, 2006). Mutations in the regulatory p85 subunit have also been detected. Any of the alterations in individual components of the PI3K/Akt pathway would result in its activation, and activation of this pathway has been reported to be among the most frequent molecular alterations in tumors (Samuels & Ericson, 2006).

# 5   Inhibition of PI Synthesis in HNSCC

PIP2, a substrate of PI3Kinase, may be metabolized from PI by two kinases, PI4Kianse and PI5Kinase, indicating the importance of inhibiting the PI metabolic pathway as an anti-tumor strategy. Our laboratory has investigated three potential mechanisms by which inhibition of PI synthesis could affect HNSCCs, anti-proliferation, inhibition of MMP (matrix metalloproteinase) production/activity, and anti-angiogenesis.

a) **Anti-proliferation** An imbalance between G1 cyclin and CDK (cyclin-dependent kinase) inhibitors (CKIs) has been found to contribute to tumorigenesis and tumor progression. Cyclin D1/PRAD1 acts as a positive regulator of the cell cycle via phosphorylaton of pRB (Rb protein) and the formation of a cyclin D1-CDK4 complex，pRB hyperphosphorylated by CDKs releases E2F, which is necessary for the activation of a gene expression network that regulates entry and progression through S phase.

CKIs are classified into two groups: members of the Ink4 family (p15, p16, p18, and p19) for cyclin D/CDK4 or cyclin D/CDK6, and the cip/kip family (p21, p27, and p57) for cyclin D/CDK4 and cyclin E/CDK2. Overexpression of cyclin D1 in HNSCC is an important prognostic marker, predicting sensitivity to chemotherapy and radiotherapy. Furthermore, imbalances between cyclin D1 and its inhibitors, p16 and p27,may be critical for HNSCC development. Strategies to block cyclin D1 function have been studied extensively; for example, the introduction of an antisense cyclin D1 expression vector into cells reduced their growth rate *in vitro* and decreased tumorigenicity in athymic nude mice(Nakashima & Clayman, 2000). In addition, wefound that inhibition of PI synthesis caused G1 arrest of HNSCC accompanied by decreased levels of cyclin D1, cyclin E and phosphorylated pRB (Baba *et al.*, 2001).

b) **Inhibition of MMP production/activity** Tumor metastasis is a complex multistep process, involving tumor growth at the primary site, entry into the circulation (intravasation), adhesion to the basement membranes (BM) of target organs, extravasation and growth at secondary sites. The intravasation and extravasation processes involve degradation of the BM by proteinases, normally MMPs. MMP-9/gelatinase B and MMP-2/gelatinase A are specific for type IV collagen, which acts as the backbone of BM, and therefore probably play a major role in degrading the BM. In HNSCC, MMP-2 and MMP-9 are associated with metastatic potential. Therefore, MMPs are attractive therapy targets and many drugs have been developed to prevent their extracellular matrix-degrading activities during metastasis and angiogenesis. We have demonstrated that inhibition of PI synthesis affects the production of MMP-2 and MMP-9 in HNSCC cell lines (Baba et al., 2000).

c) **Anti-angiogenesis** Angiogenesis, the formation of new blood vessels from pre-existing capillaries or incorporating bone marrow-derived endothelial precursor cells into growing vessels, is associated with the malignant phenotype of cancer. In addition, angiogenesis plays a role in various other diseases, such as diabetic retinopathy, age-related macular degeneration, rheumatoid arthritis, psoriasis, atherosclerosis and restenosis (Cherrington et al., 2000). Clinical association of tumor vascularity with tumor aggressiveness has been demonstrated in a wide variety of tumor types including HNSCC. Therefore, determining microvessel density in tumor tissues can be useful in predicting a patient's prognosis. Inhibition of angiogenesis can repress the growth rate of tumor cells and lead to cell death resulting from reduced nutrition and oxygen supply to the tumor. VEGF (vascular endothelial growth factor), which plays a major role in many angiogenic processes, binds to its receptor Flk-1/KDR on endothelial cells (EC), stimulating their proliferation through the phospholipase Cγ-protein kinase C-ERK (extracellular signal-regulated kinase) pathway, but not via Ras (Takahashi et al., 1999). In addition, VEGF stimulates EC migration through p38 MAPK (mitogen-activated kinase) independently of ERK (Rousseau et al., 1997). Therefore, these two major MAPK pathways are eligible targets for therapeutic reduction of angiogenesis in HNSCC.

Most clinical trials of anti-angiogenic agents have been conducted in patients with advanced tumors resistant to conventional therapies, with phase III trials comparing the efficacy of an experimental angiogenesis inhibitor plus standard chemotherapy with that of standard chemotherapy alone (Gotink & Verheul, 2010). Several recent clinical trials have shown that blocking VEGF signaling had significant clinical benefit (Ho & Kuo, 2007). SU11248, a tyrosine kinase inhibitor of the Flk-1/KDR receptor (VEGF receptor), and bevacizumab, a monoclonal antibody to VEGF, have been approved by the FDA (Ho & Kuo, 2007). Furthermore, we have demonstrated that inhibition of PI abrogated VEGF stimulation of the growth and migration of human umbilical vein ECs through the ERK-cyclin D1 and p38 pathways, respectively (Baba et al., 2004). Increased PI synthase expression is an early event in HNSCC (Kaur et al., 2010), so inhibition of PI synthesis may be a potent therapeutic strategy in patients with these tumors (Baba et al., 2010).

# 6    Cross Talk with respect to the PI3K/Akt Pathway

## 6.1    Cross Talk between EGFR and IGF1R

Growth factor switching from one pathway to another may be an adaptive mechanism, induced by blocking the dominant growth factor receptor pathway. Blockade of EGFR signaling in DU145 and PC-3 human prostate cancer cells has found to enhance the growth promoting effects of the peptide growth factor ligands basic fibroblast growth factor (bFGF) and IGF-1, respectively (Jones *et al.*, 1997). More recently, the EGFR-selective tyrosine kinase inhibitor gefitinib has been shown to inhibit the growth of EGFR-positive MCF-7-derived tamoxifen-resistant breast cancer cells, an effect that can be abrogated by exposing the cells to non-EGF ligands such as heregulin-β and IGF-II (Knowlden *et al.*, 2005). The reversal of the anti-tumor effects of gefitinib by IGF-II, acting through IGF-1R, is accompanied by reactivation of the previously reduced activity of Akt and extracellular-regulated kinase (ERK), with ERK signaling contributing to the re-establishment of tumor cell growth. Therefore, in the presence of a dominant growth pathway, cancer cells are capable of responding to other growth factors, compromising the anti-tumor activity of agents designed specifically to inhibit EGFR. Importantly, blockade of EGFR signaling frequently results in switching to the IGF-1R pathway, a common mechanism used to promote resistance to anti-EGFR treatment (Choi *et al.*, 2010). For example, gefitinib initially inhibited the growth of the EGFR-positive DU145 prostate cancer cell line and of MCF-7-derived tamoxifen- and fulvestrant resistant breast cancer cell lines, but chronic exposure to gefitinib resulted in the development of gefitinib-resistant variant sub-lines, all showing up-regulation of multiple IGF-1R signaling components when compared with their parental cell lines (Jones *et al.*, 2004). This resulted in increased production and elevated expression of the IGF-1R ligand IGF-II, increased activity of IGF-1R and increased levels of Akt activity. In addition, although the A549 lung cancer cell line is partially sensitive to gefitinib, chronic exposure resulted in a resistant variant with increased activity of elements of the IGF-1R pathway. The importance of IGF-1R signaling in cell lines with acquired gefitinib resistance was supported by the increased dependency of these cell lines on IGF-1R signaling and their greater sensitivity to growth inhibition by IGF-1R-selective TKIs (Jones *et al.*, 2004). Therefore, the dominance of the EGFR pathway in parental cells was replaced by an increased use of the IGF-1R pathway in gefitinib resistant cells.

Growth factor pathway switching may result not only from changes occurring during the development of acquired resistance, but, critically, may occur rapidly and modulate initial sensitivity to EGFR-blockade, resulting in *de novo* or intrinsic resistance to anti-EGFR agents such as gefitinib. Indeed, although the EGFR and IGF-1R pathways are classically regarded as separate entities, the overlapping of downstream signal transduction molecules indicates that these receptors can affect each other's signaling abilities, although the precise mechanisms involved in this crosstalk have not been fully elucidated. For example, gefitinib only partially blocks EGFR activity in A549 lung cancer cells, accompanied by a dramatic increase in the activity but not the expression of IGF-1R. Moreover, in these cells, IGF-1R can transphosphorylate EGFR, maintaining EGFR activity in the presence of gefitinib. Therefore, by enhancing IGF-1R activity, gefitinib limits its own efficacy in these cells. Interestingly, gefitinib was observed to enhance insulin receptor activity and levels of downstream activated Akt in *de novo* gefitinib-resistant LoVo colorectal cancer cells, which are defective in their ability to produce mature IGF-1R and predominantly express insulin receptor-isoform A (InsR-A), a member of the IGF-1R family (Jones *et al.*, 2006). Furthermore, InsR can modulate and maintain EGFR phosphorylation in these cells. Such rapid and dynamic interplay between EGFR and IGF-1R or InsR may play an important role in limiting the anti-tumor activity of gefitinib; partial and *de novo* resistance to this inhibitor has been demonstrated in A549 and LoVo cells, respectively.

Treatment of HNSCC cells and xenografts with combinations of antibodies to IGF-1R and EGFR was more effective than either agent alone at reducing cancer cell growth (Barnes *et al.*, 2007), suggesting that these combined anti-tyrosine kinase receptor directed therapies may have benefit in treating patients with HNSCC. Similarly, treatment with small molecules targeting these two pathways suppressed the growth of HNSCC cells (Slomiany *et al.*, 2007), as did the combination of cetuximab with a PI3K inhibitor (Rebucci *et al.*, 2011).

## 6.2 Cross Talk between EGFR and c-MET

The transmembrane receptor tyrosine kinase MET was shown to contribute to resistance to EGFR inhibitors in cell lines derived from head and neck, breast, gastric and lung cancers as well as in lung samples. In one study, MET amplification was detected in 9 of 43 (21%) lung tumors with acquired resistance to EGFR inhibitors, but in only 2 of 62 (3%) lung tumors with EGFR mutations from patients not previously treated with kinase inhibitors(Bean *et al.*, 2007). MET amplification causes gefitinib resistance by driving ERBB-3 dependent phosphorylation and by maintaining persistent activation of PI3K/Akt signaling in the presence of EGFR inhibition (Engelman *et al.*, 2007). In the absence of MET amplification, MET signaling can be activated by increased expression of the MET ligand hepatocyte growth factor (HGF), leading to resistance to EGFR TKIs in lung adenocarcinoma patients harboring EGFR-activating mutations, again associated with persistent PI3K/AKT activation (Yano *et al.,* 2008). Cortactin, a regulator of dynamic actin networks, was to shown to regulate MET signaling and promote resistance to EGFR inhibitors in HNSCC cell lines (Yano *et al.*, 2008). Overexpression of cortactin in these cells stabilized MET, enhanced HGF-mediated mitogenesis and activated Akt, leading to resistance to gefitinib. Interestingly, the gene encoding cortactin, *CTTN*, resides at a chromosomal locus (11q13) frequently amplified in head and neck cancers.

## 6.3 Cross Talk between EGFR and VEGFR

Tumor-induced angiogenesis plays an important role in cancer development and has been linked to EGFR resistance. EGF activation of EGFR signaling results in the secretion of proangiogenic growth factors such as VEGF, whereas blockade of EGFR inhibits the secretion of VEGF. Continuous treatment of xenograft tumors with anti-EGFR antibody resulted in the generation of six A431 human squamous cell carcinoma cell lines resistant to EGFR inhibition (Viloria-Petit *et al.*, 2001), with five of these cell lines showing elevated VEGF expression, increased angiogenic potential *in vitro* and increased tumor angiogenesis *in vivo*. Furthermore, A431 cells genetically engineered to overexpress VEGF displayed resistance to anti-EGFR antibodies *in vivo* (Viloria-Petit *et al.*, 2001*)*. Thus, resistance to EGFR antagonists may well be mediated via VEGF signaling.

Tumor-induced angiogenesis may be involved in the development and progression of HNSCC. A meta-analysis of 12 studies of VEGF protein overexpression and clinical outcome in patients diagnosed with HNSCC found that the overall risk of death within 2 years was approximately 1.9-fold higher in patients with VEGF-positive than VEGF-negative tumors (Kyzas, *et al.*, 2005). The co-overexpression of VEGF and VEGF receptor2 (VEGFR2) was correlated with a higher tumor proliferation rate and shorter survival in patients with HNSCC (Kyzas, Stefanou, *et al.*, 2005). The cross-talk between the VEGFR and EGFR signaling cascades in the biological context of HNSCC has not been fully characterized; however, ligand-VEGFR interaction activates the tyrosine kinase domain of the VEGFR, activating intracellular signaling transduction pathways, such as the PI3K/Akt pathway, involved in regulating cellular survival. Because HNSCC tumor cells also express VEGFR (Lalla *et al.*, 2003), there may be cross talk between EGFR and VEGFR through the PI3K/Akt pathway in HNSCCs, and ongoing clinical studies are exploring the combination of anti-VEGF and anti-EGFR therapies in patients with these tumors.

# 7    Cross Talk with respect to STAT3 Signaling Pathways

## 7.1    Cross Talk between EGFR and Gp130 Receptor

Although EGFR activation has been found to lead to the rapid phosphorylation of STAT3 on tyrosine 705 and the subsequent activation of STAT3-dependent gene expression, STAT3 tyrosine phosphorylation and the formation of active STAT3 DNA-binding complexes were insensitive to EGFR inhibition in many HNSCC cell lines (Sriuranpong *et al.*, 2003). Indeed, of a representative panel of 10 HNSCC-derived cell lines, 9 showed increased tyrosine phosphorylation and STAT3 activity, but only 3 showed constitutive activation of EGFR (Sriuranpong *et al.*, 2003). In searching for the mechanism responsible for the EGFR-independent activation of STAT3 in HNSCC cells, the activation of the gp130 cytokine receptor subunit was found to promote the phosphorylation of STAT3 at tyrosine 705 through the activation of intracellular tyrosine kinases of the JAK family. Surprisingly, gp130 activation was found to be initiated primarily by interleukin (IL)-6, a cytokine secreted by HNSCC cells that binds to the cell surface in an autocrine fashion. These findings suggest that the persistent activation of STAT3 in HNSCC can result from the deregulation of EGFR activity or from the EGF-independent autocrine activation of STAT3 by tumor-secreted cytokines. Furthermore, overexpression of IL-6 in HNSCC cells was found to involve increased transcription from the IL-6 promoter, which is dependent on the presence of an intact NFκB response element located 63 to 75 bp upstream of the IL-6 transcriptional initiation site. Inhibition of NFκB resulted in the marked downregulation of IL-6 mRNA and protein expression, concomitant with the decreased release of other inflammatory cytokines, such as IL-8, IL-10, granulocyte-macrophage colony-stimulating factor (GM-CSF), and granulocyte colony-stimulating factor (G-CSF). Surprisingly, the blockade of NFκB also resulted in the drastic inhibition of constitutive STAT3 activity in HNSCC cells, as reflected by the reduced tyrosine phosphorylation of STAT, and by blockage of the autocrine/paracrine activation of STAT3 (Squarize *et al.*, 2006). These findings are indicative of cross-talk between the NFκB and STAT3 signaling systems, a cross-talk initiated by the release of IL-6, which, in turn, results from the NFκB-dependent activation of the IL-6 promoter and the subsequent tyrosine phosphorylation of STAT3 by the autocrine/paracrine activation of IL-6 receptors in tumor cells.

## 7.2    Cross Talk between EGFR and c-MET

MET signaling has been shown to contribute to intrinsic resistance to EGFR tyrosine kinase inhibitors in breast cancer; MET activated c-Src in a resistant breast cancer cell line, leading to tyrosine phosphorylation of EGFR even in the presence of EGFR TKIs (Mueller *et al.*, 2008). STAT3 is phosphorylated by EGFR, EGFR-interactor Src, and c-MET, and phosphorylated STAT3 translocates to the nucleus and activates the transcription of genes involved in cell cycle progression, angiogenesis, and apoptotic resistance.

# 8    Cross Talk with respect to ERK Signaling Pathways

## 8.1    Cross Talk between EGFR and c-MET

EGFR and c-MET drive cellular proliferation by activating the Ras-Raf-MEK-ERK pathway, because c-MET is highly expressed in HNSCC, cross talk between EGFR and c-MET may occur through the ERK pathway.

## 8.2    Cross Talk between EGFR and IGF-1R

IGF-1R may stimulate cell proliferation by activating the ERK pathway, inducing resistance to EGFR inhibitors (Ahmad *et al.*, 2004; Morgillo *et al.*, 2006). This novel function of IGF-1R has been validated in NSCLC cell lines (Morgillo *et al.*, 2006) and most recently in an HNSCC model (Barnes *et al.*, 2007). Stimulation of HNSCC cell lines with IGF resulted in the heterodimerization of IGFR with EGFR, with activating phosphorylation of both receptors (Barnes *et al.*, 2007). Furthermore, treatment with the combination of an anti-IGF-1R therapeutic antibody, A12, and the anti-EGFR antibody cetuximab more effectively inhibited cellular proliferation and migration than treatment with either alone. The ability of this drug combination to inhibit EGFR-resistant HNSCCs in the preclinical and clinical settings remains to be determined.

## 8.3    Cross Talk between EGFR and VEGFR

The cross-talk between the EGFR and VEGFR signaling cascades in HNSCC has not been fully characterized. However, HNSCC cells express VEGFR. Because VEGF stimulates cell proliferation through the phospholipase Cγ-protein kinase C-ERK pathway, but not via Ras (Takahashi *et al.*, 1999), there may be cross talk between EGFR and VEGFR through the ERK pathway.

# 9    Future Prospects

Signaling of multiple receptor tyrosine kinases (RTKs) is propagated through Akt. Therefore, simultaneous inhibition of EGFR and pathway components such as Akt and mTOR could circumvent the feedback activation observed with either approach alone. The most extensive data concerning proximal and distal signaling inhibition has been observed by combining PI3K/Akt/mTOR pathway inhibitors with EGFR antagonists. Several PI3K inhibitors can restore cellular sensitivity to EGFR inhibitors. For example, the selective pI3K inhibitor PX-866 and p110α were found to abrogate gefitinib resistance in NSCLC xenografts (Ihle *et al.*, 2005). Synergistic effects of rapamycin and EGFR TKIs have been observed in several *in vitro* systems, including glioblastoma multiforme, prostate cancer, pancreatic cancer, squamous cell carcinoma, renal cell carcinoma, leukemia, cervical carcinoma and NSCLC cell lines, as well as in some xenografts (Birle & Hedley, 2006; Buck *et al.*, 2006; Costa *et al.*, 2007; Hjelmeland *et al.*, 2007; Jimeno *et al.*, 2007; Mohi *et al.*, 2004). The combination of rapamycin and erlotinib showed re-sensitization and synergistic growth inhibition in cell lines that were previously resistant to erlotinib (Buck *et al.*, 2006). Moreover, the combination of rapamycin and the irreversible EGFR TKI, HKI-272, resulted in the significant regression of lung tumors in transgenic mice possessing the secondary resistance mutation T790M (Li *et al.*, 2007). Addition of the dual PI3K/mTOR inhibitor PI-103 to erlotinib was necessary to induce growth arrest of human glioma cell lines with mutant PTEN (Fan *et al.*, 2007), suggesting that activation of the PI3K/Akt/mTOR pathway by EGFR-independent mechanisms confers resistance to EGFR inhibitors, but that this resistance can be overcome by the addition of pathway inhibitors. Collectively, these findings suggest that the combination of EGFR antagonists and PI3K/Akt pathway inhibitors may be beneficial to patients with tumors resistant to EGFR TKIs. These combinations, however, may be insufficient for the treatment of some patients with HNSCC, due to the cross talk between the ERK and STAT3 signaling pathways, as described in sections 7 and 8, and Figure 1. Because intracellular signaling of EGFR occurs via various pathways, including those involving ERK, PI3K/Akt, and STAT3, EGF-dependent induction of anti-apoptotic proteins and cell cycle inhibitors is highly variable in HNSCC cells (Rüddel *et al.*, 2010). Therefore, personalized therapy with combinations of EGFR antagonists and PI3K/Akt/mTOR inhibitors, ERK, and STAT3 pathway inhibitors is needed.

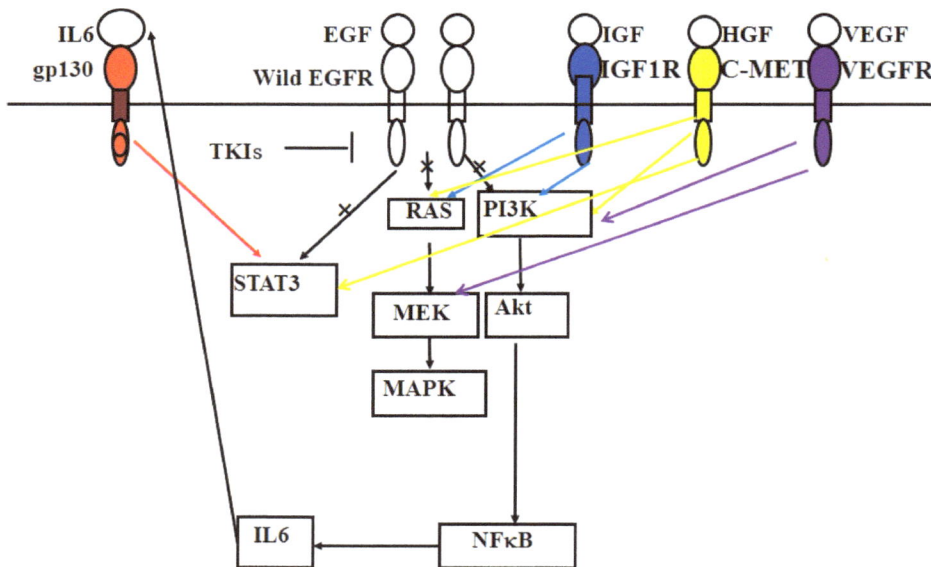

**Figure 1:** Proposed mechanism for overcoming HNSCC resistance to EGFR antagonists using PI3kinase/Akt/mTOR, STAT3 and ERK pathway inhibitors. There is molecular cross-talk between EGFR and signaling via other RTKs, including gp130, IGF1R, c-MET, and VEGFR, through PI3K/Akt and STAT3. Furthermore, in HNSCCs, molecular cross-talk between the EGFR and other RTK signaling pathways, such as IGF1R, c-MET, and VEGFR, can occurthrough ERK.

## 10    Conclusions

EGFR is expressed at a high level in HNSCC, but EGFR inhibitor monotherapy has had limited success in patients with these tumors. EGFR mutations are extremely rare in HNSCC. Three major signaling pathways have been found to mediate the downstream effects of EGFR: the PI3K/Akt, STAT3, and ERK pathways. The PI3K/Akt and STAT3 pathways are responsible for cellular survival and there is molecular cross-talk between EGFR and other RTKs that signal through PI3K/Akt and STAT3 in HNSCCs. Furthermore, the ERK pathway is responsible for cell proliferation, and there is molecular cross-talk between the EGFR and other RTK signaling pathways through ERK in HNSCCs. Hence, EGFR inhibitors alone may be unable to suppress EGFR downstream, and may affect ADCC activity(Kondo *et al.*, 2011). Therefore, personalized combination therapy targeting these signaling pathways, PI3K/Akt, STAT3, ERK, and EGFR, may provide clinical benefits for patients with HNSCC.

## Acknowledgment

This study was supported in part by a Grant-in-Aid for Scientific Research (C): 23592546 to Y. Baba.

## Conflicts of Interests

The authors disclose no conflict of interests.

## References

Ahmad, T., Farnie, G., Bundred, N. J., and Anderson, N. G. (2004). The Mitogenic Action of Insulin-Like Growth Factor I in Normal Human Mammary Epithelial Cells Requires the Epidermal Growth Factor Receptor Tyrosine Kinase. Journal of Biological Chemistry, 279(3), 1713-1719.

Anderson, J. A., Irish, J. C., McLachlin, C. M., and Ngan, B. Y. (1994). H-Ras Oncogene Mutation and Human Papillomavirus Infection in Oral Carcinomas. Archives of Otolaryngology—Head & Neck Surgery, 120(7), 755-760.

Baba, Y., Fujii, M., Tokumaru, Y., and Kato, Y. (2012). Present and Future of EGFR Inhibitors for Head and Neck Squamous Cell Cancer. Journal of Oncology, 2012, 986725.

Baba, Y., Kato, Y., Mochimatsu, I., Nagashima, Y., Kurihara, M., Kawano, T., Taguchi, T., Hata, R., and Tsukuda, M. (2004). Inostamycin Suppresses Vascular Endothelial Growth Factor-Stimulated Growth and Migration of Human Umbilical Vein Endothelial Cells. Clinical and Experimental Metastasis, 21(5), 419-425.

Baba, Y., Kato, Y., and Ogawa, K. (2010). Inostamycin Prevents Malignant Phenotype of Cancer: Inhibition of Phosphatidylinositol Synthesis Provides a Therapeutic Advantage for Head and Neck Squamous Cell Carcinoma. Cell Biology International, 34(2), 171-175.

Baba, Y., Tsukuda, M., Mochimatsu, I., Furukawa, S., Kagata, H., Nagashima, Y., Koshika, S., Imoto, M., and Kato, Y. (2001). Cytostatic Effect of Inostamycin, an Inhibitor of Cytidine 5'-Diphosphate 1,2-Diacyl-Sn-Glycerol (CDP-DG): Inositol Transferase, on Oral Squamous Cell Carcinoma Cell Lines. Cell Biology International, 25(7), 613-620.

Baba, Y., Tsukuda, M., Mochimatsu, I., Furukawa, S., Kagata, H., Nagashima, Y., Sakai, N., Koshika, S., Imoto, M., and Kato, Y. (2000). Inostamycin, an Inhibitor of Cytidine 5'-Diphosphate 1,2-Diacyl-Sn-Glycerol (CDP-DG): Inositol Transferase, Suppresses Invasion Ability by Reducing Productions of Matrix Metalloproteinase-2 and -9 and Cell Motility in HSC-4 Tongue Carcinoma Cell Line. Clinical and Experimental Metastasis, 18(3), 273-279.

Barnes, C. J., Ohshiro, K., Rayala, S. K., El-Naggar, A. K., and Kumar, R. (2007). Insulin-Like Growth Factor Receptor as a Therapeutic Target in Head and Neck Cancer. Clinical Cancer Research, 13(14), 4291-4299.

Bean, J., Brennan, C., Shih, J. Y., Riely, G., Viale, A., Wang, L., Chitale, D., Motoi, N., Szoke, J., Broderick, S., Balak, M., Chang, W. C., Yu, C. J., Gazdar, A., Pass, H., Rusch, V., Gerald, W., Huang, S. F., Yang, P. C., Miller, V., Ladanyi, M., Yang, C. H., and Pao, W. (2007). MET Amplification Occurs with or without T790M Mutations in EGFR Mutant Lung Tumors with Acquired Resistance to Gefitinib or Erlotinib. Proceedings of the National Academy of Sciences of the United States of America, 104(52), 20932-20937.

Bellacosa, A., de Feo, D., Godwin, A. K., Bell, D. W., Cheng, J. Q., Altomare, D. A., Wan, M., Dubeau, L., Scambia, G., Masciullo, V., Ferrandina, G., Benedetti Panici, P., Mancuso, S., Neri, G., and Testa, J. R. (1995). Molecular Alterations of the AKT2 Oncogene in Ovarian and Breast Carcinomas. International Journal of Cancer, 64(4), 280-285.

Bertram, J., Peacock, J. W., Fazli, L., Mui, A. L., Chung, S. W., Cox, M. E., Monia, B., Gleave, M. E., and Ong, C. J. (2006). Loss of PTEN Is Associated with Progression to Androgen Independence. Prostate, 66(9), 895-902.

Birle, D. C., and Hedley, D. W. (2006). Signaling Interactions of Rapamycin Combined with Erlotinib in Cervical Carcinoma Xenografts. Molecular Cancer Therapeutics, 5(10), 2494-2502.

Brognard, J., Sierecki, E., Gao, T., and Newton, A. C. (2007). PHLPP and a Second Isoform, PHLPP2, Differentially Attenuate the Amplitude of Akt Signaling by Regulating Distinct Akt Isoforms. Molecular Cell, 25(6), 917-931.

Buck, E., Eyzaguirre, A., Brown, E., Petti, F., McCormack, S., Haley, J. D., Iwata, K. K., Gibson, N. W., and Griffin, G. (2006). Rapamycin Synergizes with the Epidermal Growth Factor Receptor Inhibitor Erlotinib in Non-Small-Cell Lung, Pancreatic, Colon, and Breast Tumors. Molecular Cancer Therapeutics, 5(11), 2676-2684.

Burtness, B. (2005). The Role of Cetuximab in the Treatment of Squamous Cell Cancer of the Head and Neck. Expert Opinion on Biological Therapy, 5(8), 1085-1093.

Carpten, J. D., Faber, A. L., Horn, C., Donoho, G. P., Briggs, S. L., Robbins, C. M., Hostetter, G., Boguslawski, S., Moses, T. Y., Savage, S., Uhlik, M., Lin, A., Du, J., Qian, Y. W., Zeckner, D. J., Tucker-Kellogg, G., Touchman, J., Patel, K., Mousses, S., Bittner, M., Schevitz, R., Lai, M. H., Blanchard, K. L., and Thomas, J. E. (2007). A Transforming Mutation in the Pleckstrin Homology Domain of AKT1 in Cancer. Nature, 448(7152), 439-444.

Carter, C. A., Kelly, R. J., and Giaccone, G. (2009). Small-Molecule Inhibitors of the Human Epidermal Receptor Family. Expert Opinion on Investigational Drugs, 18(12), 1829-1842.

Cheng, J. Q., Ruggeri, B., Klein, W. M., Sonoda, G., Altomare, D. A., Watson, D. K., and Testa, J. R. (1996). Amplification of AKT2 in Human Pancreatic Cells and Inhibition of AKT2 Expression and Tumorigenicity by Antisense RNA. Proceedings of the National Academy of Sciences of the United States of America, 93(8), 3636-3641.

Cherrington, J. M., Strawn, L. M., and Shawver, L. K. (2000). New Paradigms for the Treatment of Cancer: The Role of Anti-Angiogenesis Agents. Advances in Cancer Research, 79, 1-38.

Choi, Y. J., Rho, J. K., Jeon, B. S., Choi, S. J., Park, S. C., Lee, S. S., Kim, H. R., Kim, C. H., and Lee, J. C. (2010). Combined Inhibition of IGFR Enhances the Effects of Gefitinib in H1650: A Lung Cancer Cell Line with EGFR Mutation and Primary Resistance to EGFR-TK Inhibitors. Cancer Chemotherapy and Pharmacology, 66(2), 381-388.

Ciardiello, F., and Tortora, G. (2003). Epidermal Growth Factor Receptor (EGFR) as a Target in Cancer Therapy: Understanding the Role of Receptor Expression and Other Molecular Determinants That Could Influence the Response to Anti-EGFR Drugs. European Journal of Cancer, 39(10), 1348-1354.

Cohen, E. E., Rosen, F., Stadler, W. M., Recant, W., Stenson, K., Huo, D., and Vokes, E. E. (2003). Phase II Trial of ZD1839 in Recurrent or Metastatic Squamous Cell Carcinoma of the Head and Neck. Journal of Clinical Oncology, 21(10), 1980-1987.

Costa, L. J., Gemmill, R. M., and Drabkin, H. A. (2007). Upstream Signaling Inhibition Enhances Rapamycin Effect on Growth of Kidney Cancer Cells. Urology, 69(3), 596-602.

Cripps, C., Winquist, E., Devries, M. C., Stys-Norman, D., and Gilbert, R.; Head, and Neck Cancer Disease Site Group. (2010). Epidermal Growth Factor Receptor Targeted Therapy in Stages III and IV Head and Neck Cancer. Current Oncology, 17(3), 37-48.

Eberhard, D. A., Johnson, B. E., Amler, L. C., Goddard, A. D., Heldens, S. L., Herbst, R. S., Ince, W. L., Janne, P. A., Januario, T., Johnson, D. H., Klein, P., Miller, V. A., Ostland, M. A., Ramies, D. A., Sebisanovic, D., Stinson, J. A., Zhang, Y. R., Seshagiri, S., and Hillan, K. J. (2005). Mutations in the Epidermal Growth Factor Receptor and in

KRAS Are Predictive and Prognostic Indicators in Patients with Non-Small-Cell Lung Cancer Treated with Chemotherapy Alone and in Combination with Erlotinib. Journal of Clinical Oncology, 23(25), 5900-5909.

Engelman, J. A., Zejnullahu, K., Mitsudomi, T., Song, Y., Hyland, C., Park, J. O., Lindeman, N., Gale, C. M., Zhao, X., Christensen, J., Kosaka, T., Holmes, A. J., Rogers, A. M., Cappuzzo, F., Mok, T., Lee, C., Johnson, B. E., Cantley, L. C., and Janne, P. A. (2007). MET Amplification Leads to Gefitinib Resistance in Lung Cancer by Activating ERBB3 Signaling. Science, 316(5827), 1039-1043.

Fan, Q. W., Cheng, C. K., Nicolaides, T. P., Hackett, C. S., Knight, Z. A., Shokat, K. M., and Weiss, W. A. (2007). A Dual Phosphoinositide-3-Kinase Alpha/mTOR Inhibitor Cooperates with Blockade of Epidermal Growth Factor Receptor in PTEN-Mutant Glioma. Cancer Research, 67(17), 7960-7965.

Forastiere, A., Koch, W., Trotti, A., and Sidransky, D. (2001). Head and Neck Cancer. The New England Journal of Medicine, 345(26), 1890-1900.

Forgacs, E., Biesterveld, E. J., Sekido, Y., Fong, K., Muneer, S., Wistuba, I. I., Milchgrub, S., Brezinschek, R., Virmani, A., Gazdar, A. F., and Minna, J. D. (1998). Mutation Analysis of the PTEN/MMAC1 Gene in Lung Cancer. Oncogene, 17(12), 1557-1565.

Frederick, B. A., Helfrich, B. A., Coldren, C. D., Zheng, D., Chan, D., Bunn, P. A., Jr., and Raben, D. (2007). Epithelial to Mesenchymal Transition Predicts Gefitinib Resistance in Cell Lines of Head and Neck Squamous Cell Carcinoma and Non-Small Cell Lung Carcinoma. Molecular Cancer Therapeutics, 6(6), 1683-1691.

Gotink, K. J., and Verheul, H. M. (2010). Anti-Angiogenic Tyrosine Kinase Inhibitors: What Is Their Mechanism of Action? Angiogenesis, 13(1), 1-14.

Gupta, A. K., McKenna, W. G., Weber, C. N., Feldman, M. D., Goldsmith, J. D., Mick, R., Machtay, M., Rosenthal, D. I., Bakanauskas, V. J., Cerniglia, G. J., Bernhard, E. J., Weber, R. S., and Muschel, R. J. (2002). Local Recurrence in Head and Neck Cancer: Relationship to Radiation Resistance and Signal Transduction. Clinical Cancer Research, 8(3), 885-892.

Harrington, L. S., Findlay, G. M., Gray, A., Tolkacheva, T., Wigfield, S., Rebholz, H., Barnett, J., Leslie, N. R., Cheng, S., Shepherd, P. R., Gout, I., Downes, C. P., and Lamb, R. F. (2004). The TSC1-2 Tumor Suppressor Controls Insulin-PI3K Signaling Via Regulation of IRS Proteins. Journal of Cell Biology, 166(2), 213-223.

Hjelmeland, A. B., Lattimore, K. P., Fee, B. E., Shi, Q., Wickman, S., Keir, S. T., Hjelmeland, M. D., Batt, D., Bigner, D. D., Friedman, H. S., and Rich, J. N. (2007). The Combination of Novel Low Molecular Weight Inhibitors of RAF (LBT613) and Target of Rapamycin (RAD001) Decreases Glioma Proliferation and Invasion. Molecular Cancer Therapeutics, 6(9), 2449-2457.

Ho, Q. T., and Kuo, C. J. (2007). Vascular Endothelial Growth Factor: Biology and Therapeutic Applications. International Journal of Biochemistry and Cell Biology, 39(7-8), 1349-1357.

Ihle, N. T., Paine-Murrieta, G., Berggren, M. I., Baker, A., Tate, W. R., Wipf, P., Abraham, R. T., Kirkpatrick, D. L., and Powis, G. (2005). The Phosphatidylinositol-3-Kinase Inhibitor PX-866 Overcomes Resistance to the Epidermal Growth Factor Receptor Inhibitor Gefitinib in A-549 Human Non-Small Cell Lung Cancer Xenografts. Molecular Cancer Therapeutics, 4(9), 1349-1357.

Inoki, K., Li, Y., Xu, T., and Guan, K. L. (2003). Rheb GTPase Is a Direct Target of TSC2 GAP Activity and Regulates mTOR Signaling. Genes & Development, 17(15), 1829-1834.

Inoki, K., Ouyang, H., Li, Y., and Guan, K. L. (2005). Signaling by Target of Rapamycin Proteins in Cell Growth Control. Microbiology and Molecular Biology Reviews, 69(1), 79-100.

Jimeno, A., Kulesza, P., Wheelhouse, J., Chan, A., Zhang, X., Kincaid, E., Chen, R., Clark, D. P., Forastiere, A., and Hidalgo, M. (2007). Dual EGFR and mTOR Targeting in Squamous Cell Carcinoma Models, and Development of Early Markers of Efficacy. British Journal of Cancer, 96(6), 952-959.

Jones, H. E., Dutkowski, C. M., Barrow, D., Harper, M. E., Wakeling, A. E., and Nicholson, R. I. (1997). New EGF-R Selective Tyrosine Kinase Inhibitor Reveals Variable Growth Responses in Prostate Carcinoma Cell Lines PC-3 and DU-145. International Journal of Cancer, 71(6), 1010-1018.

Jones, H. E., Gee, J. M., Barrow, D., Tonge, D., Holloway, B., and Nicholson, R. I. (2006). Inhibition of Insulin Receptor Isoform-A Signalling Restores Sensitivity to Gefitinib in Previously De Novo Resistant Colon Cancer Cells. British Journal of Cancer, 95(2), 172-180.

Jones, H. E., Goddard, L., Gee, J. M., Hiscox, S., Rubini, M., Barrow, D., Knowlden, J. M., Williams, S., Wakeling, A. E., and Nicholson, R. I. (2004). Insulin-Like Growth Factor-I Receptor Signalling and Acquired Resistance to Gefitinib (ZD1839; Iressa) in Human Breast and Prostate Cancer Cells. Endocrine-Related Cancer, 11(4), 793-814.

Kalish, L. H., Kwong, R. A., Cole, I. E., Gallagher, R. M., Sutherland, R. L., and Musgrove, E. A. (2004). Deregulated Cyclin D1 Expression Is Associated with Decreased Efficacy of the Selective Epidermal Growth Factor Receptor Tyrosine Kinase Inhibitor Gefitinib in Head and Neck Squamous Cell Carcinoma Cell Lines. Clinical Cancer Research, 10(22), 7764-7774.

Kaur, J., Sawhney, M., Dattagupta, S., Shukla, N. K., Srivastava, A., and Ralhan, R. (2010). Clinical Significance of Phosphatidyl Inositol Synthase Overexpression in Oral Cancer. BMC Cancer, 10, 168.

Khuri, F. R., Shin, D. M., Glisson, B. S., Lippman, S. M., and Hong, W. K. (2000). Treatment of Patients with Recurrent or Metastatic Squamous Cell Carcinoma of the Head and Neck: Current Status and Future Directions. Seminars in Oncology, 27(4 Suppl 8), 25-33.

Knowlden, J. M., Hutcheson, I. R., Barrow, D., Gee, J. M., and Nicholson, R. I. (2005). Insulin-Like Growth Factor-I Receptor Signaling in Tamoxifen-Resistant Breast Cancer: A Supporting Role to the Epidermal Growth Factor Receptor. Endocrinology, 146(11), 4609-4618.

Kondo, N., Tsukuda, M., Taguchi, T., Nakazaki, K., Sakakibara, A., Takahashi, H., Toth, G., and Nishimura, G. (2011). Gene Status of Head and Neck Squamous Cell Carcinoma Cell Lines and Cetuximab-Mediated Biological Activities. Cancer Science, 102(9), 1717-1723.

Kyzas, P. A., Cunha, I. W., and Ioannidis, J. P. (2005). Prognostic Significance of Vascular Endothelial Growth Factor Immunohistochemical Expression in Head and Neck Squamous Cell Carcinoma: A Meta-Analysis. Clinical Cancer Research, 11(4), 1434-1440.

Kyzas, P. A., Stefanou, D., Batistatou, A., and Agnantis, N. J. (2005). Potential Autocrine Function of Vascular Endothelial Growth Factor in Head and Neck Cancer Via Vascular Endothelial Growth Factor Receptor-2. Modern Pathology, 18(4), 485-494.

Lalla, R. V., Boisoneau, D. S., Spiro, J. D., and Kreutzer, D. L. (2003). Expression of Vascular Endothelial Growth Factor Receptors on Tumor Cells in Head and Neck Squamous Cell Carcinoma. Archives of Otolaryngology—Head & Neck Surgery, 129(8), 882-888.

Li, D., Shimamura, T., Ji, H., Chen, L., Haringsma, H. J., McNamara, K., Liang, M. C., Perera, S. A., Zaghlul, S., Borgman, C. L., Kubo, S., Takahashi, M., Sun, Y., Chirieac, L. R., Padera, R. F., Lindeman, N. I., Janne, P. A., Thomas, R. K., Meyerson, M. L., Eck, M. J., Engelman, J. A., Shapiro, G. I., and Wong, K. K. (2007). Bronchial and Peripheral Murine Lung Carcinomas Induced by T790M-L858R Mutant EGFR Respond to HKI-272 and Rapamycin Combination Therapy. Cancer Cell, 12(1), 81-93.

Loeffler-Ragg, J., Witsch-Baumgartner, M., Tzankov, A., Hilbe, W., Schwentner, I., Sprinzl, G. M., Utermann, G., and Zwierzina, H. (2006). Low Incidence of Mutations in EGFR Kinase Domain in Caucasian Patients with Head and Neck Squamous Cell Carcinoma. European Journal of Cancer, 42(1), 109-111.

Ma, Y. Y., Wei, S. J., Lin, Y. C., Lung, J. C., Chang, T. C., Whang-Peng, J., Liu, J. M., Yang, D. M., Yang, W. K., and Shen, C. Y. (2000). PIK3CA as an Oncogene in Cervical Cancer. Oncogene, 19(23), 2739-2744.

Madhunapantula, S. V., Sharma, A., and Robertson, G. P. (2007). PRAS40 Deregulates Apoptosis in Malignant Melanoma. Cancer Research, 67(8), 3626-3636.

Mohi, M. G., Boulton, C., Gu, T. L., Sternberg, D. W., Neuberg, D., Griffin, J. D., Gilliland, D. G., and Neel, B. G. (2004). Combination of Rapamycin and Protein Tyrosine Kinase (PTK) Inhibitors for the Treatment of Leukemias Caused by Oncogenic PTKs. Proceedings of the National Academy of Sciences of the United States of America, 101(9), 3130-3135.

Morgillo, F., Woo, J. K., Kim, E. S., Hong, W. K., and Lee, H. Y. (2006). Heterodimerization of Insulin-Like Growth Factor Receptor/Epidermal Growth Factor Receptor and Induction of Survivin Expression Counteract the Antitumor Action of Erlotinib. Cancer Research, 66(20), 10100-10111.

Mueller, K. L., Hunter, L. A., Ethier, S. P., and Boerner, J. L. (2008). Met and c-Src Cooperate to Compensate for Loss of Epidermal Growth Factor Receptor Kinase Activity in Breast Cancer Cells. Cancer Research, 68(9), 3314-3322.

Nakashima, T., and Clayman, G. L. (2000). Antisense Inhibition of Cyclin D1 in Human Head and Neck Squamous Cell Carcinoma. Archives of Otolaryngology—Head & Neck Surgery, 126(8), 957-961.

Ozawa, S., Kato, Y., Ito, S., Komori, R., Shiiki, N., Tsukinoki, K., Ozono, S., Maehata, Y., Taguchi, T., Imagawa-Ishiguro, Y., Tsukuda, M., Kubota, E., and Hata, R. (2009). Restoration of BRAK / CXCL14 Gene Expression by Gefitinib Is Associated with Antitumor Efficacy of the Drug in Head and Neck Squamous Cell Carcinoma. Cancer Science, 100(11), 2202-2209.

Rebucci, M., Peixoto, P., Dewitte, A., Wattez, N., De Nuncques, M. A., Rezvoy, N., Vautravers-Dewas, C., Buisine, M. P., Guerin, E., Peyrat, J. P., Lartigau, E., and Lansiaux, A. (2011). Mechanisms Underlying Resistance to Cetuximab in the HNSCC Cell Line: Role of AKT Inhibition in Bypassing This Resistance. International Journal of Oncology, 38(1), 189-200.

Rousseau, S., Houle, F., Landry, J., and Huot, J. (1997). p38 MAP Kinase Activation by Vascular Endothelial Growth Factor Mediates Actin Reorganization and Cell Migration in Human Endothelial Cells. Oncogene, 15(18), 2169-2177.

Rüddel, J., Wennekes, V. E., Meissner, W., Werner, J. A., and Mandic, R. (2010). EGF-Dependent Induction of BCL-xL and p21CIP1/WAF1 is Highly Variable in HNSCC Cells--Implications for EGFR-Targeted Therapies. Anticancer Research, 30(11), 4579-4585.

Samuels, Y., and Ericson, K. (2006). Oncogenic PI3K and Its Role in Cancer. Current Opinion in Oncology, 18(1), 77-82.

Saranath, D., Panchal, R. G., Nair, R., Mehta, A. R., Sanghavi, V. D., and Deo, M. G. (1992). Amplification and Overexpression of Epidermal Growth Factor Receptor Gene in Human Oropharyngeal Cancer. European Journal of Cancer Part B: Oral Oncology, 28B(2), 139-143.

Sarbassov, D. D., Guertin, D. A., Ali, S. M., and Sabatini, D. M. (2005). Phosphorylation and Regulation of Akt/PKB by the Rictor-mTOR Complex. Science, 307(5712), 1098-1101.

Shayesteh, L., Lu, Y., Kuo, W. L., Baldocchi, R., Godfrey, T., Collins, C., Pinkel, D., Powell, B., Mills, G. B., and Gray, J. W. (1999). PIK3CA Is Implicated as an Oncogene in Ovarian Cancer. Nature Genetics, 21(1), 99-102.

Slomiany, M. G., Black, L. A., Kibbey, M. M., Tingler, M. A., Day, T. A., and Rosenzweig, S. A. (2007). Insulin-Like Growth Factor-1 Receptor and Ligand Targeting in Head and Neck Squamous Cell Carcinoma. Cancer Letters, 248(2), 269-279.

Sordella, R., Bell, D. W., Haber, D. A., and Settleman, J. (2004). Gefitinib-Sensitizing EGFR Mutations in Lung Cancer Activate Anti-Apoptotic Pathways. Science, 305(5687), 1163-1167.

Soulieres, D., Senzer, N. N., Vokes, E. E., Hidalgo, M., Agarwala, S. S., and Siu, L. L. (2004). Multicenter Phase II Study of Erlotinib, an Oral Epidermal Growth Factor Receptor Tyrosine Kinase Inhibitor, in Patients with Recurrent or Metastatic Squamous Cell Cancer of the Head and Neck. Journal of Clinical Oncology, 22(1), 77-85.

Squarize, C. H., Castilho, R. M., Sriuranpong, V., Pinto, D. S., Jr., and Gutkind, J. S. (2006). Molecular Cross-Talk between the NFkappaB and STAT3 Signaling Pathways in Head and Neck Squamous Cell Carcinoma. Neoplasia, 8(9), 733-746.

Sriuranpong, V., Park, J. I., Amornphimoltham, P., Patel, V., Nelkin, B. D., and Gutkind, J. S. (2003). Epidermal Growth Factor Receptor-Independent Constitutive Activation of STAT3 in Head and Neck Squamous Cell Carcinoma Is Mediated by the Autocrine/Paracrine Stimulation of the Interleukin 6/gp130 Cytokine System. Cancer Research, 63(11), 2948-2956.

Taguchi, T., Tsukuda, M., Imagawa-Ishiguro, Y., Kato, Y., and Sano, D. (2008). Involvement of EGFR in the Response of Squamous Cell Carcinoma of the Head and Neck Cell Lines to Gefitinib. Oncology Reports, 19(1), 65-71.

Takahashi, T., Ueno, H., and Shibuya, M. (1999). VEGF Activates Protein Kinase C-Dependent, but Ras-Independent Raf-MEK-MAP Kinase Pathway for DNA Synthesis in Primary Endothelial Cells. Oncogene, 18(13), 2221-2230.

Timpson, P., Wilson, A. S., Lehrbach, G. M., Sutherland, R. L., Musgrove, E. A., and Daly, R. J. (2007). Aberrant Expression of Cortactin in Head and Neck Squamous Cell Carcinoma Cells Is Associated with Enhanced Cell Proliferation and Resistance to the Epidermal Growth Factor Receptor Inhibitor Gefitinib. Cancer Research, 67(19), 9304-9314.

Tsurutani, J., Fukuoka, J., Tsurutani, H., Shih, J. H., Hewitt, S. M., Travis, W. D., Jen, J., and Dennis, P. A. (2006). Evaluation of Two Phosphorylation Sites Improves the Prognostic Significance of Akt Activation in Non-Small-Cell Lung Cancer Tumors. Journal of Clinical Oncology, 24(2), 306-314.

van Houten, V. M., van den Brekel, M. W., Denkers, F., Colnot, D. R., Westerga, J., van Diest, P. J., Snow, G. B., and Brakenhoff, R. H. (2000). Molecular Diagnosis of Head and Neck Cancer. Recent Results in Cancer Research, 157, 90-106.

Vander Haar, E., Lee, S. I., Bandhakavi, S., Griffin, T. J., and Kim, D. H. (2007). Insulin Signalling to mTOR Mediated by the Akt/PKB Substrate PRAS40. Nature Cell Biology, 9(3), 316-323.

Viloria-Petit, A., Crombet, T., Jothy, S., Hicklin, D., Bohlen, P., Schlaeppi, J. M., Rak, J., and Kerbel, R. S. (2001). Acquired Resistance to the Antitumor Effect of Epidermal Growth Factor Receptor-Blocking Antibodies in Vivo: A Role for Altered Tumor Angiogenesis. Cancer Research, 61(13), 5090-5101.

Vogt, P. K., Gymnopoulos, M., and Hart, J. R. (2009). PI 3-Kinase and Cancer: Changing Accents. Current Opinion in Genetics and Development, 19(1), 12-17.

Wong, K. K. (2008). Searching for a Magic Bullet in NSCLC: The Role of Epidermal Growth Factor Receptor Mutations and Tyrosine Kinase Inhibitors. Lung Cancer, 60 Suppl 2, S10-s18.

Yano, S., Wang, W., Li, Q., Matsumoto, K., Sakurama, H., Nakamura, T., Ogino, H., Kakiuchi, S., Hanibuchi, M., Nishioka, Y., Uehara, H., Mitsudomi, T., Yatabe, Y., Nakamura, T., and Sone, S. (2008). Hepatocyte Growth Factor Induces Gefitinib Resistance of Lung Adenocarcinoma with Epidermal Growth Factor Receptor-Activating Mutations. Cancer Research, 68(22), 9479-9487.

# Laser Capture Microdissection in Oral Cancer Research: A Review

Tomoatsu Kaneko
*Division of Cariology, Operative Dentistry and Endodontics*
*Niigata University Graduate School of Medical and Dental Sciences, Niigata, Japan*

Takashi Okiji
*Division of Cariology, Operative Dentistry and Endodontics*
*Niigata University Graduate School of Medical and Dental Sciences, Niigata, Japan*

Jacques E. Nör
*Cariology, Restorative Sciences, and Endodontics*
*University of Michigan, Ann Arbor, MI, USA*

# 1  Introduction

Various experimental techniques are available for molecular profiling studies such as DNA microarray, differential display, serial analysis of gene expression, massive parallel signature sequencing, and suppression subtractive hybridization. However, accuracy of these systems may be compromised if the input DNA, RNA or proteins is not collected from pure population. For example, surgical samples are variable in shape and size, and are often a mixture of several kinds of tissues. Thus, the outcome of molecular biological analyses from these samples may not be accurate. The laser capture microdissection (LCM)-based molecular biological analysis has been developed as a powerful methodology that improves these problems. Because LCM allows selective retrieval of specific types of normal and diseased cells from tissue sections that can then be used for DNA, RNA or protein expression analysis. Thus, in accordance with the recent LCM technological/methodological advancement, LCM has been applied to a wide range of oral cancer research that used tissue sections. Further recent technological and methodological advances such as automated cell microdissection, cell recognition software, and immune-LCM allow us to improve the validity of molecular biological analysis in the field of oral oncology and to get more accurate diagnosis in the pathological field. For example, we have recently developed an immune-LCM method for formaldehyde-fixated, paraffin-embedded tumor tissue sections immunostained with a monoclonal antibody against Factor VIII (a marker for human endothelial cells). This immune-LCM method, in combination with reverse transcription-PCR or real time PCR analysis, is very useful to compare gene expression patterns in tumor cells versus Factor VIII-immunostained endothelial cells during the process of tumor progression and tumor angiogenesis. Thus, in this review, we focus on the presentation and discussion of existing literature that applies LCM-assisted gene expression analysis in the field of oral oncology, and provide an overview of the field of oral cancer research assisted with LCM. In addition, we present a brief protocol of cDNA synthesis following immune-LCM from paraffin-embedded tissue sections.

# 2  Equipment of LCM System

LCM was first introduced as a system that is able to retrieve defined cell population from human tissue samples and developed during the mid-1990s by Dr. Emmert-Buck and colleagues at the National Institutes of Health (NIH), Bethesda, ML, USA (Emmert-Buck *et al.*, 1996). Nowadays a variety of LCM apparatus are available such as the PixCell system (Arcturus, MDS Analytical Technology, California), Zeiss's PALM system (a subsidiary of Carl Zeiss MicroImaging, Jana, Germany), Leica LMD system (Mannheim, Germany), and mmi CellCut Plus syatem (Molecular Machines & Industries (MMI), Switzerland). Their major differences relate to how they collect dissected cells.

Three types of LCM systems are currently available. The first type is the infrared (IR)-laser based LCM system such as the PixCell II and AutoPix. The IR laser-based LCM damages the tissue very little and is good for small targets, whereas it is not suitable for dissection of thicker samples, as compared with the ultraviolet (UV)-laser based LCM system mentioned below The PixCell system was originated in a Cooperative Research and Development Agreement between NIH, the National Cancer Institute, and the National Institute for the Child and Human Development, and was manufactured/marketed by Arcturus.

The second type is the UV-laser based LCM system such as the Zeiss PALM, Leica LMD, and mmi CellCut. The UV-laser based LCM is suitable for clusters of cells and big areas of target tissues and possible to dissect thick sections such as those at 30 μm (Yamanaka *et al.*, 2012). The Zeiss PALM system (Carl Zeiss, City, Germany) uses a pulsed UV-A laser to collect samples by photonic pressure termed laser pressure catapulting. The Leica LMD system (Leica, Mannheim, Germany) uses a UV laser to cut and then dissected cells fall into a collecting tube by gravity. The mmi CellCut Plus system uses a solid-state UV laser and manufactured/marketed by MMI, which was founded in 1998 by Prof. Stefan Seeger from University of Zurich, Switzerland.

The third type is the combined IR-UV laser system such as the Arcturus Veritas, and Arcturus XT(Arcturus). These systems use IR laser capture microdissection and UV laser cutting in one single instrument. A solid-state IR laser delivers a capture technique, which preserves biomolecular integrity and is ideal for single cells or a small number of cells. The solid-state UV laser delivers unprecedented speed and precision, suited for micro dissecting dense tissue structures and for rapidly capturing large numbers of cells.

# 3    LCM-based Research in Oral Oncology

## 3.1    LCM in Oral Oncology

LCM was initially designed and developed for the analysis of solid tumors, as solid tumors have a heterogeneous cellular architecture with adjacent normal and modified stromal cells composed of a mixture of fibroblasts, smooth muscle cells, endothelial cells, and inflammatory cells (Wu X., 2003, Mbeunkui F and Johann DJ Jr., 2009). Typical analysis of the tumor tissue used surgically dissected samples with a mixture of cell types. However, in conventional gene expression analysis without using LCM, it is difficult to compare tumor tissue with normal surrounding tissue, since the dissected tumor sample is normally diluted by the inclusion of adjacent stromal cells. In contrast, the analysis with LCM is suitable for cell-specific comparisons in the tumor tissue. Thus, LCM was used to analyze various tumors including oral cancer (Leethanakul *et al.*, 2000ab; Ohyama *et al.*, 2000; Dahse *et al.*, 2002).

Oral cancer is a type of head and neck cancers developed in any part of the oral cavity or oropharynx. When oral cancer spreads (metastasizes), it usually travels through the lymphatic system and appears first in nearby lymph nodes in the neck. The new tumor at the metastatic site has the same kind of abnormal cells as the primary tumor. Although recently gained knowledge of normal and aberrant function of oncogenes and tumor suppressor genes has provided unique opportunities to understand, and ultimately to control the processes leading to malignancy, the molecular mechanisms of remain poorly understood. In oral cancer analysis, LCM also provides a great advantage. The use of LCM to harvest cells from their native tissue environment, followed by the use of high-density oligonucleotide probe arrays to identify gene expression differences between normal and malignant oral epithelial cells, provide powerful means to decode the molecular events involved in the genesis and progression of oral cancer.

## 3.2    Protein and DNA Expression Analysis

LCM is advantageous in the characterization of protein expression patterns in target tissues and cells. For example, to detect urokinase plasminogen activators in oral cancer using plasminogen–casein zymography, Arcturus PixCell II LCM system was used to extract proteins (Curino *et al.*, 2004). The results showed that the protein expression of urokinase plasminogen activators was highly increased in tumor tissue compared to adjacent non-malignant tissue in all specimens. The authors concluded that LCM combined with zymography is suited for analyzing the prognostic significance and causal involvement of the plasminogen activation system in oral cancer.

LCM can be used to DNA expression analysis. Ito *et al.* (2005) reported *p53* mutation analyses using Leica AS LMD LCM system on surgically resected human esophageal carcinomas. In the analysis, an estimated yield of 2,500 cells per sample was retrieved, and genomic DNA was obtained. They concluded that the analysis of microdissected DNA by LCM is useful for characterizing the heterogeneity of the *p53* gene mutation in multiple carcinoma lesions that cannot be accurately analyzed by the use of the whole esophageal tumor DNA.

Chang *et al.* (2008) reported a method to obtain both DNA and RNA material from a single population of LCM-harvested cells from 8-μm frozen section of oral cancer specimens. They employed a combination analysis of Veritas LCM system to retrieve 50,000 cancer cells in each specimen, and the AllPrep DNA/RNA Mini kit and the RNeasy Micro kit (Qiagen, Frederick, ML) to isolate DNA and RNA from the cells. They further examined DNA copy number gains and losses and corresponding gene expression changes in the tumor cells harvested from metastatic lymph nodes of patients with oral squamous cell carcinoma (OSCC) by using a combination analysis of Veritas LCM system and Affymetrix 250 K Nsp I SNP and U133 Plus 2.0 arrays (Affymetrix, Santa Clara, CA). They suggested that genes exhibiting copy number alteration-correlated expression have biological impact on carcinogenesis and cancer progression in OSCC (Chang *et al.*, 2010).

## 3.3   RNA Expression Analysis

The combination of LCM, RNA amplification and gene expression assays greatly facilitates the molecular characterization of specific cells and tissues.

### 3.3.1   Animal Experimental Model Analysis

In an animal experimental model, Pedersen *et al.*, reported about the analysis of global changes in keratinocyte gene expression during skin wound healing in vivo. The Arcturus PixCell II LCM system was used to isolate keratinocytes in incisional mouse skin wounds or adjacent normal skin, from 6-μm-thick cryostat sections (Pedersen *et al.*, 2003). Changes in gene expression were determined by comparative cDNA array analyses, and the approach was validated by in situ hybridization. The analysis identified 48 candidate genes not previously associated with wound reepithelialization. Moreover, the analysis revealed that the phenotypic resemblance of wound keratinocytes to squamous cell carcinoma (SCC) is mimicked at the level of gene expression, but notable differences between the two tissue-remodeling processes were also observed. Thus, they suggest that a combination of LCM and cDNA array analysis provides a powerful tool to unravel the complex changes in gene expression that underlie physiological and pathological remodeling of keratinized epithelium.

### 3.3.2   Clinical Analysis

In oral cancer tissues, a number of genes have been identified to be highly expressed/upregulated, by the use of either the LCM/oligonucleotide microarray approach (Leethanakul *et al.*, 2000a) or the LCM/cDNA library approach (Leethanakul *et al.*, 2000b). The combination of LCM and microarray is able to avoid contamination of heterogeneous cellular elements, and to compare expression levels of different genes in tumors of different stage, source and anatomical site. For example, Leethanakul *et al.* used a combination of LCM and cDNA arrays, which approach allowed a detailed analysis of gene expression and provided the first evidence for the feasibility of performing a comprehensive molecular characterization of normal, premalignant, and malignant head and neck squamous cell carcinoma (HNSCC) cells. In their study, biopsies from HNSCC patients were frozen, 8-μm thick tissue sections were cut onto RNAase free glass slides in a cryostat, and HNSCC cells were harvested from hematoxylin-stained sections using the PixCell LCM system to analyze differential gene expression. Results demonstrated that high-quality and representative cDNA libraries including more than 130 novel genes, which may have a role in the pathogenesis of HNSCC, were generated from the microdissected HNSCC tissue. In the analysis, 5000 dissected cells were sufficient to extract RNA of high integrity for the synthesis of high-quality representational cDNAs libraries. In another study, Alevizos et al. applied LCM to study differential gene expression from five cases of solid tumor tissues. The cancer tissues were snap frozen after surgical removal, and the PixCell system (LCM/GeneChip analysis) was successfully used to harvest normal and tumor cells for oligonucleotide microarray analysis and real-time PCR of collagenase, urokinase plasminogen activator, and cathepsin L (Alevizos et al., 2001). These studies clearly demonstrated that LCM-derived RNA can be analyzed on microarrays, and that array hybridization provides powerful approaches for identifying candidate genes and molecular profiling which have not been implicated in oral cancer. Moreover, the results also support the notion that such approaches are applicable to various molecular analysis of solid tumor, providing a means for obtaining information about consistent molecular alterations that advance both the understanding of the basic biology as well as the clinically relevant aspects of the molecular epidemiology of oral cancer. Thus, LCM is started to use in the analysis of the molecular changes associated with oral cancer.

Staging of cervical lymph nodes is still carried out by clinical examination of the neck region or by ultrasound, computed tomography, and magnetic resonance imaging, whereas the sensitivity of these methods is still limited due to the fact that the false negative rate is high in clinically diagnosed metastasis-negative (N0) patients. LCM has been investigated for use with gene array technology to seek for gene expression patterns in oral cancer, in an effort to find new biomarkers that will provide more accurate diagnosis, and also safer and more efficacious treatment, for oral cancer. In this regard, identification of genes and gene expression patterns in normal tissues and tumor tissues is critical. In the mid-1990s, it was difficult to perform this type of analysis, as the amount of total RNA retrieved from tissue samples by LCM was usually smaller than that required for the analysis. In 1999, however, Bertucci et al., presented protocol that allowed for the synthesis of first-strand cDNAs from small amounts of total RNA extracted from microdissected tissue samples (Bertucci et al., 1999). Moreover, DNA chip technology has been proven useful in examining global changes of gene expression upon, and in identifying target genes responsible for, a particular stimulus (Wang et al., 1999). Thus, aiming at clinical application, the combined use of LCM and gene array technologies has been developed for scanning of gene expression patterns and search for those correlating with a disease state. For example, Nguyen and colleagues applied a combination of LCM and microarray technology to investigate the differences in gene expression profiles between primary OSCC metastasized and non-metastasized to cervical lymph nodes. Specimens were embedded in Tissue-Tek OCT Compound (Sakura Finetek USA), 9-μm frozen sections were fixed with cold ethanol, and then, stained with hematoxylin. OSCC cells were obtained accurately with LCM, and total RNA was extracted to perform microarray and quantitative RT-PCR. The microarray analysis successfully selected 85 genes related to lymph node metastasis. Moreover, quantitative RT-PCR (real time PCR) for eight meaningfully expressed genes from the microarray data showed a high correlation between microarray data and quantitative RT-PCR data. Furthermore, the authors statistically constructed a prediction model, by which only one case in thirteen cases was a failure to predict. These results suggest that the diagnosis system using gene sets and LCM can be applied in diagnosis of OSCC.

In another clinical application, Lu and colleagues tried to screen tumors using phage display and LCM (Lu *et al.*, 2004). Fresh human OSCC tissue and normal mucosal (epithelium, blood vessels, and adjacent connective tissue) tissue sections were processed in the phage peptide library solution. The sections were rinsed to remove nonspecifically or weakly bound phages and dehydrated by freeze-drying (20 mtorr) for up to 10 days. Then, the phage-bound cells of interest were selected by the PixCell II LCM system. About 600 SCC cells were captured from each of the tissue samples. Then, the specific binding phages were recovered by transfection into host bacteria. The phages eluted from LCM-harvested cells were amplified and used as the input phage sub-library for the next round of biopanning. This procedure was repeated twice. After the second and third rounds of selection, tumor and mucosal tissue sections were washed to remove nonspecifically bound phages, and the binding specificity of phages selected from the previous round was assessed. Analysis of the phage numbers recovered from each whole section showed the phage solutions recovered from the second and third rounds had 8-fold and 12-fold greater affinity, respectively, for SCC tumor tissue than for normal mucosa. The results suggest that live phage-peptide conjugates can be recovered from laser capture microdissected cells in a form suitable for additional cycles of amplification. Thus, LCM will be a valuable adjunct to phage display studies.

Zhu *et al.* reported that LCM method could minimize possible contamination from infiltrated inflammatory cells (Zhu *et al.*, 2008). The cancer tissue sections immediately fixed with formalin and embedded in paraffin were stained with hematoxylin and eosin and subjected to the PALM LCM to analyze IgG1, V3, and V4f mRNA. Using in situ hybridization and LCM-correlated reverse-transcription polymerase chain reaction (RT-PCR), the authors found that rearranged IgG heavy chain transcripts were present in the oral epithelial cancer cells and in some normal epithelial cells adjacent to the tumor. These findings suggest that tumor-derived immunoglobulin may be an important new target molecule for tumor biotherapy.

### 3.4    MicroRNAexpression Analysis

LCM technologies are also useful for microRNA expression research in oral oncology. MicroRNAsare small (19 to 24 nucleotides) noncoding RNA gene products about 22 nt long that are found in diverse organisms, including animals (Lagos-Quintana, 2001, Lau *et al.*, 2001, Lee and Ambros, 2001). Since Ambros *et al.*, described specific criteria for the experimental verification of miRNAs, and conventions for naming miRNAs and miRNA genes, a number of studies are performed. As microRNA that regulate the translation and degradation of target mRNAs play a critical role in development, metabolism, and oncogenesis, it is important to clarify microRNA expression in target tissue. Liu *et al.*, investigated alterations in *miR-31* microRNA expression in head and neck squamous cell carcinoma tissues using LCM (Liu *et al.*, 2010). *miR-31* expression is known to repress several target genes to inhibit the metastasis of breast carcinomas. They reported that *miR-31* contributes to HNSCC development through hypoxia-inducible factor activation in tumor regions, wherein oxygen levels are above the threshold for 3' untranslated regionactivity.

### 3.5    Immnue-LCM Analysis

To date, formaldehyde as a 10% neutral buffered formalin is the most widely used as a fixative for various human tissues. The sections from formalin fixed samples normally show better preservation of tissue architecture, as compared with cryosections from frozen samples. As with DNA, formaldehyde reacts with RNA forming an N-methylol (N-CH2OH) followed by an electrophilic attack to form a methylene bridge between amino groups. Adenine is the most susceptible nucleotide to electrophilic attack and it is likely that the adenines within the mRNA sequence and the poly(A) tail of mRNA will be modified in the formaldehyde-fixated paraffin embedded sections to varying degrees. It is normally considered that RNA isolated from formaldehyde-fixated, paraffin embedded sections are less suitable for reverse transcription (cDNA synthesis), as compared to RNA isolated frozen tissue sections (Srinivasan *et al.*, 2002). Thus, cryo-tissue sections are commonly used for gene expression analysis using LCM (Curino *et al.*, 2004; Gandini *et al.*, 2012) and immune-LCM. However a recent report has suggested that it is possible to perform gene expression analysis from approximately one-year-old formaldehyde-fixated paraffin embedded tissue sections from human crista ampullaris (Pagedar *et al.*, 2006). We have further developed a methodology of immune-LCM of formaldehyde fixed, paraffin embedded HNSCC specimens that were immunostained for coagulation factor VIII (a marker of human endothelial cells). The Leica AS LMD, which uses a pulsed 337 nm UV laser on an upright microscope, is used (Figure 1). The laser beam can be moved with a software-controlled mirror system that allows us to select target cells and tissues: following selection of target area on a monitor by a freehand drawing tool, the computer-controlled mirror moves the laser beam along the pre-selected path and cut the target tissue. The dissected tissue sections fall into a cap of PCR tube by their gravity. The collection by gravity is very fast and it is easy to transfer the dissected tissue sections to reaction buffer. The thickness and width of the cutting line can be controlled for each tissue. Thus, this method allows us to collect good quality RNA of factor VIII-positive endothelial cells retrieved from the tumor mass. By this method, we have reported that the crosstalk between neovascular endothelial cells and tumor cells plays a major role in OSCC tumor growth and angiogenesis, and that Bcl-2 (B-cell lymphoma 2) is a key regulator of this crosstalk (Figure 2). Thus, a novel role for Bcl-2 as a pro-angiogenic signaling molecule has been presented (Kaneko *et al.*, 2007). Our step-by-step characterization of the technique based on LCM indicates that oral administration of a small-molecule inhibitor of VEGF receptors (PTK/ZK) is anti-angiogenic in early stage head and neck tumors, which are accompanied by quantifiable inhibition of the VEGF-Bcl-2-CXCL8 signaling axis (Miyazawa *et al.*, 2008). In recent analysis by using LCM, we have further reported that Bcl-2 in endothelial cells contributes to lymph node metastasis in patients with OSCC (Tarquinio *et al.*, 2012). Thus, this method using formaldehyde-fixated paraffin embedded samples may be better suited for the analysis of relatively rare cell types within a tissue, and may improve our ability to perform differential diagnosis of pathologies as compared to conventional LCM (Kaneko *et al.*, 2009).

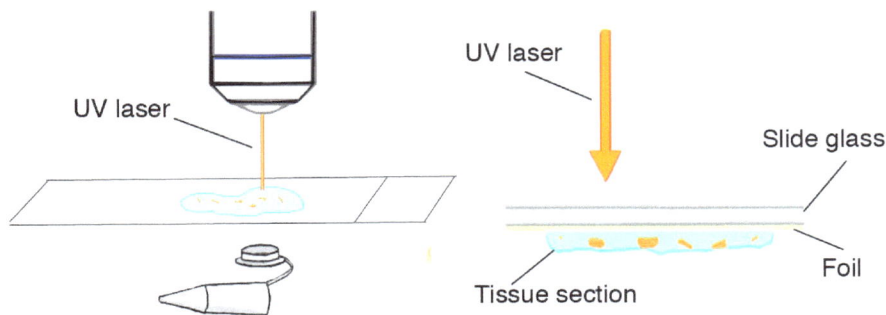

**Figure 1:** Principle of the Leica AS LMD microdissection. The tissue section that has been mounted on a PEN foiled slide is set upside down on the stage. Then, laser beam dissects the target tissue. The dissected tissue falls into collecting cap positioned under the specimen.

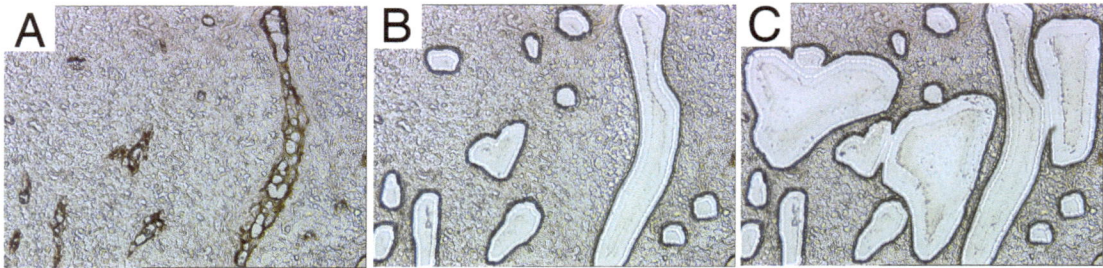

**Figure 2:** Step-by-step characterization of the technique based on immune-LCM used for retrieval of either Factor VIII-positive endothelial cells or the Factor VIII-negative surrounding tissues around Factor VIII-positive endothelial cells from formaldehyde-fixed paraffin-embedded tissue sections. **A.** Factor VIII-positive endothelial cells in a section of head and neck carcinoma. **B.** Retrieval of Factor VIII-positive endothelial cells. **C.** Retrieval of the Factor VIII-negative surrounding tissues.

## 4    Immune-LCM from Formaldehyde-fixed, Paraffin-embedded Oral Cancer Tissues

This protocol is modified from our previous report (Kaneko *et al.*, 2011).Disposable gloves should always be wornas skin often contain bacteria and molds that can be a source of contaminating RNA and RNases, The use of sterile, disposable plasticware and filtered pipette tips is recommended for RNA work to prevent cross-contamination with RNases from shared equipment.

### 4.1    Tissue fixation, Paraffin Embedding

1.    Tissues are fixed with 10% neutral buffered formaldehyde for 8 – 16 hours at 4 ˚C.

2.    Dehydrated for 30 minutes in 70% ethanol, for 1 hour in 90% ethanol, and for 30 minutes in 95% ethanol at 4 ˚C.

3.    Dehydrated 3 times for 1 hour in 100% ethanol at room temperature.

4.    Immersed 2 times in xylene for 1 hour at room temperature.

5.    Immersed 4 times in paraffin for 30 minutes at 58˚C.

6.    The specimen is embedded in paraffin and blocked.

### 4.2    Paraffin Block Storage

1.    We recommend that the paraffin blocks be stored at 4˚C, but the paraffin blocks can be stored at room temperature until processed.

2.    The blocks can be kept for 12 months, but we recommend that the blocks should be sectioned as soon as possible.

### 4.3    Sectioning, and Mounting

1. Cutting sections on a microtome with a new sterile disposable blade (8 – 10μm thick).

2. Floating paraffin ribbons on 43°C nuclease-free water (diethylpyrocarbonate (DEPC)-treated water).

3. Mounting the tissue on poly-L-lysine coated glass foiled polyethylene naphthalate (PEN) slides for laser capture microdissection(LCM, ylation).

4. Dry slides in a 35°C incubator for 6 hours.

## 4.4    Slide Storage

We recommend that the slides be stored at 4°C and LCM should be performed as soon as possible. Slides should be used within a week after preparation.

## 4.5    Staining: Nuclear Staining by Hematoxylin

1. Deparaffinize the slides 3 times with 2 min xylene washes at room temperature.

2. 100% ethanol washes 3 times for 20 sec at 4 °C.

3. 90% ethanol wash for 30 sec at 4 °C.

4. 70% ethanol wash for 1 min at 4 °C.

5. DEPC-treated water wash for 30 sec at 4 °C.

6. Gill No.3' hematoxylin (Sigma-Aldorich, Deisenhonen, Germany) for 5 – 10 sec at room temperature.

7. DEPC-treated water wash for 30 sec at 4°C.

8. Airdry the slide for 1 – 3 hours at 4 °C.

## 4.6    Staining: Immunostainig

Avidine-biotin-peroxidase complex (ABC) method is employed. 2~4 slides per session is easy to manageable.

1. Deparaffinize the slides twice with 3 min xylene washes at room temperature.

2. 100% ethanol washes 3 times for 30 sec at 4 °C.

3. 90% ethanol washes for 30 sec at 4 °C.

4. 70% ethanol washes for 1 min at 4 °C.

5. RNase-free phosphate buffered saline (PBS) washes 3 times for 30 sec at 4 °C.

6. Pre-treat these sections with 0.125% trypsin for 30 min at room temperature.

7. RNase-free PBS washes 3 times for 30 sec at 4 °C.

8. Endogenous peroxidase activity blockage with 0.3% hydrogen peroxide in methanol for 3 min at 4°C.

9. RNase-free PBS washes 3 times for 30 sec at 4 °C.

10. Incubation with a primary antibody for 16 h at 4°C, or for 30 min at room temperature

11.  RNase-free PBS washes 3 times for 30 sec at 4 ˚C.

12.  Incubation with biotinylated secondary antibody (Vector laboratories, Burlingame, CA; diluted 1:500) for 1 h at 4˚C.

13.  RNase-free PBS washes 3 times for 30 sec at 4 ˚C.

14.  Incubation with avidine-biotine-peroxidase complex (Elite ABC kit; Vector) for 1 h at 4˚C.

15.  RNase-free PBS washes 3 times for 30 sec at 4 ˚C.

16.  Development in diaminobenzidine-$H_2O_2$ solution (DAB substrate kit; Vector) for 3 min at room temperature.

17.  RNase-free PBS washes 3 times for 30 sec at 4 ˚C.

18.  Airdry the stained slides for 1 – 3 hours at 4 ˚C.

19.  Store at –70 °C ~ 4 °C until ready to perform LCM.

### 4.7    LCM (Leica AS LMD system) and Total RNA Extraction by TRIZOL® Reagent (Life Technologies™ (Invitrogen™), Carlsbad, CA)

1.  Dissection of immuno-positive cells and collection into individualtubes filled with 20 µl TRI-ZOL®Reagent, Tubes should be immediatelyplaced on ice as soon as possible.

2.  Close the tubes securely. Centrifuge the samples at 14,000 rpm for 10 sec at 4 °C.

3.  Add TRIZOL® Reagent to sufficient to 30 – 100 µl.

4.  Incubate the samples for 5 minutes at room temperature.

5.  Add chloroform in the same amount as TRIZOL® Reagent used.

6.  Close sample tubes securely. Shake tubes briefly for 30 – 60 seconds and incubate them for 5 min on ice.

7.  Centrifuge the samples at 14,000 rpm for 15 min at 4 °C.

8.  Transfer the aqueous phase to a fresh tube. (Following centrifugation, the mixture separates into three layer; a lower red phenol-chloroform phase, an interphase, and a colorless upper aqueous phase. RNA is contained exclusively in the aqueous phase.)

9.  Add isopropyl alcohol (RNA precipitant) to the tube in the same amount as the aqueous phase transferred. Incubate the samples at 4 °C for 10 minutes. Centrifuge at 13,000 rpm for 15 minutes at 4 °C. RNA will be precipitate under the tube. The RNA precipitate forms a white small dotted pellet on the side and bottom of the tube. The RNA precipitate is sometimes invisible after centrifugation,

10. Discard the supernatant gently.

11. Add 70 – 75% ethanol in DEPC-treated water to the RNA pellet and mix the sample by vortex.

12. Centrifuge at 6000 – 7500 rpm for 5 minutes at 4°C.

13. Discard the supernatant gently.

14. Add 70 – 75% ethanol in DEPC-treated water to the RNA pellet,

15. The RNA pellet can be stored at −20°C.

## 4.8    RNA Clean Up by RNeasy Mini Kit (Qiagen, Frederick, ML)

All processes of RNA clean up by RNeasy Mini Kit can be performed at room temperature

1. Add 10 µl β-Mercaptoethanol per 1 ml Buffer RLT.

2. Adjust the sample to a volume of 100 µl with RNase-free water. Add 350 µl Buffer RLT, and mix briefly.

3. Add 250 µl of 100% ethanol to the diluted RNA, and mix by pipetting without centrifuge.

4. Transfer the sample (total 700 µl) to an RNeasy Mini spin column placed in a 2 ml supplied collection tube. Centrifuge for 15 s at 8000 x g. Discard the flow-through.

5. Reuse the collection tube.

6. Add 350 µl Buffer RW1 to the RNeasy spin column. Close the lid gently, and centrifuge for 15 s at 10000 rpm to wash the spin column membrane and discard the flow-through.

7. Reuse the collection tube in step 4.

8. Add 10 µl DNase I stock solution to 70 µl Buffer RDD that is supplied with the RNase-Free DNase Set. Mix by gently inverting the tube, and centrifuge briefly to collect residual liquid from the sides of the tube.

9. Add the DNase I incubation mix (80 µl) directly to the RNeasy spin column membrane, and place at room temperature for 15 min.

10. Add 350 µl Buffer RW1 to the RNeasy spin column. Close the lid gently, and centrifuge for 15 s at 10,000 rpm. Discard the flow-through.

11. Add 500 µl Buffer RPE to the RNeasy spin column, and centrifuge for 15 s at 10,000 rpm and discard the flow-through.

12. Reuse the collection tube.

13. Add 500 µl Buffer RPE to the RNeasy spin column, and centrifuge for 2 min at 10,000 rpm.

14. Place the RNeasy spin column in a new 2 ml collection tube, and discard the old collection tube with the flow-through, and centrifuge at 13,000 rpm for 1 min.

15. Place the RNeasy spin column in a new 1.5 ml collection tube. Add 30–50 µl RNase-free water directly to the spin column membrane, and centrifuge for 1 min at 10,000 rpm to elute the RNA.

## 4.9    Single-stranded cDNA Synthesis

1. Add 1µg RNA (up to 16 µl) into 4 µl master mix (High Capacity RNA-to-cDNA Master Mix, Life Technologies™ (Applied Biosystems®)).

2. Add DEPC-treated water to sufficient to 20 µl.

3. Close PCR tubes securely, and centrifuge the tubes for 10 sec at 4 °C.

4.  Place the tubes on ice until ready to load a thermal cycler (TaKaRa PCR Thermal Cycler Dice®, Takara BIO INC, Siga, Japan).

5.  Program of the thermal cycler (Set cycler program at the reaction volume of 20 µl):

6.  cDNA synthesis and pre-denaturation: Perform 1 cycle of: 25°C for 5 min, 42°C for 30 min 85°C for 5 min.

7.  Start the reverse transcription of the cycler run.

8.  Add DEPC-treated water to sufficient to 100 µl.

9.  Store at  –70 °C until ready to perform quantitative PCR or other PCR applications.

The overall strategy described here for quantitative gene expression analysis of immunostained formaldehyde-fixated, paraffin-embedded tissue sections is summarized in Figure 3.

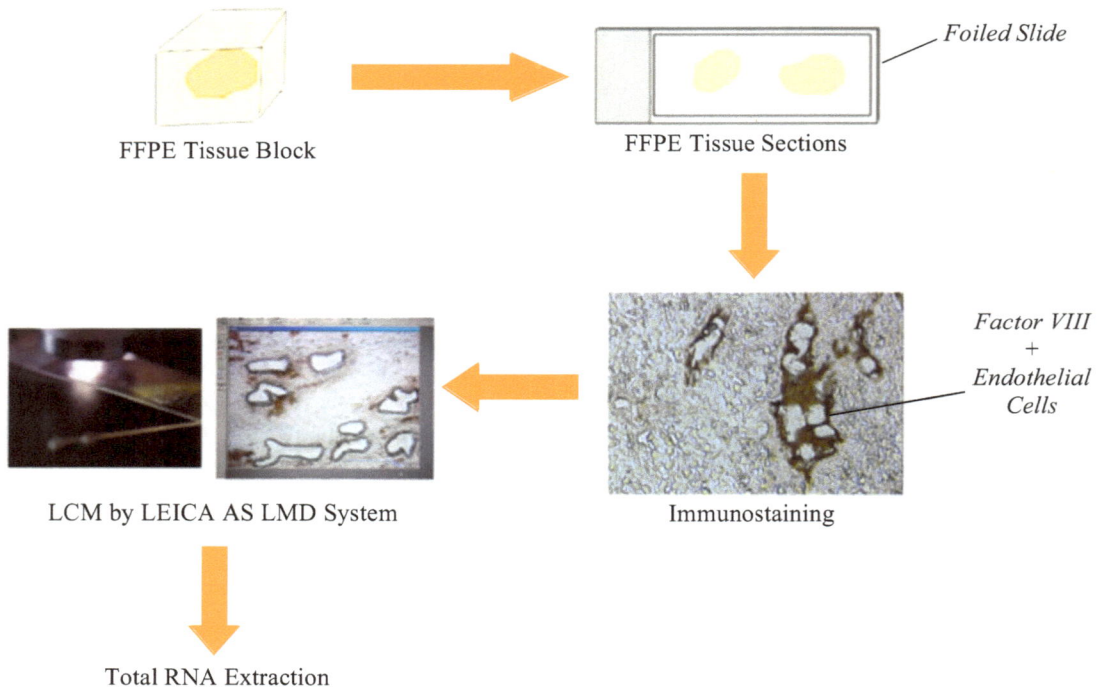

**Figure 3:** Our strategy described here for quantitative gene expression analysis following immune-LCM (LEICA AS LMD system) from formaldehyde-fixed paraffin-embedded (FFPE) tissue section.

# 5   Conclusion

Tissue based LCM is a powerful technique that combines morphology, histopathology, and molecular biological analysis. The ability of LCM to retrieve specific populations of interested cells, combined with the analysis of gene sequencing and gene expression in these sub-population of cells,has made LCM an critical device in clinical and investigative oral oncology.

# References

Alevizos, I., Mahadevappa, M., Zhang, X., Ohyama, H., Kohno, Y., Posner, M., Gallagher, G.T., Varvares, M., Cohen, D., Kim, D., Kent, R., Donoff, R.B., Todd, R., Yung, C.M., Warrington, J.A., Wong, D.T. (2001). Oral cancer in vivo gene expression profiling assisted by laser capture microdissection and microarray analysis.Oncogene, 20, 6196-6204.

Ambros, V., Bartel, B., Bartel, D.P., Burge, C.B., Carrington, J.C., Chen, X., Dreyfuss, G., Eddy, S.R., Griffiths-Jones, S., Marshall, M., Matzke, M., Ruvkun, G., Tuschl, T. (2003). A uniform system for microRNA annotation. RNA, 9, 277-279.

Bertucci, F., Van Hulst, S., Bernard, K., Loriod, B., Granjeaud, S., Tagett, R., Starkey, M., Nguyen, C., Jordan, B., Birnbaum, D. (1999). Expression scanning of an array of growth control genes in human tumor cell lines. Oncogene, 18, 3905-3912.

Curino, A., Patel, V., Nielsen, B.S., Iskander, A.J., Ensley, J.F., Yoo, G.H., Holsinger, F.C., Myers, J.N., El-Nagaar, A., Kellman, R.M., Shillitoe, E.J., Molinolo, A.A., Gutkind, J.S., Bugge, T.H. (2004). Detection of plasminogen activators in oral cancer by laser capture microdissection combined with zymography. Oral Oncology, 40,1026-1032.

Curino, A., Patel, V., Nielsen, B.S., Iskander, A.J., Ensley, J.F., Yoo, G.H., Holsinger, F.C., Myers, J.N., El-Nagaar, A., Kellman, R.M., Shillitoe, E.J., Molinolo, A.A., Gutkind, J.S., Bugge, T.H. (2004). Detection of plasminogen activators in oral cancer by laser capture microdissection combined with zymography. Oral Oncology, 40, 1026-1032.

Dahse, R., Berndt, A., Haas, K.M., Hyckel, P., Böhmer, F.D., Clauseen, U., Kosmehl, H. (2002) Laser capture microdissection in 2-D co-culture models as a tool to study tumor-stroma interactions. Biotechniques, 33, 474-475.

Emmert-Buck, M.R., Bonner, R.F., Smith, P.D., Chuaqui, R.F., Zhuang, Z., Goldstein, S.R., Weiss, R.A., Liotta, L.A. (1996). Laser capture microdissection. Science, 274, 998-1001.

Gandini, N.A., Fermento, M.E., Salomón, D.G., Blasco, J., Patel, V., Gutkind, J.S., Molinolo, A.A., Facchinetti, M.M., Curino, A.C. (2012). Nuclear localization of heme oxygenase-1 is associated with tumor progression of head and neck squamous cell carcinomas. Experimental and Molecular Pathology, 93, 237-245.

Ito, S., Ohga, T., Saeki, H., Nakamura, T., Watanabe, M., Tanaka, S., Kakeji, Y., Maehara, Y. (2005). p53 mutation profiling of multiple esophageal carcinoma using laser capture microdissection to demonstrate field carcinogenesis. International Journal of Cancer, 113, 22-28.

Kaneko, T., Okiji, T., Kaneko, R., Suda, H., Nör, J.E. (2011). Laser-capture microdissection for Factor VIII-expressing endothelial cells in cancer tissues.Methods in MolecularBiology, 755, 395-403.

Lagos-Quintana, M., Rauhut, R., Lendeckel, W., Tuschl, T. (2001). Identification of novel genes coding for small expressed RNAs. Science, 294,853-858.

Lau, N.C., Lim, L.P., Weinstein, E.G., Bartel, D.P. (2001). An abundant class of tiny RNAs with probable regulatory roles in Caenorhabditis elegans. Science, 294,858-862.

Lee, R.C., Ambros, V. (2001). An extensive class of small RNAs in Caenorhabditis elegans. Science, 294,862-864.

Leethanakul, C., Patel, V., Gillespie, J., Pallente, M., Ensley, J.F., Koontongkaew, S., Liotta, L.A., Emmert-Buck, M., Gutkind, J.S. (2000a). Distinct pattern of expression of differentiation and growth-related genes in squamous cell carcinomas of the head and neck revealed by the use of laser capture microdissection and cDNA arrays. Oncogene, 19, 3220-3224.

Leethanakul, C., Patel, V., Gillespie, J., Shillitoe, E., Kellman, R.M., Ensley, J.F., Limwongse, V., Emmert-Buck, M.R., Krizman, D.B., Gutkind, J.S. (2000b). Gene expression profiles in squamous cell carcinomas of the oral cavity: use of laser capture microdissection for the construction and analysis of stage-specific cDNA libraries. Oral Oncology, 36, 474-483.

Liu, C.J., Tsai, M.M., Hung, P.S., Kao, S.Y., Liu, T.Y., Wu, K.J., Chiou, S.H., Lin, S.C., Chang, K.W. (2010). miR-31 ablates expression of the HIF regulatory factor FIH to activate the HIF pathway in head and neck carcinoma. Cancer Research, 70, 1635-1644.

Lu, H., Jin, D., Kapila, Y.L. (2004). Application of laser capture microdissection to phage display peptide library screening. Oral Surgery, Oral Medicine, Oral Pathology, Oral Radiology & Endodontics, 98, 692-697.

Mbeunkui, F., & Johann, D.J. Jr. (2009). Cancer and the tumor microenvironment: a review of an essential relationship. Cancer Chemotherapy and Pharmacology, 63, 571-582.

Nguyen, S.T., Hasegawa, S., Tsuda, H., Tomioka, H., Ushijima, M., Noda, M., Omura, K., Miki, Y. (2007). Identification of a predictive gene expression signature of cervical lymph node metastasis in oral squamous cell carcinoma. Cancer Science. 98, 740–746.

Ohyama, H., Zhang, X., Kohno, Y., Alevizos, I., Posner, M., Wong, D.T., Todd, R. (2000). Laser capture microdissection-generated target sample for high-density oligonucleotide array hybridization. Biotechniques, 29, 530-536.

Pagedar, N.A., Wang, W., Chen, D.H., Davis, R.R., Lopez, I., Wright, C.G., Alagramam, K.N. (2006). Gene expression analysis of distinct populations of cells isolated from mouse and human inner ear FFPE tissue using laser capture microdissection--a technical report based on preliminary findings. Brain Research, 1091, 289-299.

Pedersen, T.X., Leethanakul, C., Patel, V., Mitola, D., Lund, L.R., Danø, K., Johnsen, M., Gutkind, J.S., Bugge, T.H. (2003). Laser capture microdissection-based in vivo genomic profiling of wound keratinocytes identifies similarities and differences to squamous cell carcinoma.Oncogene, 22, 3964-3976.

Srinivasan, M., Sedmak, D., Jewell, S. (2002). Effect of fixatives and tissue processing on the content and integrity of nucleic acids. American Journal of Pathology, 161, 1961-1971.

Tarquinio, S.B., Zhang, Z., Neiva, K.G., Polverini, P.J., Nör, J.E. (2012). Endothelial cell Bcl-2 and lymph node metastasis in patients with oral squamous cell carcinoma. Journal of Oral Pathology&Medicine, 41, 124-130.

Wang, Y., Rea, T., Bian, J., Gray, S., Sun, Y. (1999). Identification of the genes responsive to etoposide-induced apoptosis: application of DNA chip technology. FEBS Letters, 445, 269-273.

Wu, X., Jin, C., Wang, F., Yu, C., McKeehan, W.L. (2003). Stromal cell heterogeneity in fibroblast growth factor-mediated stromal-epithelial cell cross-talk in premalignant prostate tumors. Cancer Research, 63, 4936-4944.

Xu, C., Liu, Y., Wang, P., Fan, W., Rue, T.C., Upton, M.P., Houck, J.R., Lohavanichbutr, P., Doody, D.R., Futran, N.D., Zhao L.P., Schwartz, S.M., Chen, C., Méndez E. (2010). Integrative analysis of DNA copy number and gene expression in metastatic oral squamous cell carcinoma identifies genes associated with poor survival.Moleculer Cancer, 2010; 143.

Xu, C., Houck, J.R., Fan, W., Wang, P., Chen, Y., Upton, M., Futran, N.D., Schwartz, S.M., Zhao, L.P., Chen, C., Mendez E. (2008). Simultaneous Isolation of DNA and RNA from the Same Cell Population Obtained by Laser Capture Microdissection for Genome and Transcriptome Profiling. The Journal of Molecular Diagnostics, 10, 129–134.

Yamanaka, Y., Kaneko, T., Yoshiba, K., Kaneko, R., Yoshiba, N., Shigetani, Y., Nör, J.E., Okiji, T. (2012). Expression of angiogenic factors in rat periapical lesions. Journal of Endodontics, 38, 313-317.

Zhu, X., Li, C., Sun, X., Mao, Y., Li, G., Liu, X., Zhang, Y., Qiu, X. (2008). Immunoglobulin mRNA and protein expression in human oral epithelial tumor cells. Applied Immunohistochemistry& Molecular Morphology, 16, 32-38.

# The Use of the Micronucleus Test to Monitor Individuals at Risk of Oral Cancer

Eneida de Moraes Marcílio Cerqueira
*Toxicological Genetics Laboratory, Department of Biological Sciences*
*Feira de Santana State University, Brazil*

José Roberto Cardoso Meireles
*Toxicological Genetics Laboratory, Department of Biological Sciences*
*Feira de Santana State University, Brazil*

## 1    Introduction

Oral squamous cell carcinoma is among the ten types of malignant neoplasia of highest incidence world-wide and is particularly frequent in developing countries (Marchione *et al.*, 2007; Warnakulasuriya, 2009). In the United Kingdom, this neoplasia accounts for over 2% of all new cases of cancer in males and for more than 1% of all new cases in females (Cancer Research UK, 2012). In the United States between 2005 and 2009, 16.1 cases per 100,000 men and 6.2 per 100,000 women were diagnosed. In 2012, it is estimated that 28,540 men and 11,710 women will be diagnosed with cancer of the oral cavity and pharynx (U.S. National Institutes of Health, 2012). According to Jemal *et al.* (Jemal *et al.*, 2011), the highest oral cavity cancer rates are generally found in Melanesia, South-Central Asia, and Central and Eastern Europe and the lowest in Africa, Central America and Eastern Asia, for both males and females.

Several risk factors have been shown to be associated with this neoplasia, but cigarette smoking is considered to be the most important factor for its development, particularly when in association with alcoholic beverages (Reibel, 2003; Rodriguez *et al.*, 2004; Jemal *et al.*, 2011). Smokeless tobacco products and HPV infection are also considered to be important risk factors for oral cavity cancer (Suhas *et al.*, 2004; Syrjänen, 2005). Worldwide, considering deaths from cancers of both the oral cavity and the pharynx, smoking accounts for 42% and heavy alcohol consumption for 16% (Danaei *et al.*, 2005).

Similarly to other types of malignant neoplasia, oral squamous cell carcinoma results from alterations (point mutations and chromosomal abnormalities) in genes that control the cell cycle, and/or in genes that are involved in DNA repair. In addition to the potential for metastasis, cancer is characterized by the loss of cells' ability to evolve to death when genetic damage occurs (apoptosis) (Hanahan & Weinberg, 2000). As well as other types of malignant neoplasia, if oral squamous cell carcinoma is detected in its early stages, it can be treated successfully.

In this context, the use of biomarkers to identify genetic damage in individuals at higher risk of developing oral squamous cell carcinoma and to evaluate the malignant transformation potential of precancerous lesions is considered to be an important tool for cancer prevention. The Micronucleus Test on exfoliated cells from oral epithelium has been widely used for these purposes.

## 2    The Micronucleus Test on Exfoliated Cells from Oral Epithelium

The use of the Micronucleus Test on exfoliated cells from oral epithelium with the aim of undertaking biomonitoring on human populations exposed to genotoxic agents was first proposed by Stich *et al.* (1982). The efficacy of this test for this purpose has been highlighted in many studies (Tolbert *et al.*, 1992; Machado-Santelli *et al.*, 1994; Salama *et al.*, 1999; Cavallo *et al.*, 2005). It is worth emphasizing that increased frequencies of micronuclei precede the clinical manifestations relating to the development of oral squamous cell carcinoma. According to Stich & Rosin (1983a) and Stich (1987), the frequency of micronuclei in human cells can be used as an "endogenous dosimeter" for tissues that are targets of these agents' action.

According Salama *et al.* (1999), exfoliated oral cells are excellent for use in monitoring populations exposed to contaminants present in the environment, because these cells are in direct contact with pollutants that are ingested. Moreover, as highlighted by Zhang & Mock (1989) and Zhang (1994), they are capable of metabolizing carcinogens to reactive forms. Salama *et al.* (1999) also considered that when the test is applied to these cells, it presents greater sensitivity in detecting the effects from exposure caused by the smoking habit, than when applied to lymphocytes.

Using the Micronucleus Test is also an important strategy for monitoring preneoplastic oral lesions, thereby guiding the therapeutic approach to be adopted (Casartelli, 2000; Halder *et al.*, 2004; Kamboj & Mahajan, 2007; Saran *et al.*, 2008; Chatterjee *et al.*, 2009). Furthermore, according to Chatterjee *et al.* (2009), this test forms a very simple, practical, inexpensive and noninvasive screening technique for clinical prevention among individuals who are at risk of developing cancer.

## 2.1    Origin and Significance of Micronuclei

Micronuclei are formed by chromosomal fragments or whole chromosomes that fail to be included in the nuclei during the cell division process. They remain in the cytoplasm of interphasic cells as structures with a constitution and appearance similar to those of the nuclei (Cerqueira *et al.*, 1998). Thus, micronuclei reflect both aneugenic and clastogenic events (Figure 1).

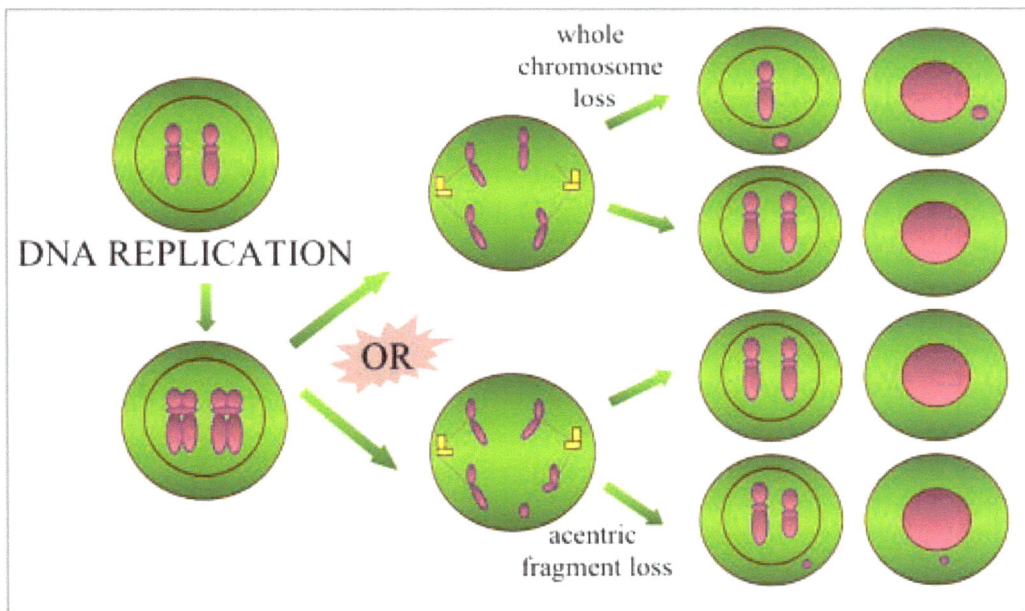

**Figure 1:** Mechanisms of micronuclei formation

## 2.2    Methodological issues

### 2.2.1    Choosing the sample

One important issue to be considered in the test is in relation to the number of individuals who should be included in the sample. Statistical software such as SPSS and Cytel Software can be used to calculate the sample size. Albertini *et al.* (2000) provided a practical description of how this calculation can be done. Segundo Au *et al.* (1991), in studies in which chromosome alterations are used as biomarkers, the minimum number of individuals to be analyzed should be 20, both for the exposed and for the control individuals. Ramírez (2000) considered that analysis on 30 individuals "ensures overall statistical representativeness for estimating sample parameters".

In case-control studies, individuals in different groups should be matched according to gender and age. The criteria for including and excluding individuals should be rigorously consonant with the focus of the study, in order to minimize the interference of confounding factors, although statistical tools may get round the possible distortions introduced by such factors.

### 2.2.2    Collecting Cells and Obtaining Smears

The oral epithelium consists of stratified squamous cells, in four distinct layers: the stratum germinativum (or stratum basale) is the most internal layer, and this is successively overlain, going towards the surface of the oral cavity, by the spinosum, granulosum and corneum strata. Maintenance of this epithelium is done at the cost of intense proliferation of the basal cells of the stratum germinativum, which become differentiated as they migrate towards the upper layers. This process takes place over a period of 7 to 21 days (Squier & Kremer, 2001). Thus, the micronucleus test on exfoliated cells of the oral mucosa is a method indicated for evaluating recent genotoxic effects.

The material can be collected using different method, depending on the tissue to be studied, but according to Bonassi et al. (2011), the collection tool may influence the frequency of micronuclei. To collect cells from the oral cavity, the following have been used: toothbrush (Lucero et al., 2000; Pastor et al., 2001); wooden spatula (Özkul et al., 1997; Bloching et al., 2000); tongue depressors (Stich & Rosin, 1983b); or cervical cell collection brushes (Meireles, 2003; Cerqueira et al., 2004; Dórea, 2012). Cleansing of the oral cavity, by means of mouthwashes using drinking water, is recommended prior to sample collection.

The material collected can be directly transferred to a slide by means of cytocentrifugation or as asmear, or it can be dripped after centrifugation on saline solution (0.9% NaCl). Some authors have recommended that the material collected should be washed before dripping, using a buffer solution (0.01 M Tris-HCl, 0.1 M EDTA and 0.02 M NaCl at pH 7.0) (Titenko-Holland et al., 1994). From our experience, we consider that direct placement of a smear on a slide with the aid of two drops of physiological saline solution is not only extremely practical but also provides a greater number of cells and spreads them out well (Meireles, 2003; Cerqueira et al., 2004; Dórea et al., 2012). The transfer method does not interfere with the frequency of micronuclei (Bonassi et al., 2011). Additional references relating to collection and processing of epithelial cells from various tissues can be found in the extensive reviews by Majer et al. (2001) and Salama et al. (1999).

### 2.2.3    Fixing and Staining the Cells

The material is generally fixed using a 3:1 solution of methanol/acetic acid (Stich & Rosin, 1983b), but other fixing agents can also be used: 80%-85% ethanol (Stich et al., 1992), 3:1 ethanol/acetic acid (Burgaz et al., 1999) or 80% methanol (Lucero et al., 2000; Cavallo et al., 2005), which may or may not depend on the staining or methodology used.

The staining method most commonly used to show up the nuclear DNA and the micronuclei, in preparation for analysis under a conventional optical microscope, as proposed by Feülgen & Rossenbeck, back in 1924. Their preparations were counterstained using 1% fast green, but staining using Giemsa (Bloching et al., 2000) and aceto-orcein (Revazova, 2001) have also been used, even though non-DNA-specific staining agents lead to overestimates (Neresyan et al., 2006). Acridine orangeor DAPI (4′, 6′-diamidino-2-phenylindole) is generally used for observations with fluorescence microscopy (Lucero et *al.*, 2000; Pastor *et al.*, 2001; Cavallo *et al.*, 2005). According to Lucero *et al.* (2000), in preparations destined for observation using fluorescence microscopy, DAPI analysis (which is DNA-specific, thereby avoiding errors introduced through counting artifacts) is advantageous in relation to stains that are not DNA-specific. When the analysis is done using confocal microscopy (Cerqueira *et al.*, 2004) or phase-contrast microscopy, only the nucleus should be stained (Tolbert *et al.*, 1992).

The FISH technique (fluorescent in situ hybridization) for analyzing micronuclei is applied using a centromeric probe and propidium iodide for counterstaining (Moore *et al.*, 1993; Titenko-Holland *et al.*, 1994; Surrallés *et al.*, 1997). This method was considered by Titenko-Holland *et al.* (1994) to be more effective than the Feülgen stain for detecting degenerative nuclear abnormalities, and makes it possible to precisely identify whether the micronucleus originated in an aneugenic event, or whether it resulted from chromosome breakage. Aneugenic or clastogenic origins for micronuclei can also be identified through using antibodies that recognized specific proteins of centromeres, but use of these antibodies on exfoliated cells runs into technical difficulties (Moore *et al.*, 1993), or difficulties based on the size of the micronuclei (Sarto *et al.*, 1987). Figure 2 illustrates the collection, processing and staining method used in our laboratory.

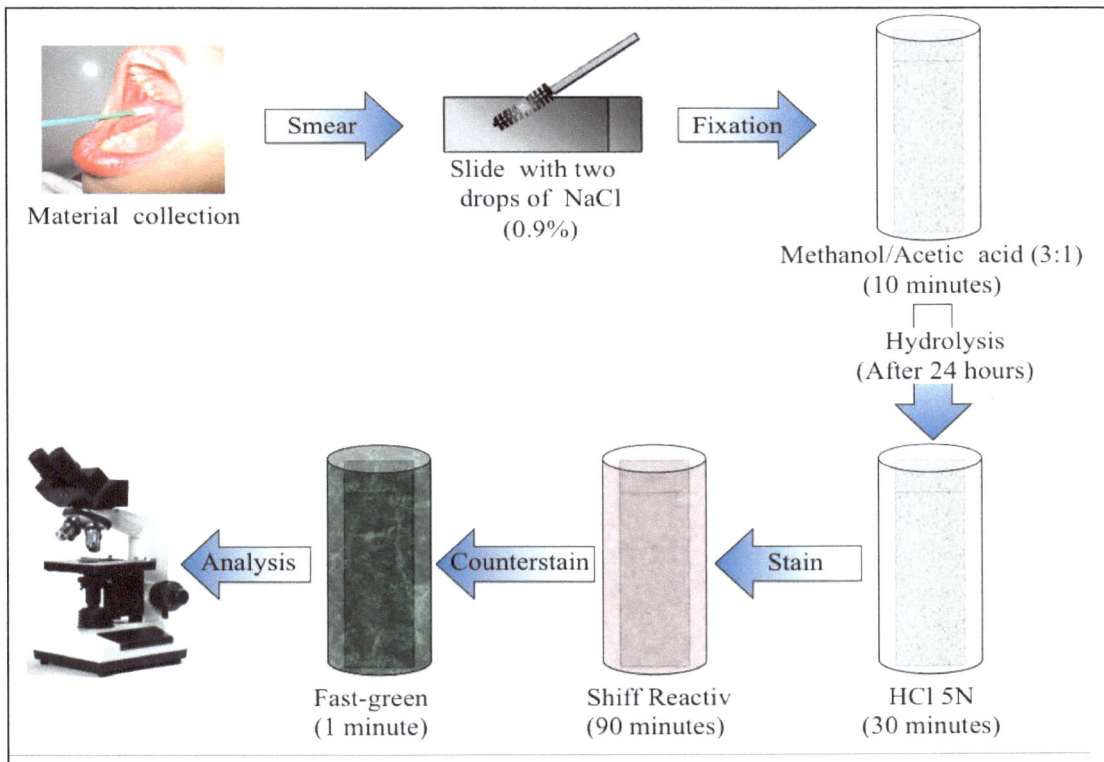

**Figure 2:** Methodology of the micronucleus test on exfoliated cells from oral epithelium

## 2.2.4    Identifying Cell Types in Buccal Exfoliated Cells

In 1985, Stich *et al.* (1985) proposed that cells presenting other nuclear alterations (karyorrhexis, multi-nucleated cells and cells presenting very large micronuclei) should be included in the count, based on their opinion that there could be some difficulty in correctly identifying micronucleated cells. Their proposal was also based on their view that the action of different carcinogens could preferentially induce different types of nuclear aberrations.

Two years later, Sarto *et al.* (1987) proposed a new analysis protocol that went against their initial proposal. They now proposed that the micronucleus count should only include cells with complete cytoplasm, with or without micronuclei, and that cells presenting degenerative nuclear phenomena such as karyorrhexis, karyolysis and pyknosis should be excluded from the analysis, along with cells presenting nuclear projections (nuclear buds and broken eggs). According to these authors, the nuclear alterations induced by these phenomena could be confounded with micronuclei (which we do not agree with, given that they are quite distinct). They also suggested that binucleated cells should also be excluded.

In 1991 and 1992, Tolbert *et al.* (1991, 1992) published two studies that suggested new criteria for cell counts in the Micronucleus Test. According to these authors, degenerative nuclear phenomena should be counted separately at the time of the micronucleus analysis, because greater occurrence of these phenomena, in itself, is indicative of apoptosis (karyorrhexis, condensed chromatin and pyknosis) and necrosis (karyolysis, karyorrhexis, condensed chromatin and pyknosis), which reveal the genotoxic and cytotoxic effects respectively of a given exposure.

Apoptosis is stimulated by exposure to mutagenic agents and acts as a protective mechanism against cancer by eliminating genetically damaged cells. High levels of occurrence of apoptosis may constitute evidence of genotoxic damage, and this would be related to the initiation of the process of malignant transformation (Tolbert *et al.*, 1992).

Pyknosis, condensed chromatin and karyorrhexis accompany keratinization, which takes place as an adaptive response to cell damage in epithelium that usually is not keratinized (Pindborg *et al.*, 1980). Karyolysis can occur in addition to these alterations, in cells undergoing necrosis, i.e. cell death, consequent to the action of exogenous agents on the cell environment (Wyllie, 1981; Galluzzi *et al.*, 2012). Occurrences of keratinization and necrosis are indicative of cytotoxicity, and these may be associated with cancer promotion via stimulation of cell proliferation (Tolbert *et al.*, 1992).

The criteria for micronucleus recognition are similar to what was described by Sarto *et al.* (1987). Micronuclei are distinctively individualized structures within the cytoplasm of interphasic cells measuring between one-fifth and one-third of the size of the main nucleus, observed in the same plane as the nucleus and presenting similar staining and chromatin distribution (Figure 4b). However, it has been suggested that a distinction should be made between micronuclei of high certainty (structures that meet all the identification criteria) and micronuclei of low certainty that are thus classified because the structure suggestive of a micronucleus does not fulfill all the requisites for inclusion (Figure 3). Nuclear projections that are described as broken eggs should also be included in the analysis. The cell count criteria proposed by these authors were ratified more recently by Thomas *et al.* (2009) in a paper in which they presented a detailed protocol for a test that they named the buccal micronucleus cytome test (BMCyt). In this protocol, the authors recommended that in addition, obviously, to making counts of cells without alterations, they should be made on the following: 1) cells with micronuclei and nuclear buds, to assess the DNA damage; 2) cells presenting karyorrhexis, karyolysis, pyknosis and condensed chromatin, to make inferences about occurrences of cell death; 3) basal cells, to assess the proliferative potential of the mucosa; and 4) binucleated cells, with information on defects in cytokinesis. The photomicrographs in

Figure 4 illustrate cell without alteration (a), cell presenting micronuclei (b) andcells with degenerative nuclear phenomena (ctof).

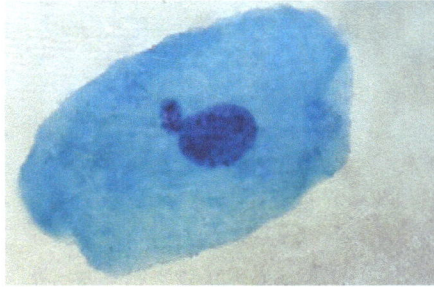

**Figure 3**: Photomicrography of cell presenting micronuclei of low certainty

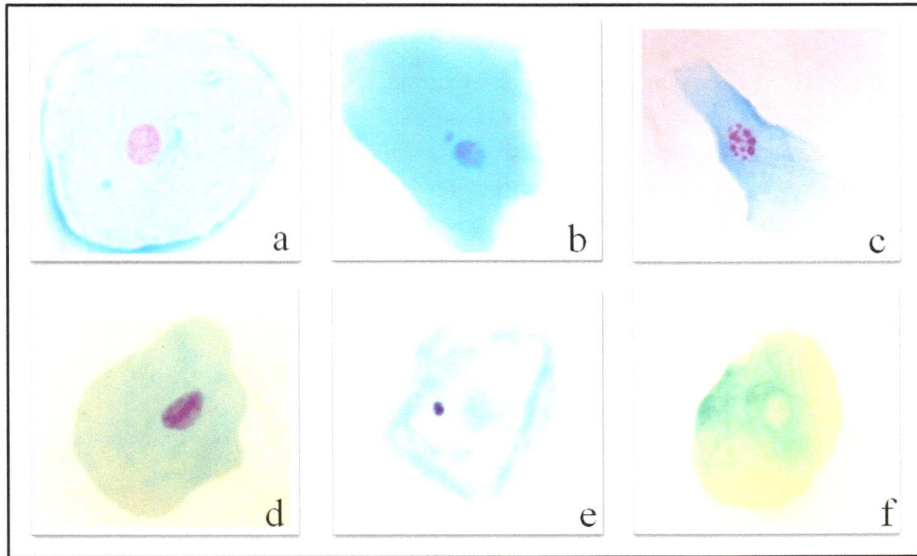

**Figure 4:** Photomicrographs of normal cell (a), cell presenting micronuclei (b) and cells with karyorrhexis (c), condensed chromatin (d), pyknosis (e) and karyolysis (f).

Attention needs to be drawn to the ambiguity relating to nuclear projections, with regard both to their significance in different cell types and to the nomenclature used to describe them, as also highlighted by Nersesyan (2005).

Nuclear projection structures known as broken eggs and buds have been analyzed in some studies (Tolbert *et al*., 1991; 1992; Torres-Bugárin *et al.,* 1998; Meireles, 2003; Santos, 2003; Cerqueira *et al*., 2004), but the real significance of their occurrence, along with the mechanisms that originate them, are little known. In some studies, their occurrence has been counted, but there has been little discussion of their importance or significance consequent to exposure to genotoxic substances.

Broken eggs were described for the first time by Tolbert *et al.* (1991) and the first reference to buds appeared in the literature in 1998, in a report by Bhattathiri (1998) on alterations induced by radiation in oral epithelial cells.

With regard to the divergences relating to the use of the terms bud and broken eggs, Nersesyan (2005) analyzed studies in which these structures were assessed in lymphocytes and drew attention to the following: 1) both structures are presented in a photo published by Fenech & Crott (2002) under the same definition of "nuclear buds"; 2) Serrano-García & Montero-Montoya (2001) described broken eggs as "buds attached to the nucleus by a stalk", and nuclear buds as "stalk-less buds"; and 3) de Almeida *et al.*(2004) presented a photo of a "stalk-less bud" that they named a "broken egg".

The term "nuclear blebbings" was used by Özkul *et al.* (1997) in reporting the exclusion of "structures similar to micronuclei, connected to the main nucleus by a bridge" from the micronucleus count, in exfoliated cells from the oral epithelium of users of Maras Powder.

From our experience with epithelial cells of the oral mucosa, we consider that the morphological distinction between nuclear buds and broken eggs is very clear (Figure5). Both of them presented continuity with the nucleus, but we take the term "bud" to indicate nuclear projections that result from strangulation in a small and limited area of the nuclear surface from which a rounded protuberance (a bud) comes out, whereas a "broken egg" comprises a structure smaller than a nucleus that is connected to it by a fine Feülgen-positive filament. In broken eggs, attention is drawn to the fact that both in these and in the nucleus, there is a chromatin concentration close to the thread which under optical microscopy is sometimes difficult to see. In such cases, analysis using confocal microscopy always reveals the presence of the filament. Moreover, the nucleus and micronucleus are rounded, whereas in cells presenting broken eggs, it is sometimes seen that both in this and in the main nucleus, the circular outline is lost and an area of straight surface remains. Cells with these characteristics were presented by Ünal *et al.* (2005) as being cells with a micronucleus. A distinction with what Tolbert *et al.* (1991) named "micronucleus of low certainty" also needs to be established. In this, as shown well in Figure 4, the extranuclear structure has a well-defined outline and does not present any continuity solution with the nucleus (which is observed in the buds) but, rather, juxtaposition.

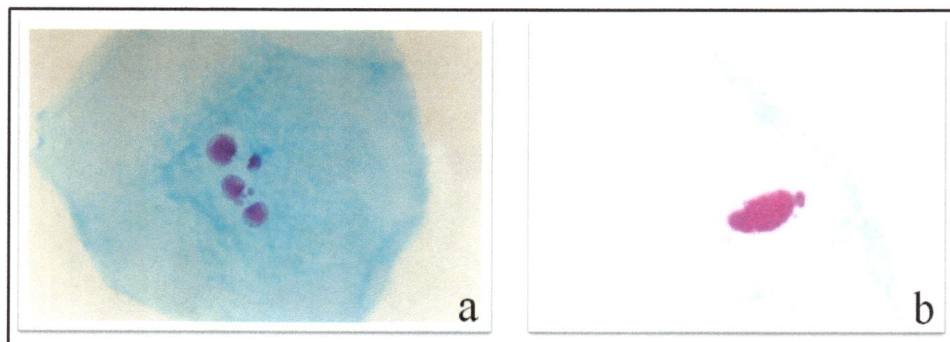

**Figure 5:** Photomicrographs of cells presenting broken eggs (a) anda nuclear buds (b)

It has been put forward that nuclear buds in lymphocytes may be the expression of the geneamplification process (Fenech & Crott, 2002; Fenech, 2002), and also that a micronucleus formation mechanism that starts with formation of a bud in the S period of the interphase might mediate removal of double minutes: acentric autonomous chromatin replication structures that express the amplification of onco-genes in malignant tumors (Shimizu *et al.*, 1998).

On the other hand, some studies in which occurrences of buds and broken eggs in lymphocytes were evaluated have correlated these structures as indicators of genotoxicity (Serrano-García & Montero-Montoya, 2001; Zeljejic & Garaj-Vrovak, 2004).

Although there is still no solidly substantiated evidence in the literature that would reveal the nature and significance of nuclear projections in lymphocytes, the results from some studies suggest that they originate both in epigenetic events (Shimizu *et al.*, 1998; Fenech & Crott, 2002; Fenech, 2002), and as a consequence of genotoxicity (Serrano-García & Montero-Montoya, 2001; Zeljejic & Garaj-Vrovak, 2004).

With regard to the real significance of nuclear buds and broken eggs in epithelial cells, the results from studies developed in the Toxicological Genetics Laboratory of Feira de Santana State University (UEFS), Brazil, strongly suggest that there is an association with the natural differentiation process of the oral epithelium. Cerqueira *et al.* (2004) observed that there was a significantly higher frequency of these structures before exposure to X-ray radiation than afterwards. In an analysis on oral mucosal cells from individuals exposed to chemical mutagens in the workplace, Meireles (2003) reported that there was a significantly higher frequency of broken eggs in the control group. Santos (2003) evaluated the genotoxic effects of exposure to pesticides and also observed that there was a significantly greater number of broken eggs in the control group than in the exposed group.

Concordant with these results, Torres-Bugarín *et al.* (1998) reported that the frequency of broken eggs was significantly higher in the negative controls than in individuals undergoing antineoplastic chemotherapy.

In a study conducted to assess the genotoxic effects of the habits of smoking and consuming alcoholic drinks, Bohrer *et al.* (2005) also described significantly higher frequencies of broken eggs among control individuals (abstemious in relation to alcohol and nonsmokers) than among either smokers or individuals who were both smokers and drinkers.

In some studies in which exfoliated cells from the oral epithelium were analyzed, no difference in the frequency of broken eggs was observed between exposed and control individuals. In evaluations on the effects of exposure to pesticides and cytostatic drugs, Gomez-Arroyo *et al.* (2000) and Torres-Bugarín *et al.* (1998; 2003) described similar frequencies of these structures between exposed and control individuals. However, in all these studies, significantly higher frequencies of micronuclei were detected in the exposed individuals. Results similar to these were obtained in a study developed in our laboratory (Cerqueira *et al.*, 2008), in which the effects of the X-ray radiation used in producing panoramic radiographs were evaluated in gingival cells. If the frequency of broken eggs were indeed indicative of genotoxicity, it would be expected that in response to this exposure, higher frequencies of both micronuclei and broken eggs would be expected.

However, going against this logic, Montero *et al.* (2003) described a significantly higher frequency of "nuclear buds", but not of micronuclei, in individuals in the central area of Mexico, a region that is recognized to be highly polluted.

Increased occurrence of broken eggs consequent to exposure to genotoxic substances was described by Montero *et al.* (2003) and Revazova *et al.* (2001), but these researchers merely presented data, without discussing the mechanisms that might lead to increased numbers of these structures consequent to the exposure.

Nersesyan *et al.* (2002a, b) evaluated occurrences of micronuclei and broken eggs in exfoliated cells from the uterine cervix of pre and postmenopausal women, in comparison with women who presented regular menstrual cycles. Significantly higher frequencies of broken eggs, but not of micronuclei, were observed among the pre and postmenopausal women. According to these authors, this suggested that occurrences of broken eggs were associated with the degenerative process in the cervical cells consequent to hormonal changes.

The hypothesis that broken eggs could be associated with degenerative processes receives backing, according to Nersesyan (2005), from a study conducted by Bindu *et al.* (2003). The latter study revealed that the frequency of micronuclei in cells of the oral epithelium in individuals subjected to radiation increased linearly with the dose (total dose of 38.5 Gy), but increased frequency of broken eggs was only observed close to the end of the radiotherapy treatment, which can be explained by degenerative changes in the tumor cells.

However, in a similar study, although Nersesyan *et al.* (1995) reported higher frequencies of micronuclei in oral epithelial cells from individuals who had been subjected to a radiation dose of 42 Gy, they did not observe any increase in the frequency of broken eggs. It has been proposed (Ramírez & Saldanha, 2002) that broken egg formation is an event that precedes micronucleus formation, but in our view there is a lack of experimental evidence to prove this supposition.

In summary, in the light of the contradictory results obtained from studies in which buds and broken eggs were analyzed in epithelial cells, we can conclude that the real significance of these abnormalities needs further investigation in order to establish this. The results from our laboratory and the data obtained by Bohrer *et al.* (2005) are concordant with the conclusion that Nersesyan (2005) reached after analyzing the literature, and strongly suggest that occurrences of these structures are not associated with genotoxicity.

## 2.2.5    Scoring Methods

With regard to the number of cells that should be counted, Albertini (2000) took the view that given the low frequencies of micronuclei in exfoliated epithelial cells, it was recommendable to count 3,000 to 5,000 cells per individual. Nonetheless, there is great variation in the numbers of cells considered in different studies. In the initial studies conducted, numbers of cells that today would be considered insufficient were counted, ranging from 300 to 500 cells (Stich & Rosin, 1983b; Stich *et al.*, 1992). At the other extreme of this scale, Beliën *et al.* (1995) took into account the low frequency of micronuclei and the intra and inter-individual variability that were detected in the results obtained from analyzing 1,000 cells from a single preparation of around 10,000 cells, and took the view that the analysis should include this total. Thus, in their view, this would require automation of the method. Since no automation methods have been established, most authors analyzed 2,000 to 3,000 or more cells (Sarto *et al.*, 1987; Lucero *et al.*, 2000; Pinto, 2000; Pastor *et al.*, 2001; Santos, 2003; Cavallo *et al.*, 2005), while others counted exactly 1,000 (Machado-Santelli *et al.*, 1994; Burgaz *et al.*, 1999; Bloching *et al.*, 2000) or 1,500 cells (Surrallés *et al.*, 1997) and yet others considered that 1,000 would be the minimum number acceptable but analyzed the maximum number of cells contained in the preparation (Meireles, 2003; Cerqueira *et al.*, 2004). Thomas *et al.* (2009) suggested that initially, a minimum of 1,000 cells should be counted in order to determine the frequencies of the various cells, and that 2,000 differentiated cells should be counted in order to calculate the frequencies of the micronuclei and nuclear projections.

Microscopic analysis should be performed by a trained person, and preferably one who has not been involved in sample collection and slide preparation. In addition, the slides should be coded and analyzed in blind tests in relation to any information that might identify the subject of the sample (Thomas *et al.*, 2009). These authors' proposed protocol includes identification criteria for the different cell types, although broken eggs are described under the name of nuclear bud.

### 2.2.6   Statistical Analysis

The results obtained using the Micronucleus Test on exfoliated cells from oral epithelium should always be subjected to adequate statistical analysis, using parametric univariate analysis (Student's t-test, ANOVA, Ancova or Pearson's correlation) or nonparametric univariate analysis: Kruskal-Wallis test, Mann-Whitney U-test, Spearman's correlation, chi-square or Wilcoxon (Thomas *et al.*, 2009.,Ceppi *et al.*, 2010). Multivariate linear regression analyses may be necessary in order to determine the influence of confounding factors.

In our studies, we have often used a conditional test to compare proportions in situations of rareevents (Bragança-Pereira, 1991). These are significance tests that form an alternative to the chi-square test along the lines of Fisher's exact test and are appropriate for evaluating cytogenetic events when a large sample of cells is necessary for detecting occurrences of a specific chromosomal aberration.

### 2.2.7   Advantages and Limitations of the Test

The Micronucleus Test on exfoliated cells is considered to be a valuable tool for identifying genetic damage consequent to exposure to mutagens because of the various advantages that it presents. These include:

- It detects the action of both clastogenic and aneugenic agents, since micronuclei result from chromosome breakage or failure to join together during fusion;

- It methodology does away with culturing procedures, which makes it less expensive than the classical chromosome analysis procedures. It can thus be applied in biomonitoring programs that include large populations;

- Genetic damage expressed as micronuclei is easy to detect and can be observed directly in cells that form the target of the mutagenic and/or carcinogenic agent studied;

- Study material from some epithelial tissues (such as from the oral, cervical and nasal epithelia) is obtained through simple noninvasive procedures;

- When the test is applied to tissues that are chronically and repeatedly exposed to mutagens, the frequency of micronuclei reflects a set of different chromosomal alterations that occur in cells of the basal layer of the epithelium.

The intrinsic disadvantage of the test is that chromosome exchanges and other rearrangements are not detected, while there is also the possibility that some fragments will be included in the main nucleus, thus becoming imperceptible, which would lead the test to underestimate the real frequency with which chromosome damage occurs.

# 3   The Micronucleus as a Biomarker for Identifying Chromosome Damage in Individuals at Higher Risk of Developing Oral Squamous Cell Carcinoma: Tobacco and Alcoholic Beverage Users

The habit of smoking is the risk factor most consistently associated with development of premalignant and malignant lesions of the oral epithelium, particularly when done concomitantly with consumption of alcoholic beverages (Llewellyn *et al.*, 2003; International Agency for Research on Cancer, 2004; Warnakulasuriya *et al.*, 2005).

In the tobacco of manufactured cigarettes and in the smoke released from them, more than 4,000 substances can be identified (Husgafvel-Pursiainen, 2004). Among these, 200 are toxic to humans and more than 50 present known carcinogenic action. Prominent among the latter are polycyclic hydrocarbons and specific nitrosamines of tobacco that are found in tar (International Agency for Research on Cancer, 2004).

Certain enzymes may metabolize the hydrocarbons of tobacco and transform them into carcinogens that are more powerful, such as aryl hydrocarbon hydroxylase (AHH), which is effective in increasing the carcinogenic potential of benzopyrene. The risk of tumor development is thus greater among smokers who produce these enzymes at higher concentrations. In addition to the action of tobacco carcinogens, the heat released by tobacco combustion worsens the aggressive action on the mucosa of the oral cavity (DeMarini, 2004).

Forms of tobacco consumption other than manufactured cigarettes have also been correlated with cancer development. Pipe and cigar smoking multiply the risk of cancer of the lips, mouth, tongue and pharynx, depending on the quantity of consumption (Silverman & Shillitoe, 1990).

The habit of tobacco-chewing, in different preparations ("areca-nut", "bidi" and "betel quid"), is considered to be a risk factor for development both of pre-malignant and malignant lesions of the oral epithelium. The use of snuff, especially when chewed, has also been correlated with development of oral squamous cell carcinoma (Lee *et al.*, 2003; Suhas *et al.*, 2004).

Evaluations on the chromosomal damage consequent to smoking, through micronucleus analysis on exfoliated cells from oral epithelium, have produced divergent results in the literature. Nonetheless, a significant number of studies have indicated that cigarette compounds are effective in inducing micronuclei.

Sarto *et al.* (1987) analyzed the aneugenic and clastogenic effects induced by tobacco on 25 individuals with such exposure (23 who smoked cigarettes and two who smoked cigars), and compared them with the same number of nonsmokers. They observed a significantly higher frequency of micronuclei consequent to chromosome breakage among the smokers.

On the other hand, using the same methodology, Stich & Rosin (1983b) did not detect any significant differences in the frequencies of micronuclei between 36 smokers (who were not alcoholic beverage consumers) and 15 nonsmokers (who were also non-drinkers).

In a study conducted in Orissa (India), Stich *et al.* (1992) analyzed occurrences of micronuclei among fishermen who habitually smoked with the lit end of the cigarette inside the mouth. Under such conditions, and given the way in which the smoke is expelled, the tongue and palate are more exposed than the cheeks. The mean frequencies of micronuclei observed in the tongue and palate were similar, but were significantly higher than those described for the cheeks.

Significantly higher frequencies of micronuclei in oral mucosal cells among smokers of manufactured cigarettes than among nonsmokers were described by Özkul *et al.* (1997) in a study that included 14 male smokers and 15 male nonsmokers.

Greater occurrence of chromosomal damage, as expressed by micronuclei, in cells of the oral mucosa, was also described by Konopacka (2003) in a study that included 50 smokers and 70 nonsmokers. The mean frequencies of micronuclei described per thousand cells were approximately three times greater among the smokers. Similar results were described by Martins & Boschini Filho (2003).

In a study that evaluated the effects of the quantity of cigarettes consumed per day with regard to induction of micronuclei, Wu *et al.* (2004) described higher frequencies of micronuclei only among individuals who smoked more than 20 cigarettes per day, in comparison with nonsmokers.

Bloching *et al.* (2000) observed significantly higher frequencies of micronuclei in cells of the oral epithelium of smokers, in comparison with a group of nonsmokers. Dose-response effects were also described. Evaluations in other studies, on occurrences of micronuclei consequent to exposure to tobacco consumed in forms other than manufactured cigarettes, have produced results that are even more consistent than those described for cigarette consumption.

In an investigation on the effects of using snuff, Tolbert *et al.* (1991) evaluated the frequency of micronuclei in exfoliated cells from the oral mucosa, among 38 women who used snufforally and 15 women who did not use tobacco. The mean numbers of micronuclei of high and low certainty among the users was twice as high as what was observed in the control group. However, the frequencies of micronuclei did not differ significantly when only the micronuclei of high certainty were considered.

Among Indians, "khaini" tobacco is commonly used. This is placed in the lower gingival groove and is left there for long period of time. In an evaluation on occurrences of micronuclei in gingival and cheek cells from users of this tobacco, Stich *et al.* (1992) registered significantly greater frequency of these structures in exfoliated cells of the gingiva. Similar results had previously been described by Stich *et al.* (1982) among users in the city of Bihar (India). The effects from using toothpaste containing "gudakhu" tobacco with regard to induction of micronuclei were also evaluated by Stich *et al.* (1992). No differences were detected between users and controls.

Dave *et al.*(1992) evaluated the cytogenetic effects induced by consumption of "areca nut" among individuals without oral lesions and users presenting fibrosis of the oral submucosa or oral cancer. Comparisons with the control group (non-users presenting normal oral mucosa) showed that there were significantly higher frequencies of sister chromatid exchanges and chromosomal aberrations in peripheral lymphocytes in the three groups of users. A similar result was reported by these authors when they evaluated occurrences of micronuclei in exfoliated cells from the oral mucosa, in the same individuals.

In a study conducted in Turkey that included 25 men who were making oral use of a powder obtained from dehydrated tobacco originating from leaves of *Nicotiana rustica* ("Maras powder"), Özkul *et al.* (1997) reported that there was a significantly higher frequency of micronuclei in the oral mucosal cells of users than in the control group.

The effects from consuming tobacco in the form of "bidi" (tobacco rolled in leaves of *Diospyros melanoxylon*and tied together with cotton thread) were assessed by Suhas *et al.* (2004) among 25individuals who were not consumers of alcoholic beverages and who solely consumed bidi, and compared them with 25 individuals without any history of exposure to any known genotoxic substance. The numbers of micronuclei were counted in cells of the oral mucosa, palate and tongue. Greater frequencies of these structures in the exposed group were recorded in cells from the oral mucosa and palate.

Genotoxic effects, expressed as greater occurrence of micronuclei in oral mucosal cells consequent to consumption of pan masala/gutkha, were described by Fareed *et al.* (2011). Similar results were obtained by El-Setouhy *et al.* (2008), among individuals who used a hookah for tobacco consumption.

However, Wu *et al.* (2004) did not detect higher frequencies of micronuclei in the oral mucosa of areca quid chewers. These authors also assessed the effects of this exposure concomitantly with consumption of manufactured cigarettes and did not observe any interaction. Thus, they suggested that the association described in the literature between oral carcinogenesis and use of areca quid might occur through routes other than genotoxicity.

An association between the habit of consuming alcoholic beverages and occurrences of oral cancer has been registered in the literature (Blot *et al.*, 1988; International Agency for Research on Cancer, 1988; Silverman & Shillitoe, 1990; Longnecker, 1995; Seitz *et al.*, 1998; Hindle *et al.*, 2000; Salaspuro, 2003). It has been suggested that alcohol probably acts as a cofactor, thereby increasing the carcinogenic potential of tobacco components for inducing cancer (Rothman &Keller, 1972; La Vecchia *et al.*, 1997; Du, 2000).

La Vecchia *et al.* (1997) suggested that alcohol may act as a solvent, thus facilitating the passage of carcinogens, especially those present in tobacco, through the cell membrane. Moreover, according to these authors, alcohol might present an association with carcinogenesis through increased metabolic activity of the liver, which could activate carcinogens, or through alterations induced directly in the metabolism of the target epithelial tissue.

With the aim of assessing the mutagenic effects of alcohol consumption, Reis *et al.* (2002) analyzed occurrences of micronuclei in exfoliated cells from the tongue and cheek mucosa of 40 nonsmokers who were chemically dependent on ethanol and 20 individuals who were abstemious in relation to alcohol and were nonsmokers. The number of micronuclei observed in the exfoliated cells from the tongue was significantly greater among the users of alcoholic beverages, but no significant difference was detected between the two groups in relation to cells from the cheek mucosa ($p > 0.05$).

Several studies evaluating the induction of chromosomal damage in lymphocytes or in exfoliated cells from the oral mucosa consequent to the habits of smoking and consuming alcoholic beverages have revealed that the alcohol present in these drinks does not, on its own, induce greater occurrence of this damage. However, in combination with the habit of smoking, additive and/or synergistic effects have been described (Stich & Rosin, 1983b; Xue *et al.*, 1992; Castelli *et al.*, 1999; Bloching *et al.*, 2000).

In exfoliated cells from the oral mucosa, Stich & Rosin (1983b) evaluated the effects of these habits on the induction of micronuclei in four groups of individuals: Group I: nonsmokers and nonusers of alcoholic beverages; Group II: smokers and non-drinkers; Group III: nonsmokers but drinkers; and Group IV: smokers and drinkers. They did not detect any significant differences in occurrences of micronuclei between the individuals in groups I, II and III, but the frequency of micronuclei in the individuals in Group IV was significantly greater than what was observed in the other three groups. Thus, their study revealed synergistic effects from the habits of smoking and alcohol consumption, on micronucleus induction.

The synergistic effect from the habits of chewing *Catha edulis* leaves, smoking manufactured cigarettes and consuming alcoholic beverages, on micronucleus induction in oral epithelial cells, was investigated by Kassie *et al.* (2001). The sample analyzed was divided into three groups: Group I was formed by 25 individuals who chewed *Catha edulis* and were smokers and drinkers; Group II was formed by an equal number of individuals who smoked and drank; and Group III was formed by 25 individuals who did not chew these leaves and neither smoked nor drank. These authors observed that: 1) the number of micronuclei among the individuals in Group I was twice what was observed among the individuals in Group II; 2) the incidence of micronuclei among the individuals in Group I was nine times greater than among the individuals in Group III; and 3) the incidence of micronuclei among the individuals in Group II was significantly greater than what was observed among the participants in Group III, thus revealing the additive effect of the habits of smoking and consuming alcoholic beverages on inducing chromosome damage.

In three studies conducted in our laboratory in which the effects of the habits of smoking and drinking were assessed, two of them did not reveal any significant differences between smokers and non-smokers (Santos, 2003; Freita *et al.*, 2005) and in the other (Meireles, 2003), the number of micronuclei was significantly greater among the smokers ($p < 0.01$). The results described by Freita *et al.* (2005) and Santos (2003) are concordant with those obtained by Bohrer *et al.* (2005), who also did not observe any significant differences in micronucleus occurrence in a study in which epithelial cells from the oral mucosa of 21 individuals who were nonsmokers and abstemious regarding alcohol, 28 smokers and 19 cigarette and alcoholic beverage consumers.

The study by Freita *et al.* (2005) included 20 individuals (6 men and 14 women), among whom eight smoked and drank; eight only smoked and four only drank. The control group was formed of equal numbers of men and women who were nonsmokers, abstemious regarding alcohol and without any history of exposure to other genotoxic agents. No associations were found, and according to these authors, this may have been due to the low exposure of the individuals analyzed: the alcoholic beverage consumption consisted predominantly of beer (83%), at the frequency of once a week (67%), and only one of the smokers declared a consumption rate greater than 20 cigarettes/day, while the majority (75%) consumed fewer than 10 cigarettes/day.

The sample analyzed by Santos (2003) was formed by 60 individuals, of whom 14 were smokers and made use of alcoholic beverages, two only smoked, 28 were nonsmokers but made use of alcoholic beverages and 16 neither smoked nor drank. Occurrences of micronuclei were not shown to be associated with either of these two habits, either singly or together, and the author concluded that the lack of association with the smoking habit could be attributed to low exposure, given that 70% of the smokers declared that their consumption was less than or equal to 10 cigarettes/day. In relation to the habit of consuming alcoholic beverages, the majority (64%) of the users declared that their consumption was greater than five glasses on one or two days per week. The lack of association with higher levels of micronuclei corroborated results from other authors in which alcohol alone did not induce genotoxicity (Stich & Rosin, 1983b; Bloching *et al.*, 2000).

Despite the divergent results obtained from studies in which occurrences of micronuclei in relation to the habits of smoking and drinking were investigated, the accumulated evidence indicates that the risk of this exposure is sufficient to discourage these habits and stimulate quitting them.

# 4   Use of the Micronucleus Test for Detecting Apoptosis in Individuals at Higher Risk of Developing Oral Squamous Cell Carcinoma: Tobacco and Alcoholic Beverage Users

Apoptosis is a genetically controlled process of cell death that occurs under normal conditions to eliminate cells that are no longer necessary to the organism or, as noted earlier, in response to genotoxic injury. Comprehension of the molecular events involved in the apoptotic process has advanced considerably over recent years, and the nucleus is considered to be an important remodeling target during this process (Schulte-Hermann, *et al.*, 2000; Miller *et al.*, 2002).

Starting from the proposal put forward by Tolbert *et al.* (1991; 1992), for a protocol for analyzing micronuclei in exfoliated cells from the oral epithelium, in which not only micronuclei were counted but also other nuclear alterations indicative of apoptosis (karyorrhexis, pyknosis and condensed chromatin) and necrosis (karyorrhexis, pyknosis, condensed chromatin and karyolysis) would be included, several other studies using this protocol have been conducted (Ramírez & Saldanha, 2002; Santos, 2003; Çelik *et al.*, 2003; Cerqueira *et al.*, 2004; Freita, *et al.* 2005; Meireles *et al.*, 2006).

In the studies that Tolbert *et al.* conducted in 1991 and 1992, to assess occurrences of micronuclei among snuff users, analyses on occurrences of pyknosis, karyorrhexis, condensed chromatin and karyolysis showed that these alterations were significantly more common among users, thus providing a good indication that this exposure produced genotoxic effects. Similar results were obtained by Freita *et al.* (2005) and Santos (2003), among individuals who were making use of cigarettes and/or alcoholic beverages. It should be emphasized that the individuals who formed the exposed group that these authors analyzed were considered to be moderate users. This highlights the sensitivity of this test for detected the effects of low exposure, when it is added to counting nuclear alterations other than micronuclei.

Induction of apoptosis in exfoliated cells from the oral mucosa of petrol/gasoline pump attendants in response to benzene exposure, and its interaction with the smoking habit, was also evaluated by Çelik, *et al.* (2003). The frequency of occurrence of karyorrhexis and karyolysis was significantly greater in the exposed group, and was also significantly greater among the smokers in this group and in the control group, in comparison with the nonsmokers in the respective groups. However, no interaction between benzene exposure and the smoking habit was observed.

In the study by Torres-Bugarín *et al.* (1998), in which occurrences of micronuclei in fire-eaters exposed to diesel were evaluated, several other nuclear alterations were counted, including those that Tolbert *et al.*(1991; 1992) considered to be indicative of apoptosis and necrosis. Like in other studies, the frequency of micronuclei was not significantly higher in the exposed group ($n = 8$) than among a group of 13 healthy individuals without any history of exposure to genotoxic agents, but the total count of other nuclear anomalies was significantly higher among the exposed individuals. Evaluation of the effects of the smoking habit between the exposed smokers ($n = 5$) and the exposed nonsmokers ($n = 3$) revealed that the smokers presented higher frequency of karyorrhexis. Comparison between the exposed smokers and a group of five smokers who had not been exposed to any other genotoxic agents showed that the exposed group presented a significantly greater number of cells with pyknosis, condensed chromatin and karyorrhexis, thus suggesting that there was some interaction between the smoking habit and exposure to diesel. Notwithstanding the small sample size evaluated by these authors, the results obtained indicated that the test had greater sensitivity for detecting genotoxicity when not only micronuclei but also other nuclear alterations were counted.

One important point to be emphasized in assessing occurrences of apoptosis in preparations for studying micronuclei is the need for correct interpretation of the nuclear alterations relating to apoptosis. Ünal *et al.* (2005), citing Çelik *et al.* (2003) and Tolbert *et al.* (1992), reported that karyolysis and karyorrhexis were evidence of apoptosis. In both studies by Tolbert *et al.* (1991; 1992) the affirmation that karyolysis is related to necrosis and not to apoptosis is very clear. In the study by Çelik *et al.* (2003), karyorrhexis and karyolysis were counted separately, but these authors reported that these alterations were considered to be indicative of apoptosis. Furthermore, although Ünal *et al.* (2005) correctly described the morphology of cells presenting karyorrhexis and karyolysis, the photographs corresponding to these were not representative of these events: two cells with karyorrhexis were indicated as presenting karyolysis.

## 5   The Micronucleus Test for Evaluating Malignant Transformation of Preneoplastic Lesions and for Biomonitoring on Individuals with Oral Squamous Cell Carcinoma

Cancer affecting the epithelium of the oral cavity is preceded by lesions that can be clinically detected, and among these, leukoplakia is the most frequently occurring type (Carnesoltas-Lázaro *et al.*, 2007; Kamboj & Mahajan, 2007). Erythroplakia, leukoerythroplakia and lichenoid dysplasia are other types of lesion that have been indicated to have the potential to evolve to malignant transformation (Rodrigues *et al.*, 2000; Kuffer & Lombardi, 2002; van der Meij *et al.*, 2006). In addition to these lesions, oral lichen planus has been the focus of studies aimed towards evaluating its potential for malignant transformation, but the results from these studies have been a source of controversy (van der Meij *et al.*, 2003; Lodi *et al.*, 2005; González-Moles *et al.*, 2006; van der Meij *et al.*, 2006).

Use of biomarkers to indicate the potential of precursor lesions to evolve to the process of malignant transformation is a preventive measure that guides therapeutic management. Within this context, several authors have considered the Micronucleus Test to be a valuable tool for biological monitoring of premalignant lesions of the oral cavity (Bloching *et al.*, 2000; Casartelli *et al.*, 2000; Halder *et al.*, 2004; Saran *et al.*, 2008).

With the aim of evaluating whether the Micronucleus Test on exfoliated cells could be used as a biomarker indicative of greater risk of development of cancer of the upper digestive tract, Bloching *et al.* (2000) analyzed cells from regions of the oral mucosa without abnormalities, in 55 individuals with carcinomas of the upper digestive tract and 16 individuals with leukoplakia, and compared the results obtained with those of 99 individuals without lesions. The frequency of micronucleus occurrence was twice as high among the individuals with lesions. These authors took the view that the results obtained indicated that micronuclei used as a biomarker were effective in assessing the risk of cancer development and could thus be of assistance in establishing preventive measures aimed towards reducing the risk of developing this disease, although this biomarker was unable to provide information regarding when or if the malignant transformation would occur.

In the study by Casartelli *et al.* (2000), the frequencies of micronucleus occurrences of micronuclei in exfoliated cells from normal oral mucosa and from areas of leukoplakia and *in situ* carcinoma were registered. The frequencies of micronuclei were significantly greater in the premalignant and malignant lesions, than in cells from the normal mucosa. These authors concluded that micronuclei could be used as a biomarker for neoplastic progression in the oral epithelium.

Halder *et al.* (2004) reached the same conclusion after evaluating occurrences of micronuclei among 50 individuals without oral lesions, 32 with premalignant lesions, 10 with a diagnosis of oral cancer for which treatment had not yet begun and eight with the same diagnosis who had already undergone surgery to treat the lesion. The mean frequencies of micronuclei recorded for these groups were 0.35%, 0.63%, 1.36% and 0.44%, respectively. According to these authors, their results evidently corroborated those described by Casartelli *et al.* (2000) and suggested that micronuclei might be a marker for oral carcinogenesis, although further studies would be necessary.

Saran *et al.* (2007) evaluated occurrences of micronuclei in oral epithelial cells from 24 individuals with oral cancer, 29 with premalignant lesions and 60without abnormalities of the mucosa. The results obtained revealed that there was a gradient of occurrences of these structures (from normal epithelium to cancer), thus indicating that the test was effective.

Ramirez and Saldanha (2002) compared micronucleus frequencies between individuals with oraland oropharyngeal carcinomas and individuals presentingoral mucosa without abnormalities. Exfoliated cells from three different regions of the oral cavity were analyzed: the region surrounding the lesion (B), the region contralateral to the lesion (A) and the region of the base of the upper gingival-labial sulcus. The results relating to comparisons within individual patients showed significant differences: micronuclei occurred most frequently in region B, followed by regions A and C. These authors emphasized the possibility that there might be a gradient of carcinogenic development (C → A → B). Comparison between individuals (patients and controls) indicated that there was a significantly higher frequency of micronucleus occurrence in the cells in the region of the lesion, in relation to the frequency of these structures in the individuals of the control group.

In a study developed in our laboratory (Dórea *et al.*, 2012), which evaluated occurrences of micronuclei in exfoliated cells from the oral epithelium of 20 individuals with oral squamous cell carcinoma and forty individuals with normal oral mucosa, micronuclei were found significantly more frequently in cells collected from lesions than in cells from normal areas, independent of the presence/absence of cancer. Given that loss of cell capacity to evolve to death consequent to occurrence of genetic damage (apoptosis) is one of the most striking characteristics of the process of malignant transformation, these authors also evaluated occurrences of degenerative nuclear alterations that indicate this process. The results obtained showed that in cells obtained from the lesions and from areas of normal mucosa in individuals with cancer, the frequency of apoptosis was significantly lower than what was seen in individuals without oral squamous cell carcinoma. This suggested that impairment of the apoptosis process affects the epithelium in a generalized manner and forms an event that precedes and favors development of malignant transformation.

Table 1 summarizes results obtained in studies using the Micronucleus Test for evaluating malignant transformation of preneoplastic lesions and for biomonitoring on individuals with oralsquamous cell carcinoma.

| Author | Kind of lesion | Endpoints analyzed |
|---|---|---|
| Bloching *et al.*, 2000 | Oral cancer and leukoplakia | Micronucleus |
| Casartelli *et al.*, 2000 | *In situ* carcinomaand leukoplakia | Micronucleus |
| Ramirez & Saldanha, 2002 | Oral and oropharyngeal carcinomas | Micronucleus |
| Halder *et al.*, 2004 | Oral cancer and premalignant lesions | Micronucleus |
| Saran *et al.*, 2008 | Oral cancer and premalignant lesions | Micronucleus |
| Dórea *et al.*, 2012 | Oral squamous cell carcinoma | Micronucleus and degenerative nuclear alterations |

**Table 1:** Studies using the Micronucleus Test in exfoliated oral cells for evaluating chromosomal damage and/or apoptosis in premalignant and malignant lesions of the oral cavity

# 5    Conclusions

- The Micronucleus Test on exfoliated cells of the oral epithelium is a valuable tool for detecting genetic damage;

- Use of a differentiated protocol, as suggested by Tolbert *et al.* (1991, 1992) increases the sensitivity of the test;

- In oral epithelial cells, broken eggs may be not associated with occurrences of chromosome damage, and thus reflect alterations relating to the normal tissue differentiation process;

- The Micronucleus Test can be used in biomonitoring for premalignant oral lesions;

- The malignant transformation process takes place accompanied by increased frequency of chromosome damage;

- The apoptotic process is disparate, even in situations of low exposure to mutagens;

- Malignant transformation is accompanied by loss of cell capacity to evolve to death in situations of DNA damage.

# References

Albertini, R. J., Anderson, D., Douglas, G.R., Hagmar, L., Hemminki, K., Merlo, F., Natarajan, A. T., Norppa, H., Shuker, D.E., Tice, R., Waters, M.D., & Aitio, A. (2000). IPCS guidelines for the monitoring of genotoxic effects of carcinogens in humans. Mutation Research, 463,111-172.

Au, W. W., Walker, D. M., Ward, J. B. Jr., Whorton, E., Legator, M. S., & Singh, V. (1991). Factors contributing to chromosome damage in lymphocytes of cigarette smokers. Mutation Reearch, 260, 137-144.

Beliën, J. A., Copper, M. P., Braakhuis, B. J., Snow, G. B., & Baak, J. P. (1995). Standardization of counting micronuclei: definition of a protocol to measure genotoxic damage in human exfoliated cells. Carcinogenesis,16, 2395-2400.

Bhattathiri, V. N., Bindu, L., Remani, P., Chandralekha, B., & Nair, K. M. (1998). Radiation-induced acute immediate nuclear abnormalies in oral cancer cells: serial cytologic evaluation.Acta Cytologica, 42, 1084-1090.

Bindu, L., Balaram, P., Mathew, A., Remani, P., Bhattathiri, V. N., & Nair, M. K. (2003). Radiation-induced changes in oral carcinoma cells_a multiparametric evaluation. Cytopathology, 14, 287-293.

Bloching, M., Hofmann, A., Lautenschläger, C., Berghaus, A., & Grummt, T. (2000). Exfoliative cytology of normal buccal mucosa to predict the relative risk of cancer in the upper aerodigestive tract using the MN-assay. Oral Oncology,36, 550-555.

Blot, W. J., McLaughlin, J. K., Winn, D. M., Austin, D. F., Greenberg, R. S., Preston-Martin, S., Bernstein, L., Schoenberg, J. B., Stemhagen, A., & Fraumeni Jr., J. F. (1988). Smoking and drinking in relation to oral and pharyngeal cancer. Cancer Research, 48, 3282-3287.

Bohrer, P. L., Filho, M. S., Paiva, R. L., da Silva, I. L., & Rados, P. V. (2005). Assessment of micronucleus frequency in normal oral mucosa of patients exposed to carcinogens. Acta Cytologica,49, 265-272.

Bonassi, S., Michael Fenech, M., Lando, C., Lin, Y., Ceppi,  M., Chang, W. P., Holland, N., Kirsch-Volders, M., Zeiger, E., Ban, S., Barale, R., Bigatti, M. P., Bolognesi, C., Jia, C., Di Giorgio, M.,  Ferguson, L. R., Fucic, A., Lima, O. G., Hrelia, P., Krishnaja, A. P., Lee, T-K., Migliore, L., Mikhalevich, L., Mirkova, E., Mosesso, P., Muller, W-U., Odagiri, Y., Scarffi, M. R., Szabova, E., Vorobtsova, I., Vral, A., & Zijno, A. (2011). The HUman MicroNucleus Project.

International database comparison for results with the cytokinesis-block micronecleus assay in human lymphocytes. I. Effect of laboratory protocol, scoring criteria, and host factors on the frequency of micronuclei. Environmental Molecular Mutagenesis, 37, 31-45.

Bragança-Pereira, C. A. (1991). Teste estatístico para comparar proporções em problemas de citogenética. In Mutagênese, carcinogênese e teratogênese : Métodos e critérios de avaliação (pp.113-121).

Burgaz, S., Karahalil, B., Bayrak, P., Taşkin, L., Yavuzaslan, F., Bökesoy, I., Anzion, R. B., Bos, R. P., & Platin, N. (1999). Urinary cyclophosphamide excretion and micronuclei frequencies in peripheral lymphocytes and in exfoliated buccal epithelial cells of nurses handling antineoplastics. Mutation Research, 439, 97-104.

Cancer Research UK. (2012) Oral cancer - UK incidence statistics (on line), 16 March 2012 (cit. June 11, 2012). Available at http://info.cancerresearchuk.org/cancerstats/types/oral/incidence/uk-oral-cancer-incidence-statistics

Carnesoltas-Lázaro, D., Domínguez-Odio, A., Frías-Vázquez, A. I., Dutok-Sánchez, C. M., & García-Heredia, G. (2007). Alteraciones citogenéticas bucoepiteliales em pacientes portadores de leucoplasia. Revista Mexicana de Patologia Clinica, 54, 104-111.

Casartelli, G., Bonatti, S., De Ferrari, M., Scala, M., Mereu, P., Margarino, G., & Abbondandolo, A. (2000). Micronucleus frequencies in exfoliated buccal cells in normal mucosa, precancerous lesions and squamous cellcarcinoma. Analytical & Quantitative Cytology & Histology, 22, 486-492.

Castelli, E., Hrelia, P., Maffei, F., Fimognari, C., Foschi, F. G., Caputo, F., Cantelli-Forti, G., Stefanini, G. F., & Gasbarrini, G. (1999). Indicators of genetic damage in alcoholics: reversibility after alcohol abstinence. Hepatogastroenterology,46, 1664-1668.

Cavallo, D., Ursini, C. L, Perniconi, B., Francesco, A. D., Giglio, M., Rubino, F. M., Marinaccio, A., & Iavicoli, S. (2005). Evaluation of genotoxic effects induced by exposure to antineoplastic drugs in lymphocytes and exfoliated cells of oncology nurses and pharmacy employees. Mutation Research,587, 45-51.

Çelik, A., Çavas, T., & Ergene-Gözükara, S. (2003). Cytogenetic biomonitoring in petrol station attendants: micronucleus test in exfoliated buccal cells. Mutagenesis, 18, 417-421.

Ceppi, M., Biasotti, B., Fenech, M., & Bonassi, S. (2010). Human population studies with the exfoliated buccal micronucleus assay: Statistical and epidemiological issues. Mutation Research, 705, 11-19.

Cerqueira, E. M. M., Santoro, C. L., Donozo, N.F., Freitas, B. A., Pereira, C. A., Bevilacqua, R. G., &Machado-Santelli, G. M.(1998). Genetic damage in exfoliated cells of the uterine cervix: Association and interaction between cigarette smoking and progression to malignant transformation?Acta Cytologica, 42, 639-649.

Cerqueira, E. M. M., Gomes-Filho, I. S., Trindade, S., Lopes, M. A, Passos, J. S., & Machado-Santelli, G.M. (2004). Genetic damage in exfoliated cells from oral mucosa of individuals exposed to X-rays during panoramic dental radiographies. Mutation Research,562, 111-117.

Cerqueira, E. M. M., Meireles, J. R. C., Lopes, M. A., Junqueira, V. C., Gomes-Filho, I. S., Trindade, S., & Machado-Santelli, G. M.(2008). Genotoxic effects of X-rays on keratinized mucosa cells during panoramic dental radiography. Dentomaxillofacial Radiology, 37, 398-403.

Chatterjee, S., Dhar, S., Sengupta, B., Ghosh, A., De, M., Roy, S., Chowdhury, R. R., & Chakrabarti, S. (2009). Cytogenetic monitoring in human oral cancers and other oral pathology: The micronucleus test in exfoliated buccal cells. Toxicology Mechanisms and Methods, 19, 427-433.

Danaei, G., van der Hoorn, S., Lopez, A. D., Murray, C., & Ezzati, M. (2005). Comparative risk assessment collaborating group (Cancers). Causes of cancer in the world: comparative risk assessment of nine behavioral and environmental risk factors. Lancet, 366, 1784-1793.

Dave, B. J., Trivedi, A. H., & Adhvaryu, S. G. (1992). Role of areca nut consumption in the cause of oral cancers. A cytogenetic assessment. Cancer,70, 1017-1023.

de Almeida, T. M., Leitao, R. C., Andrade, J. D., Beçak, W., Carrilho, F. J., & Sonohara, S. (2004). Detection of micronuclei formation and nuclear anomalies in regenerative nodules of human cirrhotic livers and relationship to hepatocellular carcinoma.Cancer Genetics and Cytogenetics, 150, 16-21.

DeMarini, D. M. (2004). Genotoxicity of tobacco smoke and tobacco smoke condensate: a review. Mutation Research, 567, 447-474.

Dórea, L.T. M., Meireles, J. R. C., Lessa, J. P.R., Oliveira, M. C., Pereira, C. A. B., Campos, A. P., & Cerqueira, E. M.M. (2012). Chromosomal damage and apoptosis in exfoliated buccal cells from individuals with oral cancer. International Journal of Dentistry, 2012, 1-6

Du, X., Squier, C. A., Kremer, M. J., & Wertz, P. W. (2000). Penetration of N-nitrosonornicotine (NNN) across oral mucosa in the presence of ethanol and nicotine. Journal of Oral Pathology & Medicine, 29, 80-85.

El-Setouhy, M., Loffredo, C. A., Radwan, G., Rahman, R. A., Mahfouz, E., Israel, E., Mohamed, M. K., & Ayyad, S. B. (2008). Genotoxic effects of waterpipe smoking on the buccal mucosa cells. Mutation Research, 655, 36-40.

Fareed, M., Afzal, M., & Siddique, Y. H. (2011) Micronucleus investigation in buccal mucosal cells among pan masala/gutkha chewers and its relevance for oral cancer. Biology and Medicine, 3, 8-15.

Fenech, M. (2002). Chromosomal biomarkers of genomic instability relevant to cancer. Drug Discovery Today, 7, 1128-1137.

Fenech, M., & Crott, J.W. (2002). Micronuclei, nucleoplasmic bridges and nuclear buds induced in folic acid deficient human lymphocytes_ evidence for breakage–fusion–bridge cycles in the cytokinesis-block micronucleus assay. Mutation Research, 504, 131–136.

Feulgen, R. & Rossenbeck, H. (1924). Mikroskopisch chemischer Nachweis einer Nucleinsäure vom Typus dre thymonucleinsäure und die daralf bestehende elektive farbung von Zelkernen in mikroskopischen Präparate. Zeitschrift für Physiologische Chemie,135, 203-248.

Freita, V. S., Lopes, M. A., Meireles, J. R. C., Reis, L., & Cerqueira, E. M. M.(2005). Efeitos genotóxicos de fatores considerados de risco para o câncer bucal.Revista Baiana de Saúde Pública, 29, 189-199.

Galluzzi, L., Vitale, I., Abrams, J. M., Alnemri, E. S., Baehrecke, E. H., Blagosklonny, M. V., Dawson, T. M., Dawson, V. L., El-Deiry, W. S., Fulda, S., Gottlieb, E., Green, D. R., Hengartner, M. O., Kepp, O., Knight, R. A., Kumar, S., Lipton, S. A., Lu, X., Madeo, F., Malorni, W., Mehlen, P., Nuñez, G., Peter, M. E., Piacentini, M., Rubinsztein, D. C., Shi, Y., Simon, H-U., Vandenabeele, P., White, E., Yuan, J., Zhivotovsky, B., Melino, G., & Kroemer, G. (2012). Molecular definitions of cell death subroutines: recommendations of the Nomenclature Committee on Cell Death 2012. Cell Death and Differentiation, 19, 107–120.

Gómez-Arroyo, S., Díaz-Sánchez, Y., Meneses-Pérez, M. A., Villalobos-Pietrini, R., & De León-Rodríguez, J. (2000). Cytogenetic biomonitoring in a Mexican floriculture worker group exposed to pesticides. Mutation Research, 466, 117-124.

González-Moles, M. A., Bascones-Ilundain, C., Gil Montoya, J. A., Ruiz-Avila, I., Delgado-Rodríguez, M., & Bascones-Martiínez, A. (2006). Cell cycle regulating mechanisms in oral lichen planus: Molecular bases in epithelium predisposed to malignant transformation. Archives of Oral Biology, 51, 1093-1103.

Halder, A., Chakraborty, T., Mandal, K., Gure, P. K., Das, S., Raychowdhury, R., Ghosh, A. K., & De, M. (2004). Comparative study of exfoliated oral mucosal cell micronuclei frequency in normal, precancerous and malignant epithelium. International Journal of Human Genetics, 4, 257-260.

Hanahan D., & Weinberg, R. A. (2000). The hallmarks of cancer. Cell. 100, 57-70.

Hindle, I., Downer, M. C., Moles, D. R., & Speight, P. M. (2000).Is alcohol responsible for more intra-oral cancer? Oral Oncology,36, 328-333.

Husgafvel-Pursiainen, K. (2004). Genotoxicity of environmental tobacco smoke: a review. Mutation Research,567, 427-445.

IARC Monographs on the Evaluation of Carcinogenic Risk to Human, Alcohol Drinking, (1988), Vol. 44. Lyon, France: International Agency for Research on Cancer.

IARC Monographs on the Evaluation of the Carcinogenic Risks of Chemicals to Humans, (2004), Vol. 83. Lyon, France: International Agency for Research on Cancer.

Jemal, A., Bray, F., Center, M. M., Ferlay, J., Ward, E., & Forman, D. (2011). Global Cancer Statistics. CA: A Cancer Journal for Clinicians, 61, 69-90.

Kamboj, M., & Mahajan, S. (2007). Micronucleus_ an upcoming marker of genotoxic damage. Clinical Oral Investigations, 11, 121-126.

Kassie, F., Darroudi, F., Kundi, M., Schulte-Hermann, R., & Knasmüller, S. (2001). Khat (Catha edulis) consumption causes genotoxic effects in humans.International Journal of Cancer,92, 329-332.

Konopacha, M. (2003). Effect of smoking and aging on micronucleus frequencies in human exfoliated buccal cells. Neoplasma,50, 380-382.

Kuffer, R.,& Lombardi, T. Premalignant lesions of the oral mucosa. A discussion about the place of oral intraepithelial neoplasia (OIN). (2002). Oral Oncology, 38, 125-130.

La Vecchia, C., Tavani, A., Franceschi, S., Levi, F., Corrao, G., & Negri, E. (1997). Epidemiology and Prevention of Oral Cancer. Oral Oncology,33, 302-312.

Lee, C-H., Ko, Y-C., Huang, H-L., Chao, Y-Y., Tsai, C-C., Shieh, T-Y., & Lin, L-M. (2003). The precancer risk of betel quid chewing, tobacco use and alcohol consumption in oral leukoplakia and oral submucous fibrosis in southern Taiwan. British Journal of Cancer, 10, 366-372.

Llewellyn, C. D., Linklater, K., Bell, J., Johnson, N. W., & Warnakulasuriya, K. A. A. S. (2003). Squamous cell carcinoma of the oral cavity in patients aged 45 years and under: a descriptive analysis of 116 cases diagnosed in the South East of England from 1990 to 1997. Oral Oncology, 39, 106-114.

Lodi, G., Scully, C., Carrozzo, M., Griffiths, M., Sugerman, P. B., &Thongprasom, K. (2005). Current controversies in oral lichen planus: Report of an international consensus meeting. Part 2. Clinical management and malignant transformation. Oral surgery, oral medicine, oral pathology, oral radiology and endodontics, 100, 164-178.

Longnecker, M. (1995). Alcohol consumption and the risk of cancer in humans: an overview. Alcohol,12, 87-96.

Lucero, L.,Pastor, S., Suárez, S., Durbán, R., Gómez, C., Parrón, T., Creus, A., & Marcos, R. (2000). Cytogenetic biomonitoring of Spanish greenhouse workers exposed to pesticides: micronuclei analysis in peripheral blood lymphocytes and buccal epithelial cells. Mutation Research,464,255-262.

Machado-Santelli, G. M., Cerqueira, E. M., Oliveira, C. T. & Pereira, C. A. B. (1994). Biomonitoring of nurses handling antineoplastic drugs. Mutation Research, 322, 203-208.

Majer, B. J., Laky, B., Knasmüller, S., & Kassie, F. (2001). Use of micronucleus assay with exfoliated epithelial cells as a biomarker for monitoring individuals at elevated risk of genetic damage and in chemoprevention trials. Mutation Research,489,147-172.

Marchioni, D. M. L., Fisberg, R. M. J., Góis Filho, F., Kowalski, L. P., Carvalho, M. B., Abrahão, M., Latorre, M. R. D. O., Eluf Neto, J., & Wünsch-Filho, V. (2007). Fatores dietéticos e câncer oral: estudo caso-controle na Região Metropolitana de São Paulo, Brasil. Cadernos de Saúde Pública, 23, 553-564.

Martins, K. F.,& Boschini Filho, J. (2003). Determinação da frequência de micronúcleos e outras alterações nucleares em células da mucosa bucal de indivíduos não-fumantes e fumantes. Revista da Faculdade de Ciências Médicas de Sorocaba, 5, 43-53.

Meireles, J. R. C. (2003). Danos genéticos em células esfoliadas da mucosa oral de indivíduos ocupacionalmente expostos a agentes mutagênicos e/ou carcinogênicos. Dissertação. (Mestrado em Genética). Universidade Federal da Paraíba, João Pessoa, Brasil.

Meireles, J. R. C., Lopes, M. A., Alves, N. N., & Cerqueira, E. M. M. (2006). Apoptose em células esfoliadas da mucosa bucal de indivíduos ocupacionalmente expostos a agentes mutagênicos e carcinogênicos. Revista Brasileira de Cancerologia, 52, 337-342.

Miller, M. L., Andringa, A., Dixon, K., & Carty, M. P. (2002). Insights into UV-induced apoptosis: ultrastructure, trichrome stain and spectral imaging. Micron, 33, 157-166.

Montero, R., Serrano, L., Dávila, V., Segura, Y., Arrieta, A., Fuentes, R., Abad, I., Valencia, L., Sierra, P., & Camacho, R. (2003).Metabolic polymorphisms and the micronucleus frequency in buccal epithelium of adolescents living in an urban environment. Environmental Molecular Mutagenesis, 42, 216-222.

Moore,L. E., Titenko Holland, N., & Smith, M. T. (1993). Use of fluorescence in situ hybridization to detect chromosome-specif changes in exfoliates human bladder and oral mucosa cells. Environmental Molecular Mutagenesis, 22, 130-137.

Nersesyan, A. K., Vardazaryan, N. S., & Arutyunyan, R. M. (2002a). Micronuclei and other nuclear anomalies in exfoliated cells of gynaecological cancer patients. Polish Journal of Environmental Studies,11,Suppl II, 58-61.

Nersesyan, A. K., Zilfian, V. N., & Koumkoumadjian, V. A. (1995). The study of micronuclei frequency in buccal mucosa cells of oral cancer patients under radiotherapy. In Proceedings of XVI International Cancer Congress (pp. 95-98).

Nersesyan, A., Kundi, M., Atefie, K., Schulte-Hermann, R., & Knasmüller, S. (2006). Effect of staining procedures on the results of micronucleus assays with exfoliated oral mucosa cells. Cancer Epidemiology Biomarkers & Prevention, 15, 1835-1840.

Nersesyan, A.K. (2005). Nuclear buds in exfoliated human cells.(Letter to the Editor). Mutation Research,588, 64-68.

Nersesyan, A.K.; Vardazaryan, N.S.; Arutyunyan, R.M. (2002b). Micronuclei and other nuclear anomalies in exfoliated buccal and uterine cervical cells of healthy Armenian women. Central European Journal of Occupational and Environmental Medicine, 8, 39-43.

Özkul, Y., Donmez, H., Erenmemisoglu, A., Demirtas, H., & Imamoglu, N. (1997). Induction of micronuclei by smokeless tobacco on buccal mucosa cell of habitual users. Mutagenesis, 12, 285-287.

Pastor, S., Gutiérrez, S., Creus, A., Cebulska-Wasilewska, A., & Marcos, R. (2001). Micronuclei in peripheral blood lymphocytes and buccal epithelial cells of Polish farmers exposed to pesticides. Mutatation Research,495, 147-156.

Pindborg, J. J., Reibel, J., Roed-Petersen, B., & Mehta, F. S. (1980). Tobacco-induced changes in oral leukoplakic epithelium. Cancer,45, 2330-2336.

Pinto, D., Ceballos, J. M., García, G., Guzmán, P., Del Razo, L. M., Vera, E., Gómez, H., García,A., & Gonsebatt, M. E. (2000). Increased cytogenetic damage in outdoor painters. Mutation Research, 467, 105-111.

Ramírez, A. (2000). Análise de células metanucleadas de alcoólicos portadores de carcinomas orais. Dissertação (Mestrado em Biologia/Genética). Departamento de Biologia do Instituto de Biociências da Universidade de São Paulo, São Paulo, Brasil

Ramirez, A., & Saldanha, P. H. (2002). Micronucleus investigation of alcoholic patients with oral carcinomas. Genetics and Molecular Research, 1, 246-260.

Reibel, J. (2003). Tobacco and oral diseases: an update on the evidence, with recommendations. Medical Principles and Practice, 12, 22-32.

Reis, S. R. A., Sadigursky, M., Andrade, M. G. S., Soares, L. P., Espírito Santo, A. R., & Vilas Bôas, D. S.(2002). Genotoxic effect of ethanol on oral mucosa cells.Pesquisa Odontológica Brasileira, 16,221-225.

Revazova, J., Yurchenko, V., Katosova, L., Platonova, V., Sycheva, L., Khripach, L., Ingel, F., Tsutsman, T., & Zhurkov, V. (2001). Cytogenetic investigation of women exposed to different levels of dioxin in Chapaevsk town. Chemosphere,43, 999-1004.

Rodrigues, T. L. C., Costa, L. J., Sampaio, M. C. C., Rodrigues, F. G., & Costa, A. L. L. (2000). Leucoplasias bucais: relação clínico-histopatológica. Pesquisa Odontológica Brasileira, 14, 357-361.

Rodriguez, T., Altieri, A., Chatenoud, L., Gallus, S., Bosetti, C., Negri, E., Franceschi, S., Levi, F., Talamini, R., & La Vecchia, C. (2004). Risk factors for oral and pharyngeal cancer in young adults. Oral Oncology, 40, 207-13.

Rothman, K., & Keller, A. (1972). The effects of joint exposure to alcohol and tobacco on risk of cancer in the mouth and pharynx. Journal of Chronic Diseases,25, 711-716.

Salama, S. A., Serrana, M., & Au, W. W. (1999). Biomonitoring using accessible human cells for exposure and health risk assessment. Mutation Research, 436, 99-112.

Salaspuro, M. P. (2003). Alcohol consumption and cancer of the gastrointestinal tract. Best Practice & Research Clinical Gastroenterology, 17, 679-694.

Santos, N. N. A. (2003). Danos citogenéticos e citológicos em indivíduos sobre diferentes formas de exposição à mutágenos, avaliados pelo Teste de Micronúcleo. Tese (Doutorado em Saúde Coletiva). Faculdade de Saúde Pública da Universidade de São Paulo, São Paulo, Brasil.

Saran, R., Tiwari, R. K., Reddy, P. P., & Ahuja, Y.R. (2008). Risk assessment of oral cancer in patients with pre-cancerous states of the oral cavity using micronucleus test and challenge assay. Oral Oncology, 44, 354-360.

Sarto,F., Finotto, S., Giacomelli, L., Mazzotti, D., Tomanin, R., & Levis, A.G. (1987). The micronucleus assay in exfoliated cells of the human buccal mucosa. Mutagenesis,2, 11-17.

Schulte-Hermann,R., Grasl-Kraupp,B., & Bursch, W. (2000). Dose-response and threshold effects in cytotoxicity and apoptosis, Mutation Research, 464, 13-18.

Seitz, H. K., Poschl, G., & Simanowski, U. A. (1998). Alcohol and cancer.Recent Developments in Alcoholism,14, 67 - 95.

Serrano-Garcia, L., & Montero-Montoya, R. (2001). Micronuclei and chromatid buds are the result of related genotoxic events. Environmental Molecular Mutagenesis, 38, 38-45.

Shimizu, N. Itoh, N., Utiyama, H., & Wahl, G.M. (1998). Selective entrapment of extrachromosomally amplified DNA by nuclear budding and micronucleation during S phase. Journal of Cell Biology, 140, 1307-1320.

Silverman, S. Jr., & Shillitoe, E. J. (1990). Etiology and predisposing factors. In Oral Cancer. (pp. 7-39).

Squier, C. A.,& Kremer, M. J. (2001). Biology of oral mucosa and esophagus. Journal of the National Cancer Institute. Monographs 29, 7-15.

Stich, H. F.,& Rosin, M. P. (1983a) Micronuclei in exfoliated human cells as an internal dosimeter for exposures to carcinogens. In Carcinogens and Mutagens in the Environment (pp. 17-25).

Stich, H. F. & Rosin, M. P. (1983b). Quantitating the synergistic effect of smoking and alcohol consumption with the micronucleus test on human bucal mucosa cells.International Journal of Cancer,31, 305-308.

Stich, H. F., Curtis, J. R., & Parida, B. B. (1982). Aplication of the micronucleus test to exfoliated cells of high cancer risk groups: tobacco chewers.International Journal of Cancer,30, 553-559.

Stich, H. F., Parida, B. B., & Brunnemann, K. D. (1992). Localized formation of micronuclei in the oral mucosa and tobacco-specific nitrosamines in the saliva of "reverse" smokers, khaini-tobacco chewers and gudakhu users. International Journal of Cancer,50, 172-176.

Stich, H. F., Stich, W., & Rosin, M. P. (1985). The micronucleus test on exfoliated human cells. In Basic an Applied Mutagenesis (pp. 337-342).

Stich, H.F. (1987). Micronucleated exfoliated cells as indicators for genotoxic damage and as markers in chemoprevention trials. Journal of Nutrition, Growth and Cancer, 4, 9-18.

Suhas, S., Ganapathy, K.S., Gayatri, D. M., & Ramesh, C. (2004). Application of the micronucleus test to exfoliated epithelial cells from the oral cavity of beedi smokers, a high-risk group for oral cancer. Mutation Research, 561, 15-21.

Surrallés, J., Autio, K., Nylund, L., Järventaus, H., Norppa, H., Veidebaum, T., Sorsa, M., & Peltonen, K. (1997). Molecular cytogenetic analysis of buccal cells and lymphocytes from benzene-exposed workers. Carcinogenesis,18, 817-823.

Syrjänen, S. (2005). Human papillomavirus (HPV) in head and neck cancer. Journal of Clinical Virology, 32, 59-66.

Thomas, P., Holland, N., Bolognesi, C., Kirsch-Volders, M., Bonassi, S., Zeiger, E., Knasmueller, S., & Fenech, M. (2009). Buccal micronucleus cytome assay. Nature Protocols, 4, 825-837.

Titenko-Holland, N., Moore, L. E., & Smith, M. T. (1994). Measurement and characterization of micronuclei in exfoliated human cells by fluorescence in situ hybridization with a centromeric probe. Mutation Research,312, 39-50.

Tolbert, P. E., Shy, C. M. & Allen, J. W. (1991). Micronuclei and other nuclear anomalies in buccal smears: a field test in snuff users. American Journal of Epidemiology, 134, 840-850.

Tolbert, P. E., Shy, C. M., & Allen, J. W. (1992). Micronuclei and other nuclear anomalies in buccal smears: methods development. Mutation Research, 271, 69-77.

Torres-Bugarín, O., De Anda-Casillas, A., Ramírez-Muñoz, M. P., Sánchez-Corona, J., Cantú, J. M., & Zúñiga, G. (1998). Determination of diesel genotoxicity in firebreathers by micronuclei and nuclear abnormalities in buccal mucosa.Mutation Research,413, 277-281.

Torres-Bugarin, O., Ventura-Aguilar, A., Zamora-Perez, A., Gomez-Meda, B. C., Ramos-Ibarra, M. L., Morgan-Villela, G., Gutierrez-Franco, A., & Zuniga-Gonzalez, G. (2003). Evaluation of cisplatin + 5-FU, carboplatin + 5-FU, and ifosfamide + epirubicine regimens using the micronuclei test and nuclear abnormalities in the buccal mucosa.Mutation Research, 539, 177-186.

U.S. National Institutes of Health. (2012) Surveillance Epidemiology and End Results providing information on cancer statistics to help reduce the burden of these diseases on the U.S. population (on line). November 2011. (cit. June 11, 2012). Available at http://seer.cancer.gov/statfacts/html/oralcav.html

Ünal, M., Çelik, A., Ateş, N. A., Micozkadioğlu, D., Derici, E., Pata, Y. S., & Akbaş, Y. (2005). Cytogenetic biomonitoring in children with chronic tonsillitis: Micronucleus frequency in exfoliated buccal epithelial cells.International Journal of Pediatric Otorhinolaryngology, 69, 1483-1488.

van der Meij, E. H., Mast, H. & van der Waal, I. (2006). The possible premalignant character of oral lichen planus and oral lichenoid lesions: A prospective five-year follow-up study of 192 patients. Oral Oncology, 43, 742-748.

van der Meij, E. H., Schepman, K. P. & van der Waal, I. (2003). The possible premalignant character of oral lichen planus and oral lichenoid lesions: a prospective study. Oral surgery, oral medicine, oral pathology, oral radiology and endodontics, 96, 164-71.

Warnakulasuriya, S. (2009) Global epidemiology of oral and oropharyngeal cancer. Oral Oncology, 45, 309-316.

Warnakulasuriya, S., Sutherland, G., & Scully, C. (2005). Tobacco, oral cancer, and treatment of dependence. Oral Oncology,41, 244-269.

Wu, P. A., Loh, C. H., Hsieh, L. L., Liu, T. Y., Chen, C. J., & Liou, S. H. (2004). Clastogenic effect for cigarette smoking, but not areca quid chewing as measured by micronuclei in exfoliated buccal mucosal cells. Mutation Research, 562, 27-38.

Wyllie, A.(1981).Cell death: a new classification separation apoptosis from necrosis. In Cell Death in Biology and Pathology. (pp. 1-34).

Xue, K. X., Wang, S., Ma, G. J., Zhou, P., Wu, P. Q., Zhang, R. F., Xu, Z., Chen, W. S., & Wang, Y. Q. (1992). Micronucleus formation in peripheral-blood lymphocytes from smokers and the influence of alcohol and tea drinking habits.International Journal of Cancer, 50, 702-705.

Zeljezic, D., & Garaj-Vrhovac, V. (2004). Chromosomal aberrations, micronuclei and nuclear buds induced in human lymphocytes by 2,4-dichlorophenoxyacetic acid pesticide formulation. Toxicology, 200, 39-47.

Zhang, L.,& Mock, D. (1989). Gamma-glutamyl transpeptidase activity in superficial exfoliated cells during hamaster buccal pouch carcinogenesis. Carcinogenesis,10,857-860.

Zhang, L. (1994). The value of glutathione S-tranferase and gamma-glutamyltranspeptidase as markers of altered foci during hamaster pouch carcinogenesis. Carcinogenesis,15, 105 -109.

# The Metastatic State of Renal Cell Carcinoma

Petros Sountoulides
*Urology Department*
*University of Ioannina, Greece*

Linda Metaxa
*Radiology Department*
*Aristotle University of Thessaloniki, Greece*

Alexandros Theodosiou
*Urology Department*
*University of Thessaly, Greece*

# 1   Epidemiological facts for RCC

Renal cell carcinoma (RCC), tumors of the renal parenchyma that arise from the renal cortex, is considered a heterogenous group of cancers with regard to its pathological and clinical features. RCC accounts for 2 – 3% of all adult malignancies and approximately 85 – 90% of all malignant kidney tumors. Males are more frequently affected (3:2 ratio) with the highest prevalence recorded in the sixth and seventh decade of life with a higher incidence in North America and the Nordic countries. The incidence and mortality of kidney cancer have continuously increased during the last 50 years in the USA and Western Europe (Pantuck et al., 2001). In 2008 approximately 271,000 new cases of renal cancer were diagnosed (Ferlay et al., 2010). The incidence of renal cancer is increasing by around 2% per year, a fact that is mainly attributed to the abundant use of imaging studies and the resultant incidental diagnosis of usually small renal tumors (Ferlay et al., 2007).

In the European Union (EU) countries approximately 88,400 new cases of RCC occurred in 2008, with an almost 2:1 male to female ratio (56,000 male and female 32,000) According to the European Committee of cancer, in 2009 the prevalence of renal cancer was 14.5 ($N = 40,395$) for men and 6.9 ($N = 24,656$) for women. The highest prevalence of RCC was observed in countries of the Eastern Europe (Lithuania, EstoniaLatvia, Czech Republic) compared to Western and Northern European countries (Romania, Portugal, Switzerland Spain, Portugal, Netherland, Denmark, Sweden, Switzerland) (Levi et al., 2008; Ferlay et al., 2010). Although an increase in RCC has been observed globally during the last decades, in recent years RCC incidence is declining in some European countries, namely, Sweden, Poland, Finland, and the Netherlands (Karim-Kos et al., 2008).

In the USA, RCC is the seventh most common cancer in men. In 2010, 58,000 cases were diagnosed and 13,000 deaths were attributed to renal cancer. The prevalence of the disease in the USA has increased since the '70s on average by 30% for the white population and 40% for the African American population (Tripathi et al., 2006). Currently one third of patients are diagnosed with locally invasive or metastatic kidney while another 25% of patients will experience tumor recurrence following what was at the time considered curative radical nephrectomy for localized disease (Gupta et al., 2008; Athar & Gentile, 2008). The median time to relapse after nephrectomy is 15 – 18 months. Renal cancer has a strong tendency to metastasize following occasionally unpredictable patterns of spread.

RCC has the worst cancer-specific mortality among urologic tumors since more than 40% of the patients with RCC die of the disease, opposite to the 20% mortality observed in prostate or bladder carcinoma (Athar & Gentile, 2008; Pascual & Borque, 2008). Generally patients with metastatic RCC have on average 13 months of survival and the five-year survival rate is under 15% (Cohen & McGovern, 2005; Rini et al., 2009).

# 2   Diagnosis and Imaging in RCC

The widespread use of cross-sectional imaging during the last years has resulted in great changes in both the diagnosis and management of RCC. Most of the cases of RCC are currently diagnosed due to imaging studies performed for mainly unrelated reasons. As a result, what was once considered the classic the triad of presenting symptoms for renal cancer (hematuria, flank pain, palpable mass) is nowadays a rare finding and is almost exclusively seen in advanced disease (Ng et al., 2006). Other non-specific systemic symptoms of advanced disease include asthenia, weight loss, anorexia, fever and symptoms or conditions that fall into the category of paraneoplastic syndromes like Stauffers syndrome, a reversible hepatic dysfunction associated with advanced RCC. Symptoms of metastatic renal cell carcinoma include: pain, stiffness, bruit, and pathologic fracture due to bone metastases; abdominal pain, jaundice, elevations in AST and ALT, and vomiting due to liver metastases, cough, dyspnea, and abnormal chest radiograph in cases of lung metastases. Brain metastases produce diplopia, personality changes, headache, ataxia, vertigo, and seizures. A challenge in renal tumoral imaging is to differentiate benign from malignant lesions but furthermore to have an accurate delineation of the extent of the tumor for optimal treatment planning. The best scanning protocol is the one that include unenhanced CT followed by imaging during the corticomedullary and nephrographic phases of enhancement. The unenhanced images place a baseline from which to measure the amount of enhancement of the lesion. The best stage to detect the renal lesion is the nephrographic but the corticomedullary is more appropriate for imaging the renal veins for possible extension of the tumor and the other organs for potential metastases (Sheth *et al.,* 2001). Several studies confirm a 85 – 90% accuracy in T staging, up to 50% for N stage and approaching 100% for M stage disease (Türkvatan *et al.*, 2009; Liu Y *et al.,* 2012).

## 3    Histotypes of RCC

The historical Heidelberg classification identified four main histologic subtypes of RCC with distinct characteristics relevant to their microscopic morphology, karyotype and genomic alterations: clear cell RCC (60 – 80%), papillary RCC (10 – 15%), chromophobe (approximately 5%) and collecting duct carcinoma (1 – 2%) (Kovacs *et al.,* 1997) Only recently were other rare subtypes (all composing < 1% of RCC cases) included in this list, mucinous tubular and spindle-type RCC, as well as tubulocystic and translocation-linked carcinomas (Yang *et al.*, 2010; Medendorp *et al.*, 2007; Argani & Ladanyi, 2005).

Clear cell renal cell carcinomas (ccRCC) which comprise the vast majority of RCCs are usually well delineated and centered on the renal cortex. In less than 5% of cases multiple satellite tumor nodules are seen throughout the kidney (Kinouchi *et al.,* 1999). A typical case of clear cell RCC is macroscopically characterized by a solid golden-yellow appearance on cut surface, with a distinct fibrous pseudocapsule sharply separating the tumor from surrounding normal renal parenchyma. Microscopically ccRCC cells are large, with their cytoplasm appearing optically clear to deeply granular. The clear cell appearance of ccRCC cells results from the accumulation of glycogen and fat (Fleming & O'Donell, 2000).

Papillary RCC is the most usual histotype of RCC to arise in patients under chronic dialysis. It is characteristically hypovascular on imaging studies and may exhibit areas of necrosis (Renshaw & Corless, 1995). Although papillary RCC is currently regarded as a distinct subtype, it should not be considered a homogeneous group of tumors since morphologically it comprises of solid variants, variants with rare papillae and variants with clear cell cytoplasm (Renshaw *et al.,* 1997).

Chromophobe RCC is grossly well-circumscribed, with a homogeneous gray to brown cut surface. Microscopically tumor cells are arranged in nests and have sharply defined borders and abundant pale cytoplasm. The pale cytoplasmic appearance is caused by the presence of cytoplasmic vesicles that stain positive for Hale colloidal iron (Bonsib, 1996). Chromophobe RCC has a high tendency for sarcomatoid transformation, probably more than any other RCC subtype (Akhtar *et al.,* 1997). However the most clinically important issue with chromophobe RCC is its close relationship with oncocytoma. Due to the fact that those two tumors have distinctly different prognosis it is imperative that a distinction between them be attempted. This distinction is possible in the majority of cases based on the different morphologic features coupled with the Hale colloidal iron stain (Cochand-Priollet *et al.*, 1997). The prognosis for chromophobe RCC is better than that of conventional ccRCC, although distant metastases are not uncommon especially in the face of coexistent papillary component or sarcomatoid transformation (Amin *et al.*, 2008).

Collecting duct carcinoma, also known as Bellini's duct carcinoma is thought to arise from collecting (Bellini) ducts (Rumpelt *et al.*, 1991). This histotype is more common in younger males, usually centers in the medulla and is surrounded by a characteristic desmoplastic reaction. The clinical course is extremely aggressive and prognosis is very poor with the majority of patients having distant metastases at the time of diagnosis (Srigley & Eble, 1998).

Sarcomatoid RCC is usually an extremely aggressive tumor with a grade IV cytology (Wang *et al.*, 2009). Extrarenal invasion as well as multiple osseous metastases is the rule since the sarcomatoid component of the tumor differentiates in the direction of cartilage and bone. The morphologic appearance of the epithelial component (when present) is usually in keeping with a proximal tubular origin as in ccRCC while some of the cases represent sarcomatoid variants of collecting duct carcinomas, papillary carcinomas, or chromophobe cell carcinomas (Cheville *et al.*, 2004).

# 4    Aetiology of RCC

There has been considerable discussion on the aetiology of RCC, however there is no evidence to confidently support the presence of a causative factor. Amongst the alleged environmental risk factors, heavy smoking is considered suspicious for an increased risk of RCC (Hunt *et al.*, 2005). Other predisposing factors include genetic predisposition, which will be further discussed in detail, occupational factors (exposure to lead, asbestos, dry cleaning solvents, and cadmium), hypertension, acquired renal cystic disease (ARCD) and dialysis and increased BMI (Label, 2006) (Weikert *et al.*, 2008; Pascual & Borque, 2008; Renehan *et al.*, 2008; Nouh *et al.*, 2010; Ljungberg *et al.*, 2011).

# 5    Genetic Factors

The risk of RCC for a first degree relative of a patient with RCC is about 2-fold, suggesting a hereditary component. Although the majority of RCC cases (> 95%) are sporadic, there are certain defined types of RCC with a hereditary pattern. Actually there is evidence that all the common histologic subtypes of RCC are caused by different distinct genetic alterations and each corresponds to a specific familiar syndrome (Cohen & Zhou, 2005). As a result, some authors have advocated approaching kidney cancer in terms of a metabolic disease, since each of the identified to date inherited kidney cancer syndromes represent disorders in iron, oxygen, nutrient or energy sensing (Linehan *et al.*, 2010). In contrast to benign renal lesions which show a normal karyotype, all RCC subtypes are characterized by alterations in their genomics. Sporadic clear cell RCCs which originate from the proximal tubule, are characterized by germline mutations of the von Hippel-Lindau (VHL) gene, a tumor suppressor gene, located on chromosome 3p25-26. Mutations in the VHL geneis the commonest alteration related to early onset of usually multiple and bilateral clear cell RCCs (ccRCC). However recent studies on exon sequencing revealed a considerable genetic heterogeneity in ccRCC; suggesting that even though the vast majority of ccRCCs contain mutated VHL, every tumor has its unique gene signature (Dalgliesh *et al.*, 2010). Under normal circumstances the VHL gene produces a protein that inhibits hypoxia inducible factors (HIFs) and plays a critical role in hypoxia response, including stimulation of angiogenesis. Loss of function leads to accumulation of HIFs and subsequent up-regulation of vascular endothelial growth factor and other factors that promote angiogenesis and tumor growth (Pfaffenroth *et al.*, 2008). Mutations in the VHL gene cause hypoxia inducible factor to stimulate angiogenesis through mainly activation of the vascular endothelial growth factor (VEGF). Other associated alterations include genes implicated in methylation regulation in 15% of cases, underlying the importance of epigenetic modifications, and truncating mutations in chromatin remodelling complex PRMB1 in 41% of cases (Audenet *et al.*, 2012). However recent animal studies have provided evidence suggesting that VHL mutations alone are insufficient for the development of ccRCC implying that additional genetic events are essential (Kapitsinou & Haase, 2008; van Rooijen *et al.*, 2010). The VHL syndrome is a rare condition (1 in 36,000 births) inherited through an autosomal dominant trait (Stolle *et al.*, 1998). The syndrome is characterized by retinal angiomas, which are usually the earlier manifestations of the syndrome, capillary haemangioblastomas of the central nervous system, tumors of the inner ear and islet tumors of the pancreas. Penetrance of each of these manifestations is not complete, for instance RCCs will only develop in 40 – 50% of VHL mutation carriers (Ljungberg *et al.*, 2011). Recent advances in the understanding of the molecular pathways involved in the non-clear cell variants of RCC include the identification of mutations in genes involved in aberrant chromatin remodeling (Singer *et al.*, 2012). Interestingly all these genes are located on chromosome 3, in close proximity to the VHL gene. In contrast to ccRCC, papillary RCC, chromophobe RCC and renal oncocytoma are less dominated by mutations in a single gene. Hereditary papillary RCC type I is associated to activation of the c-met proto-oncogene, which encodes a growth factor receptor, and chromosome 7 alterations (Oosterwijk *et al.*, 2011). A rare but more aggressive type of papillary type II RCC has been associated with alterations in chromosome 1 and an enzyme involved in the Krebs cycle, called fumarate hydratase (Pfaffenroth *et al.*, 2008). Finally, mutations in the Birt-Hogg-Dube gene are associated with the development of familiar chromophobe RCC originating from the collecting ducts although it predisposes to other histologies as well (Cheng *et al.*, 2009; Hasumi *et al.*, 2009).

## 6    Patterns of Metastatic Spread of RCC

The development of metastatic disease is a sequential process where cancer cells depart from the primary tumor via the blood supply or lymphatic chain and deposit at proximal or distant sites. This metastatic pathway is not always predictable and certainly not for renal cancer, which is notorious for its complex lymphatic drainage. However there is a predilection for certain sites, meaning that these sites are usually the first occupied by cancer cells.

There has been evidence in support of an early dissemination model, where metastasis occurs early in the lifecycle of cancer cells (Oppenheimer, 2006). In an experimental study, engineered untransformed mouse mammary cells were found to express inducible oncogenes transgenes that were able to bypass the primary site and show up at secondary metastatic sites (Podsypanina *et al.*, 2008). In another animal study, Kaplan *et al.* (2005) also showed that cancer cells in mice models might have instructed bone marrow cells to migrate to pre-selected organs in order to establish a hospitable environment. This event preceded the appearance of cancer cells by four to six days and micrometastatic colonies formed five days later. These studies might explain the unpredictable metastatic pattern of renal tumors and account for the late appearance of metastatic disease in organs and sites that are considered outside of the "usual" metastatic pathway of RCC (Sountoulides *et al.,* 2011). With regard to RCC, it metastasizes via the hematogenous route through the paravertebral venous plexus. This is an anastomotic network of avalvular veins surrounding the bone marrow and vertebras and is connected with pelvic, intercostal, azygos and cava veins. That allows tumor seeding in both a caudal direction toward the pelvis and a cranial direction to the calotte (Torres Muros *et al.*, 2006).

Once metastases from RCC are present, the lungs are commonly affected by single (30.4%) or multiple metastases (75.6%). Lung metastases are considered a relevant therapeutic challenge. The 5-year survival rate after complete resection of pulmonary metastasis from RCC is up to 60%. (Chen *et al.,* 2008; Russo, 2010). The survival rate is higher after resection of pulmonary metastases than after resection of brain or other extrapulmonary metastases (Volkmer & Gschwend, 2002; Kavolius *et al.,* 1998). In case of lung metastasis, the number and size of nodules to be removed, a long interval between the diagnosis of RCC and the occurrence of metastasis (> 1 year) and a good performance status indicated a favorable clinical setting for pulmonary metastasectomy (Pfannschmidt *et al.,* 2002).

Skeletal metastases are relatively common in advanced renal cancer. These are highly osteolytic, destructivelesions leading to debilitating skeletal complications including severe pain, increased fracture rate and spinal cord compression. These lesions pose significant surgical challenges due to the increased risk of life-threatening hemorrhage. The most common locations of bone metastases from RCC are the spine, pelvis, femur, scapula, and the humerus. Solitary osteolytic bone metastasis may present in up to 26% of all mRCC cases and confer a 5-year survival of 11% (Ruiz-Cerda & Jimenez Cruz, 2009; Lin *et al.*, 2007). Althausen reported that those patients with solitary osseous metastasis and the longest interval between the diagnosis of RCC and the diagnosis of the metastasis have a relatively favorable prognosis and they should be treated as radically as possible (Althausen *et al.,* 1997), while Kavolius reported that resection of solitary metachronous RCC metastases from renal cell carcinoma (RCC) is associated with a 5-year survival rate of 35% to 50% (Kavolius *et al.,* 1998). Fortunately, the continuing development of anti-resorptive drugs is revolutionizing the medical management of metastatic bone disease and offers a major advantage on quality of life. The bisphosphonate zoledronic acid appears to yield a significant benefit in terms of reduction in skeletal related events compared to placebo, while the recent release of denosumab, a fully human monoclonal antibody that specifically targets the RANK-ligand offers another promising therapeutic alternative for patients with renal cancer and metastatic bone disease (Wood & Brown, 2012). Accordingto the American Society of Clinical Oncology (ASCO) and the National Comprehensive Cancer Network (NCCN), patients with bone metastasis should have zoledronic acid, pamidronate, or denosumab (with calcium and vitamin D supplementation) added to their chemotherapy regimen if they have an expected survival of 3 months or longer and have adequate renal function (Iranikhah *et al.*, 2012; Cassinello Espinosa *et al.*, 2012).

# 7   Lymph Node Involvement

Cancer specific survival is dramatically worse in patients with kidney tumors and regional lymph node involvement. The incidence of lymph node involvement for surgically resected kidney tumors with no evidence of distant metastases at diagnosis ranges from 3 – 14% (Minervini *et al.*, 2011; Blom *et al.,* 1999; Pantuck, *et al.,* 2003). Preoperative imaging using computerized tomography (CT) or magnetic resonance imaging (MRI) has proved inaccurate in positively identifying lymph nodal metastases. A recent study showed that 10% of patients with clinically negative lymph nodes on preoperative imaging had positive lymph nodes for cancer on histology after lymph node removal. This may mean that at least 10% of all renal cell cancers are understaged (Chapman *et al.,* 2008). Accordingly, given the inability of imaging studies to accurately define the lymph node status due to false-negative results, (Terrone *et al.,* 2006; Chapman *et al.,* 2008) lymph node dissection may be key in providing knowledge of the true histology of the renal-associated lymph nodes, thereby improving staging accuracy and consequently effecting the use of adjuvant chemotherapy and the patient's ultimate prognosis.

However, the concept of lymph node dissection in kidney cancer is still controversial both regarding whether or not lymph node dissection should be performed at all, and as to the extent of the dissection. According to the guidelines of both the UICC/AJCC and the EAU, lymphadenectomy for renal cell cancer has not provided a proven benefit, suggesting that it should be restricted to the perihilar tissue for staging purposes (Ljungberg *et al.,* 2007). It is not uncommon however for pathologists to find "no nodes" in radical nephrectomy specimens, further confounding the problem. Also, the practice patterns of urologists in the United States verify the lack of consensus on the role or even the definition of LND for tumors of the kidney. Results of one survey showed that at the time of radical nephrectomy for a localized renal tumor, 26% of urologists do not perform a formal lymph node dissection, whereas 41% perform a limited node dissection and 33% perform a full retroperitoneal lymph node dissection extending from the crus of the diaphragm to the bifurcation of the aorta or vena cava (Kim *et al.,* 2006).

The absence of an accepted standardized approach to retroperitoneal lymph node dissection contributes to the uncertainty about the benefits of lymph node dissection for renal tumors. In addition, recent evidence of the complex and unpredictable pattern of lymph node drainage of the kidney further contribute to the lack of consensus regarding the template for lymph node dissection. According to findings from studies in cadavers, extensive lymphadenectomy might well need to include the nodes around the celiac artery along with the contralateral paraaortic lymph nodes (Assouad *et al.,* 2006). The potential morbidity of this approach, given the presence of positive nodes in so few patients is far too high to justify a routine or extended node dissection in all patients afflicted with renal tumors.

Removal of all the lymph nodes that drain the kidney is technically demanding, adds hours to the operating time and can be the cause of serious complications. Currently there is no documented survival benefit from lymphadenectomy. More so as it has been shown that as many as 40% of patients with nodal metastases at the time of nephrectomy are alive 5 years after surgery (Karakiewicz *et al.,* 2007). Reasons for this may be that lymphadenectomy is done inconsistently, it is usually only done in patients that already have advanced disease, and there is little consensus on the proper surgical template. Some authors advocate a complete retroperitoneal dissection, while others favor a more limited template in order to reduce morbidity and mortality. Therefore, performing lymph node dissection during radical nephrectomy for RCC is not currently considered the standard of care (Ljungberg *et al.,* 2007). However the role of lymphadenectomy in locally advanced disease is still under question mainly due to the lack of prospective, well-recruited, trials with adequate number of events.

# 8   Rare Metastatic Sites

## 8.1   Orbit

Ocular metastases from RCCs are extremely rare and are more likely to involve the iris, ciliary body and choroids, although eyelid, lacrimal sac and orbital metastases have also been described. All the tumors with a tendency of metastasizing through the blood have a high possibility to metastasize into areas with a great flow of blood. This is why the posterior pole of the oculus, which has higher posterior choroidal blood flow, is the most common localization of those lesions (Galetović et al., 2010). During the last years only 23 cases have been reported. In 7 cases the eye or orbital metastasis was the first manifestation of a previously unknown RCC, while in 14 cases there was a history of nephrectomy for RCC. The diagnosis in most of the cases was done following excision biopsy that revealed metastatic RCC (Galetović et al., 2010; Sabatini & Ducic, 2009; Rodney et al., 2009; Shoaib et al., 2008; Vozmediano-Serrano et al., 2006; Shome et al., 2007; Mudiyanselage et al., 2008; Mancini et al., 2008).

### 8.2    Parotid Gland

Major salivary gland metastases from distant primary tumors are exceedingly uncommon. An extensive literature search revealed 26 cases of RCC metastatic to the parotid gland. In 14 of these patients, parotid metastasis was the initial sign of the kidney tumor while in the rest, parotid metastasis occurred following nephrectomy. The longest interval from nephrectomy to solitary parotid metastasis was 19 years (Deeb et al., 2012). The most common presenting symptom is that of a palpable parotid mass, while in one case there was facial paralysis. In all cases fine-needle aspiration (FNA) biopsy was diagnostic (Seijas et al., 2005; Spreafico et al., 2008; Dequanter et al., 2005; Kundu et al., 2001; Moudouni et al., 2006). The mechanism by which RCC reaches the parotid gland is, again, via hematogeneous route.

### 8.3    Nasal and Paranasal Cavities

The nose is another very uncommon site for RCC metastases. Approximately 50 cases of nasal recurrences of RCC have been reported in the literature. The maxillary sinuses are the paranasal sinuses most commonly afflicted by metastatic tumors, followed in frequency by the ethmoid and sphenoid, while there is only one reported case of an isolated metastasis to the nasal septum and one case of metastasis to the frontonasal region 15years after nephrectomy for RCC (Kumar et al., 2007). The most frequent patients' complaints are nasal obstruction, swelling and pain, although epistaxis is the most alarming symptom because of the high vascular stroma of these metastatic deposits (Lee et al., 2005; Pereira Arias et al., 2002). In 15 of the cases there was no known history of renal mass, while the rest of them had previously undergone nephrectomy at a time interval ranging from 6 months to 17 years prior to the diagnosis of the metastatic lesion.

### 8.4    Tongue and Tonsils

The tongue is a frequent target for RCC metastasis although isolated spread to the floor of the mouth is rare. Lesions in the tongue or floor of the mouth can cause severe pain, bleeding, difficulty eating and even complete oral obstruction. Unfortunately, oral cavity metastasis from RCC is usually a manifestation of widespread disease (Yoshitomi et al., 2011). The literature review revealed 30 cases of RCC metastatic to the tongue. Out of these, only six cases presented initially with tongue metastases before the diagnosis of primary RCC (Azam et al., 2008; Cochrane et al., 2006). Treatment of tongue metastasis is usually palliative and aims to provide patient comfort by means of pain relief while preventing bleeding, infection and breathing difficulties. Surgical excision is recommended as palliative treatment with emphasis on preservation of tongue structure and function (Azam et al., 2008; Cochrane et al., 2006; Basely et al., 2009; Torres-Carranza et al., 2006; Massaccesi et al., 2009; Wadasadawala et al., 2011; Yoshitomi et al., 2011). Only six cases of tonsil metastases from RCC have been reported. All patients had nephrectomy for RCC 6months to 10years prior to the tonsil metastasis and two of them were previously diagnosed with bone and lung metastasis from RCC (StaÅ„czyk *et al.*, 2006; Massaccesi *et al.*, 2009; GarcÃa Lozano *et al.*, 1998; Menauer & Issing *et al.*, 1998).

## 8.5   Thyroid Gland

Although secondary involvement of the thyroid by RCC is uncommon, more than 150 cases of recognized cases of RCCs metastatic to the thyroid have been reported. Metastatic disease from the kidney to the thyroid gland can occur more than 20 years after nephrectomy, with an average time interval of approximately 7.5 years. Only in five cases were metastases to the thyroid gland the first manifestation of RCC (Bugalho *et al.*, 2006; Nixon *et al.*, 2011; Lee *et al.*, 2007). There are hypotheses that might explain the relatively high incidence of metastases from the kidney to the thyroid gland. The rich blood supply of the thyroid gland is an obvious reason, although some researchers have also suggested that the abnormal thyroid gland is more vulnerable to metastatic growth due to a decrease in oxygen and iodine content alteration (Testini *et al.*, 2008). Metastases to the thyroid can present with symptoms of hypothyroidism, breathing difficulties because of gland enlargement causing airway obstruction, trouble or pain swallowing, and cough due to the vasogastric effect (Garfield *et al.*, 2007). Diagnosis is confirmed by thyroid scintigraphy, thyroid ultrasonography, and cytology of the material obtained through FNA (Buła *et al.*, 2010).

## 8.6   Heart

There have been rare reports of solitary late metastasis to the heart with the right ventricle being the preferred chamber involved. Isolated metastasis of RCC to the left ventricle of the heart is considered an extremely unique incident. Historically, up to 10% of patients with RCC have tumor thrombus involving the renal vein and inferior vena cava and in up to 1% tumor thrombus extends into the right atrium. There are no more than 25 reports of cardiac metastases of RCC. In 3 cases, a malignant pericardial effusion was the sole evidence of metastatic disease (Zustovich *et al.*, 2008; Tokuyama *et al.*, 2011; Juraszynski *et al.*, 2010). In 3 cases left ventricular metastasis occurred 18 to 23 years after nephrectomy (Talukdera *et al.*, 2010; Bradley *et al.*, 1995; Aburto *et al.*, 2009). In 2 cases there was right ventricular metastasis from RCC, which was incidentally diagnosed after an episode of syncope (Alghamdi & Tam, 2006), and during the evaluation of hematuria (Otahbachi *et al.*, 2009). Finally one case involved metastasis to the interventricular septum which caused cardiac paradox (Faizel *et al.*, 2006).

## 8.7   Gallbladder

The gallbladder is a very rare metastatic site of RCC with only 33 reported cases of RCC metastatic to the gallbladder (Chung *et al.*, 2012). All cases involved polypoid-like masses that can easily be mistaken with benign gallbladder polyps (Fang *et al.*, 2010). Final diagnosis was made only after cholecystectomy and histopathology examination of the lesions.

## 8.8   Pancreas

Pancreatic metastases from RCC are relatively rare, with a reported incidence ranging from 1.6% to 11% in large series of patients (Adsay *et al.*, 2004, Washington *et al.*, 1995). Of the primary tumors that can metastasize to the pancreas, renal cell carcinoma (RCC) is the most common, followed by lung cancer, breast cancer, adenocarcinoma, and melanoma. A lot of papers mention that RCC has a high affinity for the parenchyma of the pancreas and an electivity to grow there, but the mechanism has not been extensively explained (Ballarin *et al.*, 2011).

### 8.9    Skin

Skin metastases of RCC are not easy to diagnose due to the low suspicion index for these skin lesions, both because these lesions mimic common dermatological disorders and due to the usually long interval since nephrectomy. Skin metastases have been reported to occur in around 3% of renal tumors. Several cases of calvarial metastases from clear cell RCC have been reported in the literature (Gaetani *et al.*, 2005; Cohen, 2001; Martínez-Rodríguez *et al.*, 2008), but only one case of papillary RCC with cutaneous metastases (Srinivasan *et al.*, 2010). Skin metastases mainly occur in the head, neck and trunk, in that order. The diagnosis is only made after histopathology examination of the cutaneous lesion. Skin metastases are usually late manifestations of the disease, are associated to synchronous metastases to other sites and carry a poor prognosis (Survival shorter than six months) (García Torrelles *et al.*, 2007; Arrabal-Polo *et al.*, 2009; Jilani *et al.*, 2010; Johnson *et al.*, 2011; Mahmoudi *et al.*, 2012; Terada, 2012; Chauhan *et al.*, 2011).

### 8.10    Genitalia

Ovarian metastases are found in 0.5% of cases of renal cancer and are thought to occur by retrograde venous embolization through the renal vein to the ovarian vessels. In total only 24 cases of metastasis to the ovaries from RCC have been reported with 6 of the cases initially considered as primary ovarian clear cell cancers (Toquero *et al.*, 2009; Albrizio *et al.*, 2009; Stolnicu *et al.*, 2007; Jalón Monzón *et al.*, 2008; Udoji & Herts, 2012, Guney *et al.*, 2010). With regard to metastatic testicular involvement, the incidence of secondary testicular tumors ranges from 0.3% to 3.6% (Schmorl *et al.*, 2008). To our knowledge only six cases of testicular metastases from RCC have been reported within the last seven years, in one case there was a contralateral chromophobe RCC metastatic to the testis, six years after nephrectomy (Ulbright *et al.*, 2008; Wu *et al.*, 2010).

### 8.11    Muscle and Joints

Metastatic RCC to muscles is a very rare incident indeed. According to Satake, (Satake *et al.*, 2009) until 2009 only 32 cases of skeletal muscle metastasis from RCC had been reported; our search added another four. Five cases of acute monarthritis secondary to asymptomatic RCC have been described, where the patients were initially diagnosed with septic arthritis. However the finding of hot spots on isotope bone scans and biopsy samples showing secondary neoplasms confirmed the lesions to represent metastatic sites of RCCs. MRI has proven helpful in delineating the features and extent of muscle invasion by the tumor (Picchio *et al.*, 2010; Hur *et al.*, 2007; Placed *et al.*, 2010; Trumm *et al.*, 2011).

# 9    Management of Metastatic Disease

Metastatic RCC is still considered a non-curable disease state despite the huge efforts in recent years to come up with effective treatment. Thus the best chance of cure lies in the early detection of the disease when the tumor is either organ-confined or locally advanced and therefore amenable to radical surgical excision. At the same time, the constantly changing algorithm of treatment for advanced and metastatic RCC represents the field with the most dramatic changes in oncology in the last few years.

Regarding its medical management, metastatic RCC is considered refractory to treatment with traditional systemic cytotoxic chemotherapies, and until recently management options were limited to immunotherapy and palliative care. RCC has long been considered an immunosuppressive tumor and as such cytokine therapy had for decades been considered as acceptable therapeutic option albeit with limited long-term disease free survival rates, not exceeding 10 months (Yang *et al.*, 2003; Coppin *et al.*, 2005; Motzer *et al.*, 1999). Recently however the encouraging initial results from clinical trials of targeted therapies which derive their efficacy through affecting angiogenesis, (anti-angiogenetic agents and m-TOR inhibitors) signaled a turn in the management of mRCC (Wagstaff, 2006). This paradigm shift in the medical management of metastatic RCC is still evolving and will likely produce more robust results in the future as novel more potent and better tolerated agents are sought and the role of combination and sequential anti-VEGF schemes is defined (Choueiri, 2011).

## 10    Cytokine Therapy

It was only until recently that immunotherapy, in the form of cytokine therapy, was considered the mainstay of treatment for advanced RCC, even though the somewhat vague term "immunotherapy" comprises a vast array of different therapeutic approaches. Cytokine therapy mainly in the form of interleukin-2 and interferon-α has been used alone and in combination for the treatment of advanced RCC.

Although *Interleukin-2* (IL-2) was until 2005 the only drug approved by the Food and Drug Administration (FDA) for the treatment of advanced RCC, significant questions concerning IL-2–based immunotherapy still remain open. Interleukin's proposed mechanism of action involves both direct effects on cancer cells as well as a general stimulation of the immune system. In more detail, IL-2 acts by stimulating cytotoxic T lymphocytes (CTLs), natural killer (NK) cells and CD8 cells that induce an anti-tumor immune response (Olencki & Bukowski, 2000). IL-2's direct effects on cancer cells include cell cycle perturbations and production of cytotoxic reactive oxygen species, e.g., NO (Porta *et al.*, 2007). Although IL-2 probably kills cancer cells with more than one mechanism it also acts, in terms of both activity and toxicity, as completely different drugs depending on the dose and route of administration (Porta *et al.*, 2007). The therapeutic efficacy and safety of high-dose interleukin (HD IL-2) for metastatic RCC has been examined in the setting of large randomized clinical studies. In the study by McDermott *et al.* (2005) although HD IL-2 showed better response rates compared to low dose (23% versus 10%), no significant difference in progression-free survival or overall survival was observed. Moreover high-dose i.v.IL-2 was associated with significant toxic side effects. Similar results were reached in the study conducted by the National Cancer Institute (NCI) were mRCC patients received either HD or LD IL-2. Overall response rates were 21% for the HD group, versus 13% for the LD group with again a significant price to pay in terms of toxicity, but no difference in overall survival despite the longer duration of responses in patients receiving high-dose IL-2 (Yang *et al.*, 2003). Today HD-IL-2 is considered as first-line treatment option for good risk patients with mRCC (Patard, 2009) (Figure 1). Taken together, overall complete and durable responses with IL-2 have been achieved in no more than 5% of patients. Apart from the disappointing results of IL-2, its administration was associated with a substantial increase in the incidence of grade III-IV toxicities in the high dose group. IL-2 has been linked to the life-threatening capillary leak syndrome and is not indicated in cases of brain metastases, cardiac, pulmonary or renal dysfunction and poor performance status (Fyfe *et al.*,1995; Yang *et al.* 2003; McDermott *et al.*, 2005). Interferons (IFNs) are members of a family of regulatory proteins produced by eukaryotic cells in response to viral infections and to several other biologic or synthetic inducers (Porta *et al.*, 2007). The precise mechanisms supporting IFN-induced antitumor activity are still not completely known. IFNs have a broad range of biological effects including immune stimulation, antiangiogenesis, direct antiproliferative and pro-apoptotic effects as well as effects of cell differentiation that could potentially induce a clinically significant antitumor response in vivo (Lindner, 2002; Nanus *et al.,* 1990, Porta *et al.,* 2007). *Interferon-α* was the interferon more extensively used for the management of mRCC following early evidence of antitumor activity against RCC and thus became the standard preparation used in clinical practice. The efficacy and the possible survival benefit of interferon for patients with mRCC have been evaluated in clinical trials. Interferon compared to medroxyprogesterone (MPA) demonstrated a significant overall survival advantage with an added median survival time of 2.5 months compared to MPA. The estimated 1-year survival rates were 43% for the interferon arm versus 31% for the MPA arm (no authors, 1999). In another study where 160 patients with mRCC were randomized to either interferon-α2a or vinblastine, overall survival was significantly better for those under interferon (15.8 months versus 8.8 months). Complete response rates, although low, were also in favor of interferon (8.9% versus 1.2%) (Pyrhönen *et al.,* 1999). Cytokines have also been used in combination in order to augment the modest survival benefits of either IL-2 or interferon monotherapies. However clinical studies have shown that the combination of cytokines did not provide with a significant clinical advantage in terms of survival or even quality of life. In other words despite its modest efficacy, cytokine monotherapy is superior to cytokine combination therapy. Negrier *et al.,* (1998) and Atzpodien *et al.,* (1993) and the combined approach is associated with limited efficacy and modest success rates in the majority of mRCC cases (Kruck *et al.,* 2008). Drug-related toxicity is a significant issue with cytokine therapy, high-dose IL-2 in particular can be extremely toxic, requiring inpatient administration with intensive supportive care (Coppin *et al.,* 2005). However, the toxicity of IL-2 can be significantly reduced by subcutaneous administration (Geertsen *et al.,* 2004). A recently published study (PERCY Quattro trial) evaluated both cytokines (interferon alfa-2a, interleukin 2) and the combination of both with regard to their possible survival benefit for a total of 492 intermediate prognosis RCC patients. Although there were no significant survival differences between the interferon-α treated patients or between the interleukin-2 treated patients, grade 3-4 toxicities were significantly more frequent in cytokine-treated patients than in medroxyprogesterone-treated patients. The authors concluded that intermediate risk mRCC patients gain no survival advantage with either interleukin-2 or interferon-α, instead these agents induce a significant risk of toxicity (Negrier *et al.,* 2007). The results of this study were reflected in the recent European Association of Urology guidelines, suggesting that patients with favorable risk profile and clear-cell subtype histology are potential candidates for cytokine therapy (Ljungberg *et al.,* 2010).

## 11    Molecular Pathways in RCC and Targeted Therapies

The limitations of cytokine treatment intensified research into a more thorough understanding of the underlying molecular biology of RCC. The recent understanding of the fundamentals of kidney cancer biology and the discovery of the implicated pathways, particularly the vascular endothelial growth factor (VEGF) pathway and the mammalian target of rapamycin (mTOR) led to the development of therapies with inhibitory activity against these pathways. As a result, systemic therapy for metastatic renal cell carcinoma (mRCC) that was once limited to interleukin-2 and interferon (IFN)-α, has been recently enriched with the simultaneous emergence of several active compounds that have become available for first- and second-line use.

## 12    Molecular Biology

Under normal conditions, hypoxia inducible factors (HIFs) bind to the von Hippel-Lindau (VHL) protein which is involved in proteolysis as part of an ubiquitin ligase complex and is constantly degraded. In almost all cases of VHL syndrome and in around 70% of sporadic RCC cases the VHL gene is inactivated. The resultant alteration in the VHL proteins leads to disruption of this interaction between the HIF and the VHL protein, impaired degradation of HIF, and accumulation of the HIF transcription factors under normal (non-hypoxic) conditions. HIF accumulation can also result from activation of the mammalian target of rapamycin (mTOR) downstream of cellular stimuli and the PI3-K/Akt pathway (Oosterwijk *et al.*, 2011). Under normal circumstances the mTOR pathway regulates cell growth, and its upregulation in tumors contributes to protein degradation and angiogenesis (Sarbassov *et al.*, 2005). Those accumulated HIFs translocate into the nucleus where they lead to massive transcription of hypoxia inducible genes including vascular endothelial growth factor (VEGF) and platelet-derived growth factor (PDGF). These factors in turn, bind to their corresponding receptors on the surface of endothelial cells and result to neovascularization.

Therefore molecular therapies target these two, essential to the pathophysiology of clear cell RCC, pathways: the hypoxia response pathway associated with inactivation of the VHL tumor suppressor gene and the mTOR signaling pathway. Agents targeting these pathways include inhibitors of multiple tyrosine kinase receptors (TKIs) including VEGF-R and PDGFR (sorafenib, sunitinib, pazopanib, axitinib), antibodies that directly inhibit VEGF (Bevacizumab), and factors that exclusively inhibit the kinase activity of the mTOR complex 1 (temsirolimus and everolimus).

The clinical implementation of targeted molecular therapies has provided encouraging results for patients with mRCC. Molecular-targeted therapies have better efficacy and tolerability than cytokine therapy, and many are administered orally (Hutson, 2011). The administration of these agents (TKIs) has provided with impressive objective response rates as high as 45%, has led to almost doubling of the progression-free survival (PFS) while up to 30% of patients achieve partial remissions (PR) (Staehler *et al.*, 2010; Rini *et al.*, 2009). However, one has to bear in mind that whether these treatments directly target the tumor cells remains uncertain, as at pharmacologically relevant doses of sunitinib no effect on RCC cells was noted (Huang *et al.*, 2010). Furthermore there is evidence in support of growth of tumor cells along large mature vessels, allowing the potential for escaping TKI treatment and evidently progression of cancer despite treatment (Audenet *et al.*, 2012).

## 13    Tyrosine Kinase Inhibitors (TKIs)

Sunitinib (Sutent®, Pfizer Inc., NY, USA) is an orally bioavailable small molecule multi-tyrosine kinase inhibitor of the VEGF receptors (VEGFR-1, -2, and -3), platelet-derived growth factor receptor-a and b (PDGFR-a/b) and c-KIT, FLT-3 and RET (Motzer *et al.*, 2007). Initial phase II trials of administration of 50 mg of sunitinib daily for 4 weeks demonstrated objective partial responses of approximately 40% (Motzer *et al.*, 2006). Sunitinib was compared to IFN-ain a phase III trial of once-daily 50 mg sunitinib versus IFN-a in 750 patients. Sunitinib demonstrated a superior progression-free survival time (11 months vs. 5 months, HR: 0.42; $p < 0.000001$) The initial report included an increased objective response rate (ORR; 28 vs. 5%), and the final analysis found prolonged OS in the sunitinib group compared with the IFN-a group (26.4 vs. 21.8 months; HR: 0.821; $p = 0.051$) and final ORRs of 47% for sunitinib and

12% for IFN-a ($p < 0.001$) (Motzer et al., 2009). In 2006, sunitinib received approval from the US FDA and the EMA as a first-line therapy to treat advanced mRCC. Sunitinib is now recommended as first-line therapy for good and intermediate risk patients with mRCC and in the second line setting for patients who have failed prior cytokine therapy (Ljungberg et al., 2010; Patard et al., 2011) (Figure 1 and Figure 2) Sorafenib (Nexavar®, Bayer Pharmaceuticals, Berlin, Germany) is a small molecule orally bioavailable multi-kinase inhibitor that decreases tumor cell proliferation by targeting intracellular (Raf-1/B-Raf) and cell surface kinases (VEGFR-1,-2 and -3, FLT-3, PDGF-b, RET, FGFR-1, KIT) (Lyons et al., 2001). In 2006, sorafenib was approved by the EMA for the treatment of mRCC after the failure of IL-2- or IFN-a-based first-line therapy. The recommended dosage of sorafenib is 400 mg twice daily, taken either 1 h before or 2 h after food intake.

Sorafenib was evaluated in a randomized phase III trial in 903 patients with mRCC, the majority (> 80%) of whom had failed previous IL-2- or IFN-a-based first-line therapy (Escudier et al., 2009)Median PFS was significantly improved in patients receiving sorafenib compared with those receiving placebo (5.5 months versus 2.8 months). The first interim analysis of OS showed that sorafenib reduced the risk of death by 28% compared with placebo, while final analysis demonstrated a significant improvement in OS with sorafenib (17.8 vs. 14.3 months; HR: 0.78; $p = 0.029$), after censoring placebo patients who had crossed over to sorafenib (Bukowski et al., 2009). Based on the results of this trial, sorafenib is recommended as a second-line agent in cytokine-refractory or cytokine-unsuitable patients (Patard, 2008; Ljungberg et al., 2010) (Figure 2). Pazopanib (Votrient®, GlaxoSmithKline, London, UK) is a broad spectrum tyrosine kinase inhibitor, inhibiting VEGFR1,-2 and -3, PDGFR-a and -b and c-Kit (Sonpavde & Hutson, 2007). Pazopanib's efficacy has been recently tested in a phase III trial of both treatment naïve patients and also for patients who failed therapy with cytokines or bevacizumab (Figure 2). In both groups of patients pazopanib achieved significant benefits with regard to PFS compared to placebo (overall: 9.2 vs. 4.2 months; HR: 0.46; $p < 0.0001$; treatment-naive (54%): 11.1 vs. 2.8 months; HR: 0.40; p < 0.0001; and cytokine-pretreated (46%): 7.4 vs. 4.2 months; HR: 0.54; $p < 0.001$). A tumor response rate of 30% for pazopanib was observed, compared to 3% with placebo ($p < 0.001$), in 435 treatment-naïve and cytokine-pretreated mRCC patients although OS was not positively affected (Sternberg et al., 2010). These results led to pazopanib (800 mg) receiving FDA approval in 2009 for the treatment of advanced mRCC either as a first line treatment regimen or in cases of cytokine failure (Patard et al., 2011). Pazopanib is currently compared to sunitinib for patients with mRCC who have received no prior systemic therapy in an ongoing randomized clinical trial (COMPARZ) (Pazopanib Versus Sunitinib in the Treatment of Locally Advanced and/or Metastatic Renal Cell Carcinoma (COMPARZ). NCT00720941). Axitinib, an inhibitor of VEGFRs 1–3 is administered orally at a dosage of 5 mg twice daily. Axitinib has shown anti-tumor activity with a favorable noncumulative toxicity profile in clinical trials of patients with advanced mRCC previously treated with cytokines, chemotherapy or other targeted agents. For cytokine-refractory advanced RCC axitinib demonstrated an ORR of 44.2%, median time to progression of 15.7 months and median OS of 29.9 months (Rixe et al., 2007). Rini et al. (2009) reported an ORR of 22.6%, a median PFS of 7.4 months, and a median OS of 13.6 months in 62 patients with sorafenib-refractory mRCC. The results of the Phase III AXIS trial comparing axitinib and sorafenib as second-line therapies for mRCC were presented recently (Rini et al., 2011) demonstrating that for patients with disease progression on first line therapy, axitinib has the potential for a standard second-line treatment (Calvo et al., 2012) (Figure 2). Bevacizumab (Avastin®, Roche, Basel, Switzerland) is a humanized monoclonal antibody that inhibits angiogenesis by directly binding the VEGF ligand and neutralizing all forms of circulating VEGFs. The recommended dose is 10 mg/kg bodyweight every 2 weeks in combination with IFN-a at 9 MIU three times per week. Bevacizumab was licensed as a first-line therapy in combination with IFN-a for patients with mRCC in 2007 in the EU and in 2009 in the USA.

The efficacy of bevacizumab in combination with IFN-a as first-line treatment was reported in a randomized study (AVOREN) of 649 previously untreated mRCC patients. Median PFS was significantly longer in the bevacizumab plus IFN-a group compared with the IFN-a alone plus placebo control group (10.2 vs 5.4 months; HR: 0.60; $p < 0.0001$). However, no improvement was reported in OS based on the final analysis conducted after 444 deaths, with a median OS of 23.3 months in the bevacizumab plus IFN-a arm and 21.3 months in the IFN-a plus placebo arm (Rini et al., 2008; Rini et al., 2010). Bevacizumab was also tested in the settings of combination treatment for advanced RCC in the TORAVA trial where 171 untreated mRCC patients were randomized to receive a combination of bevacizumab (10 mg/kg every 2 weeks) and temsirolimus (25 mg weekly), sunitinib (50 mg/day for 4 weeks followed by 2 weeks off), or IFN-a (9 MIU three-times per week). Analysis found a PFS of 29.5% (median: 8.2 months), 35.7% (median: 8.2 months) and 61.0% (median: 16.8 months), respectively. However, 51% of patients treated with the combination of temsirolimus and bevacizumab had to discontinue the scheme due to toxicity (Negrier et al., 2011). Bevacizumab plus IFN-a is recommended as first-line treatment option, for patients with mRCC with favorable or intermediate disease profile offering a prolonged progression free survival (Rini et al., 2008; Escudier et al., 2007, Patard 2009).

## 14   m-TOR inhibitors

Another pathway involved in RCC development, growth, proliferation, angiogenesis, and potential for metastasis is the mammalian target of rapamycin (mTOR).

Temsirolimus (Torisel®/CCI-779, Pfizer Inc., NY, USA) is an intravenously administered mTOR inhibitor of the PI3K/Akt/mTOR pathway resulting in G1 growth arrest of the treated tumor. Temsirolimus also reduces the level of proangiogenic growth factors HIF-1, HIF-2a, VEGF and PDGF (Kruck et al., 2012). Temsirolimus was approved as a first-line therapy in 2007 for mRCC patients with at least three of six poor prognostic risk factors. The recommended dose for Temsirolimus is 25 mg over a 30–60-min period once a week. Premedication with intravenous antihistamine is recommended to minimize the risk of allergic reactions. Temsirolimus was tested in a randomized phase III trial of temsirolimus (25 mg) monotherapy versus temsirolimus (15 mg) plus IFN-a (6 MIU) in 626 patients with mRCC and poor prognosis. Patients who received temsirolimus alone had significantly longer median PFS compared with those who received IFN-a alone or a combination of temsirolimus and IFN-a. The median OS in the IFN-a, temsirolimus and combination therapy groups was 7.3, 10.9 and 8.4 months, respectively and subgroup analysis found no differences in OS between clear and non-clear-cell renal carcinoma (Hudes et al., 2007) There is recent evidence to support that temsirolimus leads to meaningful improvements in overall survival and thus should be the first-line option for patients with poor risk features (Bullock et al., 2010). Temsirolimus has been recommended as first-line treatment option for treatment-naïve patients with non-clear cell histology and poor MSKCC prognostic factors and prognosis (Patard, 2009; Ljungberg et al., 2010) (Figure 1).

Everolimus (Afinitor®/RAD001, Novartis, Basel, Switzerland) is a synthetic, orally bioavailable analog of the mTOR inhibitor rapamycin that inhibits downstream targets of the PI3K/Akt/mTOR pathway. Everolimus was officially licensed in 2009 by the FDA for the treatment of mRCC and is available in a 5-mg or 10-mg tablet; the recommended dose for advanced mRCC treatment is 10 mg once daily

(Kruck *et al.,* 2012). Everolimus significantly prolonged PFS relative to placebo (4.0 vs. 1.9 months; HR: 0.30; $p < 0.0001$) in patients with mRCC who had progressed with prior anti-VEGF therapy. The final results of the study indicated extended PFS (4.9 vs 1.9 months; HR: 0.33; $p < 0.001$ by independent central review and 5.5 vs 1.9 months; HR: 0.32; $p < 0.001$ by investigators) (Motzer *et al.*, 2008; Motzer *et al.*, 2010). Everolimus is now the recommended second-line systemic therapy for patients who have progressed on prior VEGF-targeted therapy (Patard, 2008; Patard *et al.,* 2011) (Figure 2). Etaracizumab, Vorinostat, tivozanib, regorfanib, XL880 and Infliximab, antitumor vaccines and checkpoint inhibitors anti-CTLA4 and anti-PD1 are other agents currently under study.

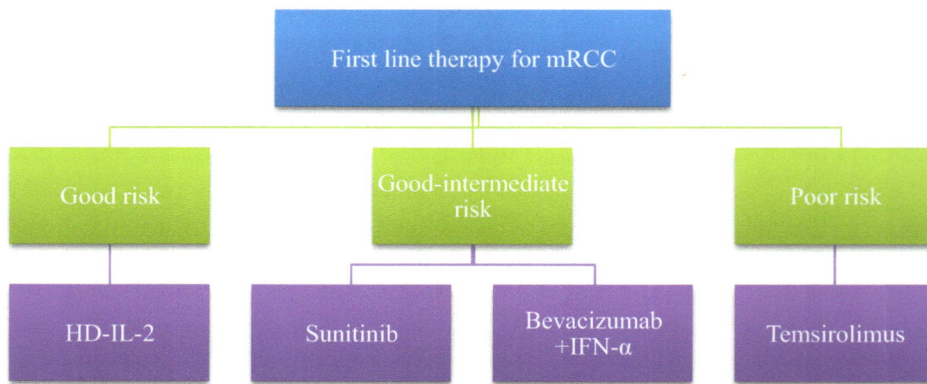

**Figure 1:** Therapeutic options for first-line treatment of mRCC.

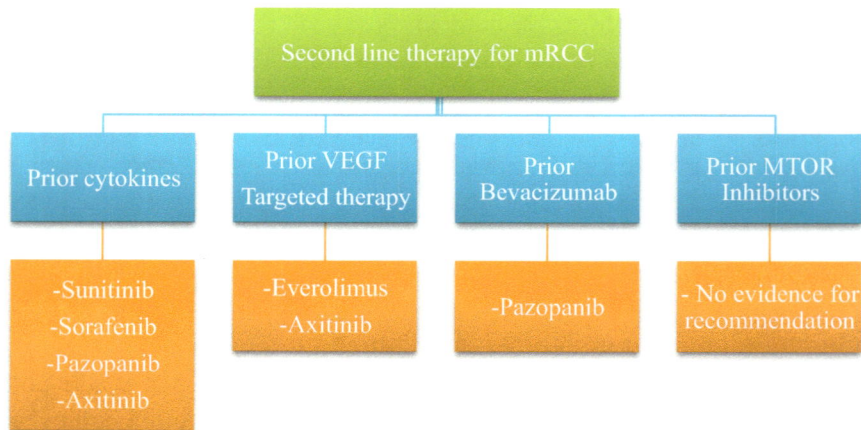

**Figure 2:** Therapeutic options for second-line treatment of mRCC.

## 15    Adverse Effects of Molecular Treatments

Molecular therapies for mRCC are often accompanied by potentially serious side effects. Patients treated with tyrosine kinase inhibitors (TKI's) may experience adverse effects such as fatigue, hypertension, diarrhea, nausea, proteinuria, cardiac toxicity, hypothyroidism, pancytopenia, hand-foot syndrome, mucositis and gastrointestinal toxicities. Interestingly, a diastolic blood pressure ≥90 mmHg appears to be associated with a better response to treatment with axitinib and sunitinib (Rini *et al.*, 2011; Rixe, 2007; Escudier *et al.*, 2011).The most commonly reported grade 3 adverse events associated with sorafenib are hypertension (12%), fatigue (11%), diarrhea (9%) and hand–foot syndrome (9%) (Motzer *et al.*, 2007; Motzer *et al.*, 2009). There is evidence that TKI treatment is the cause of alterations of the immune status of RCC patients, as sunitinib is found to inhibit the proliferation of primary human T-cells both from healthy volunteers and from RCC patients (Gu Y *et al.*, 2010). Also the incidence of hematologic adverse events from sunitinib treatment in Japanese patients was higher compared to Western populations, implying a relationship between ethnic origin and frequency of severe treatment toxicity due to different genetic backgrounds (Uemura *et al.*, 2010). The VEGF antibody-cytokine combination presents a different pattern of toxicity, including gastrointestinal perforation, bleeding, thromboembolic events, proteinuria, anorexia and fever. The mTOR's adverse event profile includes hyperglycemia, hyperlipidemia, asthenia, hematological toxicity, pneumonitis, infections, and mucositis (Kirchner *et al.*, 2010; Bhojani *et al.*, 2008). The most common adverse events observed during everolimus treatment are nausea (38.5%), anorexia (38.5%), diarrhea (30.8%) (Motzer *et al.*, 2008) Due to the increased risk of side effects, it is highly recommended that these treatments be undertaken only under the guidance of oncology specialists with expertise in the toxicity, interactions and monitoring of patients.

# 16   Sequential and combination therapy

The clinical introduction of novel targeted therapies has shifted research into the evaluation of the optimal drug sequence and also the potential benefits from combination therapy. As more information regarding the underlying molecular mechanisms of RCC becomes available, new targeted agents, and new combinations will be studied with the goal of providing survival advantage with minimal toxicity. Despite the availability of multiple treatment options, several challenges remain: selecting the best first-line or subsequent therapy for a given patient, the optimal sequencing of the various agents available and identifying well tolerated and effective drug combinations.

There is recent clinical evidence to suggest that targeting different pathways through sequential therapy may offer an advantage in terms of overcoming resistance to individual agents (Moreno Garcia *et al.*, 2012; Escudier *et al.*, 2009). Sequential treatment with targeted therapies is currently considered the standard of care for patients with metastatic renal cell carcinoma (mRCC). This stepwise approach initially involves the administration of a first-line vascular endothelial growth factor receptor-tyrosine kinase inhibitor (VEGFr-TKI). In the event of disease progression under first line treatment there are studies suggesting that failure to a previous anti-VEGF therapy might not preclude failure to a VEGFR agent with a different mechanism of action and molecular target, given that the targets are overlapping but not identical (Stein & Flaherty, 2007). In many cases of disease progression during TKI therapy, switching to a different TKI can bring the disease under control again. Therefore sequence therapy with tyrosine kinase inhibitors is an effective alternative to the TKI/mTOR inhibitor sequence. Several trials have shown substantial clinical benefits from a TKI–TKI sequence including sunitinib, sorafenib and axitinib in mRCC patients failing treatment with prior VEGFr-targeted TKIs (Eichelberg *et al.*, 2008; Sablin *et al.*, 2009; Dudek *et al.*, 2009). Patients with mRCC who will experience disease progression during initial VEGF-TKI therapy may alternatively switch to treatment with everolimus or axitinib (Motzer *et al.*, 2008). Sequential treatment with multiple targeting agents provides disease control and additional PFS.

Clinical guidelines recommend the use of everolimus, an mTOR inhibitor, in patients with VEGFr-TKI-refractory mRCC (Patard et al., 2011). Recent positive results of the phase III AXIS trial led to recent approval in the United States of the VEGFr-TKI axitinib for use in patients with mRCC who failed one previous therapy (Figure 2). Ongoing studies comparing first-line everolimus followed by second-line sunitinib versus the opposite sequence (RECORD-3 study) and comparing the optimal sequence of sorafenib given prior or after sunitinib (SWITCH trial) are awaited with interest. Currently there is not sufficient evidence for a clear recommendation for second-line alternatives after disease progression under mTOR inhibitors. In contrast to the first-line setting based on large Phase III studies, insufficient data are available to determine the optimal sequence after single or multiple systemic treatment failures in advanced RCC (Kruck et al., 2012). Antiangiogenic drug combination has been recently proposed in a theoretical effort to enhance the positive effects of monotherapy and overcoming drug resistance by either inhibiting several steps of the same pathway (vertical blockade) or by targeting in parallel two different pathways (horizontal blockade) (Sosman & Puzanov, 2009). A variety of drug combinations, (bevacizumab + sunitinib, bevacizumab + sorafenib, sunitinib or sorafenib + IFN-a-2b, temsirolimus + bevacizumab) have been tested in phase I studies (Feldman et al., 2009; Gollob et al., 2007; Azad et al., 2008; Patnaik et al., 2007). In general results were not encouraging due to either lack of synergistic or additive efficacy of the drugs or due to severe drug-related toxicity precluding the use of certain drug combinations (Feldman et al., 2009; Patnaik et al., 2007). Expert opinion considers antiangiogenic drug combinations investigational and not currently recommended outside the context of clinical trials.

Beyond overall survival and progression free survival, it is also fundamental to distinguish which therapies offer a major benefit in terms of quality of life. There are some studies reporting an advantage in quality of life when VEGFR inhibitors (sunitinib and sorafenib) are administered (Cella et al., 2008; Escudier et al., 2009), however no placedo-controlled trial has reported a health-related quality of life benefit according to a recent systematic review of randomized trials (Coppin et al., 2012). Since durable complete responses still remain elusive, improving overall survival is the main challenging objective although this effort is to an extent hampered by the lack of biomarkers predictive of response to treatment (Audenet et al., 2012). Cytoreductive nephrectomy was considered to be beneficial in terms of survival prolongation compared to cytokine therapy alone according to two randomized studies (Mickisch et al., 2001) (Flanigan et al., 2001) and is the current standard of care for mRCC. In the era of molecular targeted therapies such studies have not yet been conducted, although the vast majority of patients in the sunitinib and sorafenib trials underwent nephrectomy (Escudier et al., 2007; Motzer et al., 2007). There is evidence supporting that standard cytoreductive nephrectomy should probably be reconsidered at least for poor prognosis patients according to MSKCC criteria (Bex & Powles, 2012; Logan et al., 2008). Current practice patterns in this issue are based on individual clinical indications while results from ongoing studies (CARMENA trial, SURTIME trial) are eagerly awaited.

# 17   Prognostic Factors in mRCC

In general, pathologic prognostic features that have been proposed in RCC include nuclear grade, histologic subtype, and molecular biomarkers. Since the impact of histologic subtype on prognosis has been addressed previously the role of molecular markers will be discussed in more detail. The association of particular molecular markers with progression and outcome means that certain markers can be used to identify the likelihood for progression and can be incorporated into nomograms for patient counseling and for patient stratification in clinical trials. Molecular biomarkers that have been investigated in RCC prognostics include carbonic anhydrase IX (CA-IX), p53, p21, PTEN, Vimentin, pAKT, IMP3, B7H1/B7H4, Hif-1α and Survivin. Genetic biomarkers include VHL mutation, deletion, and/or hypermethylation.

The prognostics for the metastatic state of RCC are somewhat different from early stage disease. For instance although nuclear grade has been recognized as an independent predictor of survival in early stage disease, it has not been shown to correlate with survival in the metastatic setting (Patard *et al.,* 2005; Frank *et al.,* 2002). Prognostic molecular biomarkers have been identified by both DNA microarray and tissue array techniques. In a study on 150 metastatic clear cell RCC cases, using tissue array techniques investigators isolated CAIX, p53, PTEN, and vimentin as independent prognostic factors for survival. Increased immunohistochemical staining of p53 and vimentin was predictive of poor survival, while increased staining with CAIX and PTEN were associated with more favorable outcomes (Kim *et al.,* 2005). Increased CAIX tumor expression has also been found to be an independent predictor of prolonged survival in mRCC patients treated with IL-2, (Atkins *et al.,* 2005)while other investigators believe that CAIX expression as a predictive marker requires additional investigation (Leibovich *et al.,* 2007). Tumor expression of the insulin-like growth factor-II mRNA binding protein, IMP3, has been linked to poor outcome perhaps due to its association with poor prognostic features including tumor necrosis and sarcomatoid differentiation. Hoffmann *et al.* found a 42% increased risk of death from RCC in patients whose tumor IMP3 expression was positive (Hoffmann *et al.,* 2008). With regard to genetic markers, loss of heterozygosity (LOH) of chromosomes 8p, 9p and 14q have been associated with higher grade and stage in clear cell RCC and papillary RCC (Beroud *et al.,* 1996). LOH of chromosome 9p has been correlated with progression in locally advanced clear cell RCC and papillary RCC (Moch *et al.,* 1996; Schraml *et al.,* 2000). Finally on genetic biomarkers, although alterations in the VHL gene (mutations, deletions, hypermethylation) have been identified in 60% of patients with clear cell RCC, the question whether VHL loss correlates with survival has received variable answers (Patard *et al.,* 2008; Choueiri *et al.,* 2008).

## 18  Conclusions and Future Directions

Metastatic RCC is known to be an aggressive, potentially lethal and highly resistant disease. Nevertheless, the introduction of new targeted therapies based on an improved understanding of RCC tumor biology has produced encouraging outcomes with substantial improvement on overall survival for patients with advanced RCC. However despite some dramatic initial responses, targeted treatment rarely cannot be considered curative as advanced cancers become resistant to VEGF and mTOR agents in the long term.

The future holds promise that the genomic approach to RCC classification, will allow the identification of prognostic markers and predictive indicators of response to treatment while technological developments, such as large-scale analysis and high-speed sequencing, will allow the systematic screening of tumors to fully determine the somatic genetic architecture of RCC (Audenet *et al.,* 2012; Wright & Kapoor A, 2011). Metastatic RCC represents a field of constant and rapid evolvement and progress during the last few years. Today patients with RCC have several alternative treatment options that warrant survival prolongation with acceptable morbidity. Still, certain issues need further refinement. Among those is the place for cytoreductive nephrectomy in the era of targeted molecular treatments, the timing and ideal sequencing of targeted therapies, the optimal combination of these agents and the understanding of the mechanisms of drug resistance. What ongoing research on RCC allows us to expect from the future is the possibility of personalized treatment for renal cancer patients.

# References

Aburto J, Bruckner AB, Blackmon HS, Beyer AE & Reardon JM. (2009). Renal cell carcinoma metastatic to the left ventricle. Tex Heart Inst J, 36(1):48-49.

Adsay NV, Andea A, Basturk O, Kilinc N, Nassar H, Cheng JD. (2004). Secondary tumors of the pancreas: an analysis of a surgical and autopsy database and review of the literature. Virchows Arch 444: 527-535

Akhtar M, Tulbah A, Kardar AH, Ali MA. (1997) Sarcomatoid renal cell carcinoma: the chromophobe connection. Am J Surg Pathol, 21:1188-1195 .

Albrizio M, La Fianza A, Gorone MS (2009). Bilateral metachronous ovarian metastases from clear cell renal carcinoma: a case report. Cases J,5(2):7083.

Alghamdi A, Tam J (2006). Cardiac metastasis from a renal cell carcinoma. Can J Cardiol, 22(14):1231-1232.

Althausen P, Althausen A, Jennings LC, Mankin HJ (1997).Prognostic factors and surgical treatment of osseous metastases secondary to renal cell carcinoma. Cancer, 80(6):1103-1109.

Amin MB, Paner GP, Alvarado-Cabrero I, Young AN, Stricker HJ, Lyles RH, Moch H (2008). Chromophobe renal cell carcinoma: histomorphologic characteristics and evaluation of conventional pathologic prognostic parameters in 145 cases.Am J Surg Pathol, 32(12):1822-34.

Argani P, Ladanyi M (2005). Translocation carcinomas of the kidney. Clin Lab Med, 25:363-78

Arrabal-Polo MA, Arias-Santiago SA, Aneiros-Fernandez J, Burkhardt-Perez P, Arrabal-Martin M & Naranjo-Sintes R. (2009). Cutaneous metastases in renal cell carcinoma: a case report. Cases J, 25(2):7948.

Assouad J, Riquet M, Foucault C, Hidden G, Delmas V (2006). Renal lymphatic drainage and thoracic duct connections: implications for cancer spread. Lymphology, 39:26-32

Athar U, Gentile TC. (2008) Treatment options for metastatic renal cell carcinoma: a review. Can J Urol, 15: 3954–66.

Atkins M, Regan M, McDermott D, et al. (2005). Carbonic anhydrase IX expression predicts outcome of interleukin 2 therapy for renal cancer. Clin Cancer Res, 11(10):3714–3721.

Atzpodien J, Kirchner H, Hänninen EL, Deckert M, Fenner M, Poliwoda H (1993). Interleukin-2 in combination with interferon-alpha and 5-fluorouracil for metastatic renal cell cancer. Eur J Cancer, 29A Suppl 5:S6-8.

Audenet F, Yates DR, Cancel-Tassin G, Cussenot O, Rouprêt M. (2012) Genetic pathways involved in carcinogenesis of clear cell renal cell carcinoma: genomics towards personalized medicine. BJU Int,109(12):1864-70.

Azad NS, Posadas EM, Kwitkowski VE, et al. (2008). Combination targeted therapy with sorafenib and bevacizumab results in enhanced toxicity and antitumor activity. J Clin Oncol, 26:3709-14

Azam F, Abubakerr M, Gollins S. (2008). Tongue metastasis as an initial presentation of renal cell carcinoma: a case report and literature review. J Med Case Reports 2:249.

Ballarin R., Spaggiari M., Cautero N., Ruvo N., Montalti R., Longo C., Pecchi A., Giacobazzi P., Marco G., Amico G., Gerunda GE., Benedetto F. (2011). Pancreatic metastases from renal cell carcinoma: The state of the art. World J Gastroenterol, 21; 17(43): 4747-4756.

Basely M, Bonnel S, Maszelin P, Verdalle P, Bussy E, de Jaureguiberry JP (2009). A rare presentation of metastatic renal clear cell carcinoma to the tongue seen on FDG PET. Clin Nucl Med, 34(9):566-569.

Béroud C, Fournet J-C, Jeanpierre C, et al. (1996). Correlations of allelic imbalance of chromosome 14 with adverse prognostic parameters in 148 renal cell carcinomas. Genes Chromosomes Cancer, 17:215–224.

Bex A, Powles T (2012). Selecting patients for cytoreductive nephrectomy in advanced renal cell carcinoma: who and when. Expert Rev Anticancer Ther, 12(6):787-97.

Bhojani N, Jeldres C, Patard JJ, et al. (2008). Toxicities associated with the administration of sorafenib, sunitinib, and temsirolimus and their management in patients with metastatic renal cell carcinoma. Eur Urol, 53:917-30.

Blom JHM, van Poppel H, Marechal JM et al. (1999). Radical nephrectomy with and without lymph node dissection: preliminary results of the EORTC randomized phase III protocol 30881. Eur Urol, 36: 570–75

Bonsib SM(1996). The relationship between cytoplasmic vesicles and colloidal iron stain. J Urol Pathol, 4:9-14

Bradley MS, Bolling FS. (1995). Late renal cell carcinoma metastasis to the left ventricular outflow tract. Ann Thorac Surg, 60(1):204-206.

Bugalho MJ, Mendonça E, Costa P, Santos JR, Silva E, Catarino AL, Sobrinho LG (2006).A multinodular goiter as the initial presentation of a renal cell carcinoma harbouring a novel VHL mutation. BMC Endocrine Disorders, 6:6.

Bukowski RM, Eisen T, Szczylik C, et al. (2007). Final results of the randomized phase III trial of sorafenib in advanced renal cell carcinoma: survival and biomarker analysis. J Clin Oncol, 25: abstract 5023.

Buła G, Waler J, Niemiec A, Koziołek H, Bichalski W & Gawrychowski J (2010). Diagnosis of metastatic tumours to the thyroid gland by fine needle aspiration biopsy. Endokrynol Pol, 61(5):427-429.

Bullock A, McDermott DF, Atkins MB (2010).Management of metastatic renal cell carcinoma in patients with poor prognosis. Cancer Manag Res, 24;2:123-32

Calvo E, Ravaud A, Bellmunt J (2012). What is the optimal therapy for patients with metastatic renal cell carcinoma who progress on an initial VEGFr-TKI? Cancer Treat Rev. 2012 Jul 23. (Epub ahead of print)

Cassinello Espinosa J, González Del Alba Baamonde A, Rivera Herrero F, Holgado Martín E (2012). SEOM guidelines for the treatment of bone metastases from solid tumours. Clin Transl Oncol, 14(7):505-11.

Cella D, Li JZ, Cappelleri JC, Bushmakin A, Charbonneau C, Kim ST, Chen I, Motzer RJ (2008).Quality of life in patients with metastatic renal cell carcinoma treated with sunitinib or interferon alfa: results from a phase III randomized trial. J Clin Oncol, 26(22):3763-3769.

Chapman T, Sharma S, Zhang S, Wong M, Kim H (2008). Laparoscopic lymph node dissection in clinically node-negative patients undergoing laparoscopic nephrectomy for renal carcinoma . Urology, 71, 2: 287-91

Chauhan A, Ganguly M, Nath P & Chowdhary GS (2011).Cutaneous metastasis to face and neck as a sole manifestation of an unsuspected renal cell carcinoma. Int J Dermatol, 50(1):81-4.

Chen F, Fujinaga T, Shoji T, Miyahara R, Bando T, Okubo K, Hirata T, Date H (2008). Pulmonary resection for metastasis from renal cell carcinoma.Interact Cardiovasc Thorac Surg, 7(5):825-828.

Cheng L, Zhang S, MacLennan GT, Lopez-Beltran A, Montironi R. (2009) Molecular and cytogenetic insights into the pathogenesis, classification, differential diagnosis, and prognosis of renal epithelial neoplasms. Hum Pathol , 40(1):10-29.

Cheville JC, Lohse CM, Zincke H, Weaver AL, Leibovich BC, Frank I, Blute ML(2004). Sarcomatoid renal cell carcinoma: an examination of underlying histologic subtype and an analysis of associations with patient outcome. Am J Surg Pathol, 28(4):435-41.

Choueiri TK (2011). VEGF inhibitors in metastatic renal cell carcinoma: current therapies and future perspective. Curr Clin Pharmacol, 6(3):164-8.

Choueiri TK, Vaziri SA, Jaeger E, et al. (2008). von Hippel-Lindau gene status and response to vascular endothelial growth factor targeted therapy for metastatic clear cell renal cell carcinoma. J Urol, 180(3):860–865.

Chung PH, Srinivasan R, Linehan WM, Pinto PA, Bratslavsky G (2012). Renal cell carcinoma with metastases to the gallbladder: four cases from the National Cancer institute (NCI) and review of the literature. Urol Oncol. Jul-Aug 30(4):476-81

Cochand-Priollet B, Molinié V, Bougaran J, Bouvier R, Dauge-Geffroy MC, Deslignières S, Fournet JC, Gros P, Lesourd A, Saint-André JP, Toublanc M, Vieillefond A, Wassef M, Fontaine A, Groleau L(1997).Renal chromophobe cell carcinoma and oncocytoma. A comparative morphologic, histochemical, and immunohistochemical study of 124 cases. Arch Pathol Lab Med, 121(10):1081-6.

Cochrane TJ, Cheng L, Crean S. (2006). Renal cell carcinoma: A rare metastasis to the tongue–a case report. Dent Update, 33(3):186-187.

Cohen D, Zhou M (2005).Molecular genetics of familiar renal cell carcinoma syndromes. Clin Lab Med, 25:259-77

Cohen HT, McGovern FJ (2005). Renal-cell carcinoma. N Engl J Med, 353:2477–2490.

Cohen PR. (2001). Metastatic tumors to the nail unit: subungual metastases. Dermatol Surg, 27(3):280-293.

Coppin C, Porzsolt F, Awa A, Kumpf J, Coldman A, Wilt T (2005). Immunotherapy for advanced renal cell cancer. Cochrane Database Syst Rev, (1):CD001425.

Coppin C, Kollmannsberger C, Le L, Porzsolt F, Wilt TJ (2011). Targeted therapy for advanced renal cell cancer (RCC): a Cochrane systematic review of published trials. BJU Int, 108(10):1556-63

Dalgliesh GL, Furge K, Greenman C et al. (2010). Systematic sequencing of renal carcinoma reveals inactivation of histone modifying genes. Nature, 463:360-3

Deeb R, Zhang Z, Ghanem T. (2012). Metastatic Renal Cell Carcinoma to the Parotid Gland in the Setting of Chronic Lymphocytic Leukemia. Case Reports in Medicine ID 265708, 17-26

Dequanter D, Lothaire P, Andry AG (2005). Secondary malignant tumors of the parotid. Otolaryngol Chir Cervicofac, 122(1):18-20.

Dudek AZ, Zolnierek J, Dham A, Lindgren BR, Szczylik C (2009). Sequential therapy with sorafenib and sunitinib in renal cell carcinoma. Cancer, 115(1): 61–67.

Eichelberg C, Heuer R, Chun FK et al. (2008). Sequential use of the tyrosine kinase inhibitors sorafenib and sunitinib in metastatic renal cell carcinoma: a retrospective outcome analysis. Eur. Urol, 54(6): 1373–1378.

Escudier B, Goupil MG, Massard C, Fizazi K (2009). Sequential therapy in renal cell carcinoma. Cancer, 115(10 Suppl):2321-2326.

Escudier B, Pluzanska A, Koralewski P, et al. (2007). Bevacizumab plus interferon alfa-2a for treatment of metastatic renal cell carcinoma: a randomised, double-blind phase III trial. Lancet, 370:2103–11.

Escudier B, Eisen T, Stadler WM, et al. (2009). Sorafenib for treatment of renal cell carcinoma: final efficacy and safety results of the phase III treatment approaches in renal cancer global evaluation trial. J Clin Oncol, 27:3312–8.

Escudier BJ, Bellmunt J, Negrier S et al. (2010). Phase III trial of bevacizumab plus interferon alfa-2a in patients with metastatic renal cell carcinoma (AVOREN): final analysis of overall survival. J Clin Oncol, 28:2144-50

Escudier B, Gore M (2011). Axitinib for the management of metastatic renal cell carcinoma. Drugs R. D, 11(2): 113–126.

Fang X., Gupta N., Shen S., Tamboli P., Charnsangavej C., Rashid A., Wang H. (2010). Intraluminal Polypoid Metastasis of Renal Cell Carcinoma in Gallbladder Mimicking Gallbladder Polyp. Arch Pathol Lab Med 134:1003–1009.

Feldman DR, Baum MS, Ginsberg MS, et al. (2009).Phase I trial of bevacizumab plus escalated doses of sunitinib in patients with metastatic renal cell carcinoma. J Clin Oncol, 27:1432-9

Ferlay J, Autier P, Boniol M, Heanue M, Colombet M, Boyle P (2007). Estimates of the cancer incidence and mortality in Europe in 2006. Ann Oncol, 18:581-92

Ferlay J, Parkin DM, Steliarova-Foucher E. Estimates of cancer incidence and mortality in Europe in 2008. Eur J Cancer 2010;46:765–81.

Karim-Kos HE, de Vries E, Soerjomataram I, Lemmens V, Siesling S, Coebergh JW (2008). Recent trends of cancer in Europe: A combined approach of incidence, survival and mortality for 17 cancer sites since the 1990s. Eur J Cancer, 44:1345–1389.

Flanigan RC, Salmon SE, Blumenstein BA, et al. (2001). Nephrectomy followed by interferon alfa-2b compared with interferon alfa-2b alone for metastatic renal-cell cancer. N Engl J Med, 345:1655-9.

Fleming S, O'Donnell M(2000). Surgical pathology of renal epithelial neoplasms: recent advances and current status. Histopathology, 36(3):195-202.

Frank I, Blute ML, Cheville JC, Lohse CM, Weaver AL, Zincke H (2002). An outcome prediction model for patients with clear cell renal cell carcinoma treated with radical nephrectomy based on tumor stage, size, grade and necrosis: the SSIGN score. J Urol, 168(6):2395–2400.

Fyfe G, Fisher RI, Rosenberg SA, Sznol M, Parkinson DR, Louie AC (1995). Results of treatment of 255 patients with metastatic renal cell carcinoma who received high-dose recombinant interleukin-2 therapy. J Clin Oncol, 13(3):688-96.

Gaetani P, Di Ieva A, Colombo P, Tancioni F, Aimar E, Debernardi A, Baena RR (2005). Calvarial metastases as clinical presentation of renal cell carcinoma: report of two cases and review of the literature. Clin Neurol Neurosurg,107(4):329-333.

Galetović D, Bućan K, Karlica D, Lesin M & Znaor L. (2010). Bilateral choroidal metastases of kidney carcinoma. Acta Med Croatica, 64(3):221-4.

García Torrelles M, Beltrán Armada JR, Verges Prosper A, Santolaya García JI, Espinosa Ruiz JJ, Tarín Planes M, Sanjuán de Laorden C. (2007). Skin metastases from a renal cell carcinoma. Actas Urol Esp, 31(5):556-558.

Garcia Lozano MC, Fernandez Gomez J, Lloret Selles E, Delgado Quero A, Galdeano, Granda E. (1998). Metastasizing hypernephroma in palatine tonsil. An Otorrinolaringol Ibero Am.25 (6):565-76.

Garfield DH, Hercbergs A, Davis PJ. (2007). Hypothyroidism in patients with metastatic renal cell carcinoma treated with sunitinib. J Natl Cancer Inst, 99(12):975-976

Geertsen PF, Gore ME, Negrier S, Tourani JM, von der MH (2004). Safety and efficacy of subcutaneous and continuous intravenous infusion rIL-2 in patients with metastatic renal cell carcinoma. Br J Cancer, 90:1156–62.

Gollob JA, Rathmell WK, Richmond TM et al. (2007). Phase II trial of sorafenib plus interferon alfa-2b as first- or second-line therapy in patients with metastatic renal cell cancer. J Clin Oncol, 25:3288-95

Gu Y, Zhao W, Meng F et al. (2010). Sunitinib impairs the proliferation and function of human peripheral T cell and prevents T-cell mediated immune response in mice. Clin Immunol, 135:55-62

Guney S, Guney N, Ozcan D, Sayilgan T, Ozakin E (2010). Ovarian metastasis of a primary renal cell carcinoma: case report and review of literature. Eur J Gynaecol Oncol, 31(3):339-41.

Gupta K, Miller JD, Li JZ, Russell MW, Charbonneau C (2008) Epidemiologic and socioeconomic burden of metastatic renal cell carcinoma (mRCC): a literature review. Cancer Treat Rev, 34: 193–205.

Hasumi Y, Baba M, Ajima R, et al. (2009). Homozygous loss of BHD causes early embryonic lethality and kidney tumor development with activation of mTORC1 and mTORC2. Proc Natl Acad Sci USA, 106:18722-7

Hoffmann NE, Sheinin Y, Lohse CM, et al. (2008).External validation of IMP3 expression as an independent prognostic marker for metastatic progression and death for patients with clear cell renal cell carcinoma. Cancer, 112(7):1471–1479.

Huang D, Ding Y, Li Y et al. (2010). Sunitinib acts primarily on tumor endothelium rather than tumor cells to inhibit the growth of renal cell carcinoma. Cancer Res, 70:1053-62

Hudes G, Carducci M, Tomczak P, Dutcher J, Figlin R, Kapoor A, Staroslawska E, Sosman J, McDermott D, Bodrogi I et al. (2007). Temsirolimus, interferon alfa, or both for advanced renal-cell carcinoma. N Engl J Med, 356(22):2271-2281.

Hunt JD, van der Hel OL, McMillan GP, Bofetta P, Brennan P (2005). Renal cell carcinoma in relation to cigarette smoking: meta-analysis of 24 studies. Int J Cancer,114:101-8

Hur J, Yoon CS, Jung WH. (2007). Multiple skeletal muscle metastases from renal cell carcinoma 19 years after radical nephrectomy. Acta Radiol 48(2):238-241.

Hutson TE (2011). Targeted therapies for the treatment of metastatic renal cell carcinoma: clinical evidence. Oncologist, 16 Suppl 2:14-22.

Iranikhah M, Wilborn TW, Wensel TM, Ferrell JB (2012). Denosumab for the prevention of skeletal-related events in patients with bone metastasis from solid tumor. Pharmacotherapy, 32(3):274-84.

Jalón Monzón A, Alvarez Múgica M, Bulnes Vázquez V, González Alvarez RC, García Rodríguez J, Martín Benito JL, Ferrer Barriendo J & Regadera Sejas FJ. (2008). Ovarian metastasis of a primary renal cell carcinoma. Arch Esp Urol , 61(4):534-537.

Jilani G, Mohamed D, Wadia H, Ramzi K, Meriem J, Houssem L, Samir G, Ben Nawfel R (2010). Cutaneous metastasis of renal cell carcinoma through percutaneous fine needle aspiration biopsy: case report. Dermatol Online, J 16(2):10.

Juraszynski Z, Szpakowski E, Biederman A. (2010). Giant metastatic intrapericardial tumor 20 years after nephrectomy. Ann Thorac Surg, 90(1):292-3.

Johnson RP, Krauland K, Owens NM, Peckham S (2011). Renal medullary carcinoma metastatic to the scalp.Am J Dermatopathol, 33(1):e11-13.

Kaplan RN, Riba RD, Zacharoulis S, Bramley AH, Vincent L, Costa C, MacDonald DD, Jin DK, Shido K, Kerns SA, Zhu Z, Hicklin D, Wu Y, Port JL, Altorki N, Port ER, Ruggero D, Shmelkov SV, Jensen KK, Rafii S, Lyden D (2005). VEGFR-1 positive haematopoietic bone marrow progenitors initiate the pre-metastatic niche. Nature, 438 (7069):820-827.

Kapitsinou PP, Haase VH (2008). The VHL tumor suppressor and HIF: insights from genetic studies in mice. Cell Death Differ, 15:650-9

Karakiewicz PI, Trinh Q-D, Bhojani N et al. (2007). Renal cell carcinoma with nodal metastases in the absence of distant metastatic disease: prognostic indicators of disease-specific survival. Eur Urol, 51:1616-24

Kavolius JP, Mastorakos DP, Pavlovich C, Russo P, Burt ME, Brady MS (1998).Resection of metastatic renal cell carcinoma. J Clin Oncol, 16(6):2261-2266.

Kim HL, Lam J, Belldegrun A (2006). Surgical management of renal cell carcinoma: role of lymphadenectomy in renal cell carcinoma surgery, role of lymph node dissection in renal cell carcinoma, in Vogelzang N, Scardino P, Shipley W, et al. (Eds): Comprehensive Textbook of Genitourinary Oncology. Philadelphia, Lippincott Williams and Wilkins, 2006, pp 739–743.

Kim HL, Seligson D, Liu X, et al. (2005). Using tumor markers to predict the survival of patients with metastatic renal cell carcinoma. J Urol, 173(5):1496–1501

Kinouchi T, Mano M, Saiki S, Meguro N, Maeda O, Kuroda M, Usami M, Kotake T (1999). Incidence rate of satellite tumors in renal cell carcinoma. Cancer, 86(11):2331-6.

Kirchner H, Strumberg D, Bahl A, Overkamp F (2010).Patient-based strategy for systemic treatment of metastatic renal cell carcinoma. Expert Rev Anticancer Ther, 10(4):585-96.

Kovacs G, Akhtar M, Beckwith BJ, et al. (1997).The Heidelberg classification of renal cell tumours. J Pathol, 183:131-3

Kruck S, Kuczyk MA, Gakis G, KramerMW, Stenzl A, Merseburger AS (2008). Novel therapeutic options in metastatic renal cancer—review and post ASCO 2007 update. Rev Recent Clin Trials, 3: 212–6.

Kruck S, Bedke J, Kuczyk MA, Merseburger AS (2012).Second-line systemic therapy for the treatment of metastatic renal cell cancer.Expert Rev Anticancer Ther, 12(6):777-85

Kumar P, Virk RS,  Gupta A (2007). An unusual presentation of metastatic renal cell carcinoma to the frontonasal region: a case report. The Internet Journal of Head and Neck Surgery. Volume 1 Number 1,

Kundu S, Eynon-Lewis NJ, Radcliffe GJ (2001).Extensive metastatic renal cell carcinoma presenting as facial nerve palsy. J Laryngol Otol, 115(6):488-490.

Label DA. (2006). Risk factors, classification and staging of renal cell cancer. Med Oncol, 23(4):443-54

Lee HM, Kang HJ, Lee SH. (2005) Metastatic renal cell carcinoma presenting as epistaxis. Eur Arch Otorhinolaryngol, 262:69–71

Lee WM, Batoroev KY, Odashiro NA & Nguyen G. (2007). Solitary metastatic cancer to the thyroid: a report of five cases with fine-needle aspiration cytology. CytoJournal 4:5.

Leibovich BC, Sheinin Y, Lohse CM, et al. (2007). Carbonic anhydrase IX is not an independent **predictor of outcome for** patients with clear cell renal cell carcinoma. J Clin Oncol, 25(30):4757–4764.

Levi F, Ferlay J, Galeone C et al. (2008). The changing pattern of kidney cancer incidence and mortality in Europe. BJU Int, 101:949–958

Lin PP, Mirza AN, Lewis VO, Cannon CP, Tu SM, Tannir NM, Yasko AW (2007).Patient survival after surgery for osseous metastases from renal cell carcinoma. J Bone Joint Surg Am, 89(8):1794-1801.

Lindner DJ (2002). Interferons as antiangiogenic agents. Curr Urol Rep, 4(6): 510-514

Linehan WM, Srinivasan R, Schmidt LS (2010).The genetic basis of kidney cancer:  a metabolic disease. Nat Rev Urol, 7:277-85

Liu Y, Song T, Huang Z, Zhang S, Li Y (2012). The accuracy of multidetector Computed Tomography for preoperative staging of renal cell carcinoma. Int Braz J Urol. 38: 00-00

Ljungberg B, Hanbury DC, Kuczyk MA, Merseburger AS, Mulders PF, Patard JJ, Sinescu IC (2007). European Association of Urology Guideline Group for renal cell carcinoma.Renal cell carcinoma guideline. Eur Urol, 51(6):1502-10

Ljungberg B, Cowan NC, Hanbury DC, et al. (2010). EAU guidelines on renal cell carcinoma: the 2010 update. Eur Urol, 58:398-40

Logan T, McDermott DF, Dutcher JP et al. (2008).Exploratory analysis of the influence of nephrectomy status on temsirolimus efficacy in patients with advanced renal cell carcinoma and poor-risk features (abstract). J Clin Oncol, 26(suppl):5050

Lyons JF, Wilhelm S, Hibner B, Bollag G (2001). Discovery of a novel Raf kinase inhibitor. Endocr Relat Cancer, 8(3):219-225

Mahmoudi HR, Kamyab K, Daneshpazhooh M (2012). Cutaneous metastasis of renal cell carcinoma: a case report. Dermatol Online J,15;18(5):12.

Mancini V, Battaglia M, Lucarelli G, Di Lorenzo V, Ditonno P, Bettocchi C & Selvaggi FP. (2008).Unusual solitary metastasis of the ciliary body in renal cell carcinoma. Int J Urol, 15(4):363-5.

Martínez-Rodríguez R, Rodríguez-Escovar F, Bujons Tur A, Maroto P, Palou J, Villavicencio H (2008). Skin metastasis during follow-up of a clear cell renal carcinoma. Arch Esp Urol, 61(1):80-82.

Massaccesi M, Morganti AG, Serafini G, Di Lallo A, Deodato F, Picardi V & Scambia G. (2009). Late tonsil metastases from renal cell cancer: a case report. Tumori, 95(4):521-524.

McDermott DF, Regan MM, Clark JI, Flaherty LE, Weiss GR, Logan TF, Kirkwood JM, Gordon MS, Sosman JA, Ernstoff MS, Tretter CP, Urba WJ, Smith JW, Margolin KA, Mier JW, Gollob JA, Dutcher JP, Atkins MB (2005). Randomized phase III trial of high-dose interleukin-2 versus subcutaneous interleukin-2 and interferon in patients with metastatic renal cell carcinoma. J Clin Oncol, 23(1):133-41.

Medendorp K, van Groningen JJ, Schepens M et al. (2007). Molecular mechanisms underlying the MiT translocation sub-group of renal cell carcinomas. Cytogenet Genome Res, 118:157-65

Menauer F, Issing WJ (1998). Unusual metastasis of renal cell carcinoma.A case report with review of the literature. Laryngorhinootologie, 77(9):525-7.

Mickisch GH, Garin A, van Poppel H, et al., European Organisation for Research and Treatment of Cancer (EORTC) Genitourinary Group (2001). Radical nephrectomy plus interferon-alfa-based immunotherapy compared with interferon alfa alone in metastatic renal-cell carcinoma: A randomized trial. Lancet, 358:966-70.

Minervini A, Lilas L, Morelli G et al. (2011). Regional lymph node dissection in the treatment of renal cell carcinoma: is it useful in patients with no suspected adenopathy before or during surgery? BJU Int , 88 : 169-72

Moch H, Presti JC Jr, Sauter G, et al. (1996). Genetic aberrations detected by comparative genomic hybridization are associated with clinical outcome in renal cell carcinoma. Cancer Res, 56:27–30.

Moreno Garcia V, Basu B, Molife LR, Kaye SB (2012). Combining antiangiogenics to overcome resistance: rationale and clinical experience. Clin Cancer Res, 18(14):3750-61.

Motzer RJ, Mazumdar M, Bacik J, Berg W, Amsterdam A, Ferrara J (1999). Survival and prognostic stratification of 670 patients with advanced renal cell carcinoma. J Clin Oncol, 17:2530-40

Motzer RJ, Hutson TE, Tomczak P, et al. (2007). Sunitinib versus interferon alfa in metastatic renal-cell carcinoma. N Engl J Med, 356: 115–24.

Motzer RJ, Escudier B, Oudard S, et al. (2008). Efficacy of everolimus in advanced renal cell carcinoma: a double-blind, randomised, placebo-controlled phase III trial. Lancet, 372:449–56.

Motzer RJ, Rini BI, Bukowski RM, Curti BD, George DJ, Hudes GR, Redman BG, Margolin KA, Merchan JR, Wilding G, Ginsberg MS, Bacik J, Kim ST, Baum CM, Michaelson MD (2006). Sunitinib in patients with metastatic renal cell carcinoma. JAMA, 295(21):2516-24.

Motzer RJ, Hutson TE, Tomczak P, et al. (2009). Overall survival and updated results for sunitinib compared with interferon alfa in patients with metastatic renal cell carcinoma. J Clin Oncol, 27:3584–90.

Motzer RJ, Escudier B, Oudard S et al. (2010). Phase 3 trial of everolimus for metastatic renal cell carcinoma : final results and analysis of prognostic factors. Cancer, 116(18): 4256–4265.

Moudouni SM, Tligui M, Doublet JD, Haab F, Gattegno B & Thibault P (2006). Late metastasis of renal cell carcinoma to the submaxillary gland 10 years after radical nephrectomy. Int J Urol, 13(4):431-432.

Mudiyanselage SY, Prabhakaran VC, Davis GJ, Selva D. (2008).Metastatic renal cell carcinoma presenting as a circumscribed orbital mass. Eur J Ophthalmol, 18(3):483-5.

Nanus DM, Pfeffer LM, Bander NH, Bahri S, Albino AP (1990). Antiproliferative and antitumor effects of alpha-interferon in renal cell carcinomas: correlation with the expression of a kidney-associated differentiation glycoprotein. Cancer Res, 50(14):4190-4.

Negrier S, Escudier B, Lasset C, Douillard JY, Savary J, Chevreau C, Ravaud A, Mercatello A, Peny J, Mousseau M, Philip T, Tursz T (1998). Recombinant human interleukin-2, recombinant human interferon alfa-2a, or both in metastatic renal-cell carcinoma. Groupe Français d'Immunothérapie. N Engl J Med, 338(18):1272-8.

Negrier S, Perol D, Ravaud A, Chevreau C, Bay JO, Delva R, Sevin E, Caty A, Escudier B; For The French Immunotherapy Intergroup (2007). Medroxyprogesterone, interferon alfa-2a, interleukin 2, or combination of both cytokines in patients with metastatic renal carcinoma of intermediate prognosis: results of a randomized controlled trial. Cancer 2007, 110(11):2468-77.

Négrier S, Gravis G, Pérol D et al. (2011). Temsirolimus and bevacizumab, or sunitinib, or interferon a and bevacizumab for patients with advanced renal cell carcinoma (TORAVA): a randomised Phase 2 trial. Lancet Oncol. 12(7), 673–680.

Nixon JI, Whitcher M, Glick J, Palmer LF, Shaha RA, Shah PJ, Patel GS, Ganly I. (2011). Surgical management of metastases to the thyroid gland. Ann Surg Oncol, 18(3):800-804.

Ng CS. (2006)Radiologic diagnosis and staging of renal and bladder cancer. Semin Roentgenol, 41(2):121-38

(No authors listed) (1999). Interferon-alpha and survival in metastatic renal carcinoma: early results of a randomised controlled trial. Medical Research Council Renal Cancer Collaborators. Lancet, 353(9146):14-7.

Nouh MA, Kuroda N, Yamashita M, et al. (2010). Renal cell carcinoma in patients with end-stage renal disease: relationship between histological type and duration of dialysis. BJU Int, 105:620-7

Olencki, T. and Bukowski, R.M. (2000) Interleukin-2 in metastatic renal cell carcinoma.In Renal Cell Carcinoma. Molecular Biology, Immunology and Clinical Management.Bukowski, R.M. and Novick, A.C., Eds. Humana Press, Totowa, NJ. pp. 301–318.

Oosterwijk E, Rathmell WK, Junker K, Brannon AR, Pouliot F, Finley DS, Mulders PFA, Kirkali Z, Uemura H, Belldegrun A (2011). Basic research in kidney cancer. Eur Urol, 60:622-33

Oppenheimer SB. (2006) Cellular basis of cancer metastasis: A review of fundamentals and new advances. Acta Histochemica, 108(5):327-334.

Osman F, Geh JI, Griffith MJ (2006).An unusual cause of cardiac paradox. European Journal of Echocardiography Volume 8, Issue 2 Pp. 91-92.

Otahbachi M, Cevik C, Sutthiwan P (2009). Right ventricle and tricuspid valve metastasis in a patient with renal cell carcinoma. Anadolu Kardiyol Derg, 10;9(4):E11-2.

Pantuck, AJ, Zisman A, Dorey F, Chao D H, Han K-R, Said J Gitlitz BJ, Figlin RA, Belldegrun AS. (2003). Renal cell carcinoma with retroperitoneal lymph nodes: role of lymph node dissection. J Urol, 169(6):2076-83.

Pantuck AJ, Zisman A, Belldegrun AS. (2001). The changing natural history of renal cell carcinoma. J Urol; 166, 1611–23

Pantuck AJ, Belldegrun AS, Figlin RA (2007). Cytoreductive nephrectomy for metastatic renal cell carcinoma: Is it still imperative in the era of targeted therapy? Clin Cancer Res, 13(2 Pt 2):693s-6s.

Pascual D, Borque A. (2008).Epidemiology of kidney cancer. Adv Urol, 782381.

Patard JJ, Leray E, Rioux-Leclercq N, et al. Prognostic value of histologic subtypes in renal cell carcinoma: a multicenter experience. J Clin Oncol. 2005;23(12):2763–2771.

Patard JJ (2008). European association of urology guidelines for systemic therapy in metastatic renal cell carcinoma:What is recommended and why? Eur Urol Suppl 2008;7:46-54.

Patard JJ, Fergelot P, Karakiewicz PI, et al. (2008). Low CAIX expression and absence of VHL gene mutation are associated with tumor aggressiveness and poor survival of clear cell renal cell carcinoma. Int J Cancer, 123(2):395–400.

Patard JJ, Pignot G, Escudier B, Eisen T, Bex A, Sternberg C, Rini B, Roigas J, Choueiri T, Bukowski R, Motzer R, Kirkali Z, Mulders P, Bellmunt J (2011). ICUD-EAU International Consultation on kidney cancer 2010: treatment of metastatic disease. Eur Urol, 60:684-690

Patnaik A, Ricart A, Cooper J et al. (2007).A phase I, pharmacokinetic and pharmacodynamics study of sorafenib (S), a multi-targeted kinase inhibitor in combination with temsirolimus (T), an mTOR inhibitor in patients with advanced solid malignancies (abstract). J Clin Oncol, 28:2131-6

Pereira Arias JG, Ullate Jaime V, Valcárcel Martín F, Onaniel Pérez VJ, Gutiérrez Díez JM, Ateca Díaz-Obregón R & Berreteaga Gallastegui JR (2002). Epistaxis as initial manifestation of disseminated renal adenocarcinoma. Actas Urol Esp, 26(5):361-5.

Pfaffenroth EC, Linehan WM (2008). Genetic basis for kidney cancer: opportunity for disease-specific approaches to therapy. Expert Opin Biol Ther, 8:779-90

Pfannschmidt J, Hoffman H, Muley T, Krysa S, Trainer C, Dienemann H (2002). Prognostic factors or survival after pulmonary resection of metastatic renal cell carcinoma. Ann Thorac Surg,74:1653-7

Picchio M, Mascetti C, Tanga I, Spaziani E (2010). Metastasis from renal cell carcinoma presenting as skeletal muscle mass: a case report. Acta Chir Belg,110(3):399-401.

Placed IG, Alvarez-Rodriguez R, Pombo-Otero J, VÃ¡zquez-BartolomÃ P, Hermida-Romero T & Pombo-Felipe F (2010). Metastatic renal cell carcinoma presenting as shoulder monoarthritis: diagnosis based on synovial fluid cytology and immunocytochemistry. Acta Cytol, 54(5):730-3.

Podsypanina K, Du YC, Jechlinger M, Beverly LJ, Hambardzumyan D, Varmus H (2008).Seeding and propagation of untransformed mouse mammary cells in the lung. Science, 321(5897):1841-1844.

Porta C, Paglino C, Imarisio I, Bonomi L (2007).Cytokine-based immunotherapy for advanced kidney cancer: past results and future perspectives in the era of molecularly targeted agents. ScientificWorldJournal, 9;7:837-49.

Pyrhönen S, Salminen E, Ruutu M, Lehtonen T, Nurmi M, Tammela T, Juusela H, Rintala E, Hietanen P, Kellokumpu-Lehtinen PL (1999). Prospective randomized trial of interferon alfa-2a plus vinblastine versus vinblastine alone in patients with advanced renal cell cancer. J Clin Oncol, 17(9):2859-67.

Rumpelt HJ, Störkel S, Moll R, Schärfe T, Thoenes W (1991).Bellini duct carcinoma: further evidence for this rare variant of renal cell carcinoma.Histopathology, 18(2):115-22.

Renehan AG, Tyson M, Egger M, Heller RF, Zwahlen M (2008). Body mass index and incidence of cancer: a systematic review and meta-analysis of prospective observational studies. Lancet,371:569-78

Renshaw AA, Corless CL (1995). Papillary renal cell carcinoma.Histology and immunohistochemistry.Am J Surg Pathol, 19(7):842-9.

Renshaw AA, Zhang H, Corless CL, Fletcher JA, Pins MR (1997).Solid variants of papillary (chromophil) renal cell carcinoma: clinicopathologic and genetic features. Am J Surg Pathol, 21(10):1203-9.

Rini BI, Halabi S, Rosenberg JE, Stadler WM, Vaena DA, Ou SS, Archer L, Atkins JN, Picus J, Czaykowski P Dutcher J, Small EJ. (2008). Bevacizumab plus interferon alfa compared with interferon alfa monotherapy in patients with metastatic renal cell carcinoma: CALGB 90206. J Clin Oncol, 26(33):5422-5428.

Rini BI, Halabi S, Rosenberg JE et al. (2010). Phase III trial of bevacizumab plus interferon a versus interferon a monotherapy in patients with metastatic renal cell carcinoma: final results of CALGB 90206. J Clin Oncol, 28(13): 2137–2143.

Rini BI, Cohen DP, Lu DR, et al. (2011). Hypertension as a biomarker of efficacy in patients with metastatic renal cell carcinoma treated with sunitinib. J Natl Cancer Inst, 103:763-73

Rini BI, Campbell SC, Escudier B (2009).Renal cell carcinoma. Lancet, 373:1119-32

Rini BI, Wilding G, Hudes G et al. (2009). Phase II study of axitinib in sorafenibrefractory metastatic renal cell carcinoma. J Clin Oncol 27(27), 4462–4468.

Rini BI, Escudier B, Tomczak P et al. (2011). Axitinib versus sorafenib as second-line therapy for metastatic renal cell carcinoma (mRCC): results of Phase III AXIS trial. ASCO Meeting Abstracts 29(Suppl. 15),4503.

Rixe O, Billemont B, Izzedine H (2007). Hypertension as a predictive factor of sunitinib activity. Ann Oncol, 18:1117

Rixe O, Bukowski RM, Michaelson MD et al. (2007). Axitinib treatment in patients with cytokine-refractory metastatic renal-cell cancer: a Phase II study. Lancet Oncol, 8(11): 975–984 .

Rodney AJ, Gombos DS, Fuller GN, Pagliaro LC & Tannir NM. (2009) Choroidal and conjunctival metastases from renal cell carcinoma.Am J Clin Oncol, 32(4):448-9.

Ruiz-Cerda JL, Jimenez Cruz F (2009) . (Surgical treatment for renal cancer metastases). Actas Urol Esp, 33(5):593-602.

Russo P (2010). Multi-modal treatment for metastatic renal cancer: the role of surgery. World J Urol, 28:295-301

Sabatini P, Ducic Y. (2009). Bilateral lacrimal gland masses: unusual case of metastatic renal cell carcinoma. J Otolaryngol Head Neck Surg, 38(1):E1-2.

Sablin MP, Negrier S, Ravaud A et al. (2009). Sequential sorafenib and sunitinib for renal cell carcinoma. J Urol, 182(1): 29–34 .

Sarbassov D, Ali S, Sabatini D (2005). Growing roles for the mTOR pathway. Curr Opin Biol, 17:596-603

Satake N, Ohno Y, Yoshioka K, Sakamoto N, Takeuchi H, Tachibana M (2009). Case of renal cell carcinoma metastasized to iliopsoas muscle. Nippon Hinyokika Gakkai Zasshi, 100(3):495-499.

Schmorl P, Ostertag H, Conrad S (2008). Intratesticular metastasis of renal cancer. Urologe A ,47(8):1001-1003.

Schraml P, Muller D, Bednar R, et al. (2000). Allelic loss at the D9S171 locus on chromosome **9p13 is associated with** progression of papillary renal cell carcinoma. J Pathol, 190:457–461.

Seijas BP, Franco FL, Sastre RM, García AA,  López-Cedrún Cembranos JL (2005). Metastatic renal cell carcinoma presenting as a parotid tumor. Oral Surg Oral Med Oral Pathol Oral Radiol Endod,  99(5):554-557.

Sheth S, Scatarige J, Horton K, Corl F,  Fishman E  (2001). Current Concepts in the Diagnosis and Management of Renal Cell Carcinoma: Role of Multidetector CT and Three-dimensional CT.  RadioGraphics, 21: S237–S254

Shoaib KK, Haq IU, Ali K, Mukhtar MA & Nazir M. (2008).Choroidal metastasis from renal cell carcinoma presenting with cataract. J Coll Physicians Surg Pak, 18(6):380-1.

Shome D, Honavar SG, Gupta P, Vemuganti GK, Reddy PV. (2007). Metastasis to the eye and orbit from renal cell carcinoma--a report of three cases and review of literature. Surv Ophthalmol, 52(2):213-23.

Singer EA, Gupta GN, Srinivasan R. (2012). Targeted therapeutic strategies for the management of renal cell carcinoma. Curr Opin Oncol, 24(3):284-90.

Spreafico R, Nicoletti G, Ferrario F, Scanziani R, Grasso M (2008). Parotid metastasis from renal cell carcinoma: a case report and review of the literature. ACTA Otorhinolaryngologica Italica, 28(5):266-268.

Srigley JR, Eble JN (1998). Collecting duct carcinoma of kidney.Semin Diagn Pathol, 15(1):54-67.

Srinivasan N, Pakala A, Al-Kali A, Rathi S, Ahmad W. (2010). Papillary renal cell carcinoma with cutaneous metastases. Am J Med Sci, 339(5):458-61.

Sosman J, Puzanov I (2009). Combination targeted therapy in advanced renal cell carcinoma. Cancer, 115:2368-75

Sountoulides P, Metaxa L, Cindolo L. (2011) Atypical presentations and rare metastatic sites of renal cell carcinoma: a review of case reports. J Med Case Rep, 2;5:429.

Sonpavde G, Hutson TE (2007). Pazopanib: a novel multitargeted tyrosine kinase inhibitor. Curr Oncol Rep, 9(2), 115–119.

Stanczyk R, Omulecka A & Pajor A. (2006) . (A case of renal clear cell carcinoma metastasis to the oropharynx). Otolaryngol Pol, 60(1):97-100.

Staehler M, Haseke N, Zilinberg E, Stadler T, Karl A, Siebels M, Dürr HR, Siegert S, Jauch KW, Bruns CJ, Stief CG (2010). Complete remission achieved with angiogenic therapy in metastatic renal cell carcinoma including surgical intervention. Urol Oncol, 28(2):139-44.

Stein MN, Flaherty KT (2007). CCR drug updates: sorafenib and sunitinib in renal cell carcinoma. Clin Cancer Res, 13(13):3765-3770.

Sternberg CN, Davis ID, Mardiak J, Szczylik C, Lee E, Wagstaff J, Barrios CH, Salman P, Gladkov OA, Kavina A, Zarbá JJ, Chen M, McCann L, Pandite L, Roychowdhury DF, Hawkins RE (2010). Pazopanib in locally advanced or metastatic renal cell carcinoma: results of a randomized phase III trial. J Clin Oncol, 28(6):1061-8.

Stolle C, Glenn G, Zbar B, Humphrey JS, Choyke P, Walther M, Pack S, Hurley K, Andrey C, Klausner R, Linehan WM (1998).Improved detection of germline mutations in the von Hippel-Lindau disease tumor suppressor gene.Hum Mutat, 12(6):417-23.

Stolnicu S, Borda A, Radulescu D, Puscasiu L, Berger N, Nogales FF (2007). Metastasis from papillary renal cell carcinoma masquerading as primary ovarian clear cell tumor. Pathol Res Pract, 203(11):819-822.

Talukdera MQ, Deoa SV, Maleszewskib JJ, Parka SJ & Talukder MQ (2010).Late isolated metastasis of renal cell carcinoma in the left 5 ventricular myocardium.Interact Cardiovasc Thorac Surg, 11(6):814-816.

Terada T. (2012). Cutaneous metastasis of renal cell carcinoma: a report of two cases. Int J Clin Exp Pathol,  5(2):175-8.

Terrone C, Cracco C, Porpiglia F, et al. (2006). Reassessing the current TNM lymph node staging for renal cell carcinoma. Eur Urol 49: 324–331

Testini M, Lissidini G, Gurrado A, Lastilla G, Ianora AS, Fiorella R (2008). Acute airway failure secondary to thyroid metastasis from renal carcinoma. World J Surg Oncol, 6:14.

Tokuyama Y, Iwamura M, Fujita T, Sugita A, Maeyama R, Bessho H, Ishikawa W, Tabata K, Yoshida K, Baba S. (2011). Myocardial metastasis from renal cell carcinoma treated with sorafenib. Hinyokika Kiyo, 57(10):555-8.

Toquero L, Aboumarzouk MO, Abbasi Z (2009). Renal cell carcinoma metastasis to the ovary: a case report. Cases J, 14(2):7472.

Torres-Carranza E, Garcia-Perla A, Infante-Cossio P, Belmonte-Caro R, Loizaga-Iriondo JM & Gutierrez-Perez JL. (2006). Airway obstruction due to metastatic renal cell carcinoma to the tongue. Oral Surg Oral Med Oral Pathol Oral Radiol Endod, 101(3):e76-78.

Tripathi RT, Heilbrun LK, Jain V, Vaishampayan UN (2006). Racial disparity in outcomes of a clinical trial population with metastatic renal cell carcinoma. Urology, 68:296–301

Trumm CG, Rubenbauer B, Piltz S, Reiser MF, Hoffmann RT  (2011). Screw placement and osteoplasty under computed tomographic-fluoroscopic guidance in a case of advanced metastatic destruction of the iliosacral joint. Cardiovasc Intervent Radiol, 34 Suppl 2:S288-93.

Türkvatan A, Akdur PO, Altinel M, Olçer T, Turhan N, Cumhur T, Akinci S, Ozkul F. (2009). Preoperative staging of renal cell carcinoma with multidetector CT. Diagn Interv Radiol, 15(1):22-30.

van Rooijen E, Voest EE, Logister I, et al. (2010). von Hippel-Lindau tumor suppressor mutants faithfully model pathological hypoxia-driven angiogenesis and vascular retinopathies in zebrafish. Dis Model Mech, 3:343-53

Uemura H, Shinohara N, Yuasa T, et al. (2010). A phase II study of sunitinib in Japanese patients with metastatic renal cell carcinoma: insights into the treatment, efficacy and safety. Jpn J Clin Oncol, 40:194-202

Udoji E, Herts BR (2012). Renal cell carcinoma metastatic to the ovary. J Urol,188(2):603-4.

Ulbright TM,Young RH. (2008). Metastatic carcinoma to the testis: a clinicopathologic analysis of 26 nonincidental cases with emphasis on deceptive features. Am J Surg Pathol, 32(11):1683-1693.

Volkmer BG, Gschwend JE (2002). (Value of metastases surgery in metastatic renal cell carcinoma). Urologe A, 41(3):225-230.

Vozmediano-Serrano MT, Toledano-Fernández N, Fdez-Aceñero MJ, Gil-Díez JL & García-Saenz S. (2006). Lacrimal sac metastases from renal cell carcinoma. Orbit, 25(3):249-51.

Wadasadawala T, Kumar P, Agarwal J & Ghosh-Laskar S (2011).Palliation of dysphagia with radiotherapy for exophytic base tongue metastases in a case of renal cell carcinoma. Indian J Urol, 27(4):550-2.

Wang X, MacLennan GT, Zhang S, Montironi R, Lopez-Beltran A, Tan PH, Foster S, Baldridge LA, Cheng L (2009). Sarcomatoid carcinoma of the upper urinary tract: clinical outcome and molecular characterization. Hum Pathol, 40(2):211-7.

Wagstaff J(2006). New horizons in the treatment of renal cell cancer. Ann Oncol Suppl, 17 Suppl 10:x19-22.

Washington K,  McDonagh D. (1995). Secondary tumors of the gastrointestinal tract: surgical pathologic findings and comparison with autopsy survey. Mod Pathol, 8: 427-433.

Weikert S, Boeing H, Pischon T et al. (2008).Blood pressure and risk of renal cell carcinoma in the European prospective investigation into cancer and nutrition. Am J Epidemiol, 167: 438-46

Wood SL, Brown JE (2012). Skeletal metastasis in renal cell carcinoma: current and future management options. Cancer Treat Rev, 38(4):284-91.

Wright I, Kapoor A (2011).Current systemic management of metastatic renal cell carcinoma - first line and second line therapy. Curr Opin Support Palliat Care, 5(3):211-21.

Wu HY, Xu LW, Zhang YY, Yu YL, Li XD, Li GH. (2010). Metachronous contralateral testicular and bilateral adrenal metastasis of chromophobe renal cell carcinoma: a case report and review of the literature. J Zhejiang Univ Sci B, 11(5):386-389.

Yang G, Breyer BN, Weiss DA, MacLennan GT (2010).Mucinous tubular and spindle cell carcinoma of the kidney. J Urol, 183:738-9

Yang JC, Sherry RM, Steinberg SM, Topalian SL, Schwartzentruber DJ, Hwu P, Seipp CA, Rogers-Freezer L, Morton KE, White DE, Liewehr DJ, Merino MJ, Rosenberg SA (2003). Randomized study of high-dose and low-dose interleukin-2 in patients with metastatic renal cancer. J Clin Oncol, 21(16):3127-32.

Yoshitomi I, Kawasaki G, Mizuno A, Nishikido M, Hayashi T, Fujita S, Ikeda T. (2011). Lingual metastasis as an initial presentation of renal cell carcinoma. Med Oncol, 28(4):1389-94.

Zustovich F, Gottardo F, De Zorzi L, Cecchetto A, Dal Bianco M, Mauro En, Cartei G (2008). Cardiac metastasis from renal cell carcinoma without inferior vena involvement: a review of the literature based on a case report. Two different patterns of spread. Clin Oncol, 13(3):271-274.

# Primary Placement Technique, Usefulness, and Complications of Jejunostomy

Yasushi Rino

*Departments of Surgery*
*Yokohama City University, Japan*

# 1   Introduction

Enteral feeding via insertion of a percutaneous endoscopic gastrostomy (PEG) tube is standard procedure in many institutions and is the recommended procedure for long-term maintenance of good nutrition in patients with disorders that involve severe dysphagia and generalized weakness or immobility. Esophagectomy or total gastrectomy results in reduction of food intake, leading to malnourishment and weight loss (Derogar *et al.*, 2012; Saeki *et al.*, 2008). It is therefore important that enteral feeding is established at an early stage, in order to minimize further malnutrition, and jejunostomy is now regarded as the standard treatment. Jejunostomy is performed in patients undergoing esophagectomy to improve their nutrition status in many institutes, and if complications, including leakage and stenosis of anastomosis, recurrent nerve palsy, pneumonia etc, occur after esophagectomy, the patient cannot take anything by mouth over the long-term. In such cases, jejunostomy tube placement is performed in order to improve their nutrition status and quality of life (QOL).

Rino *et al.* (2011) developed the skin-level jejunostomy tube (SLJT) placement to improve nutrition in patients undergoing esophagectomy since March 2008.They selected the Entristar™ skin-level gastrostomy tube (G-tube) for jejunostomy due to their familiarity with its use in gastrostomy. The G-tube is a short 20 Fr diameter tube with internal and external retention bolsters to secure its position and minimize movement. The feeding and/or decompression ports are fitted with an antireflux valve that may be closed with a cap when it is not in use. As with all skin-level devices, the Entristar™ device is normally inserted as a replacement tube, when a mature tract has already been established during a previous percutaneous endoscopic gastrostomy (PEG) procedure. The technique is simpler than the standard jejunostomy. The rapidity with which it can be introduced, and the multiple benefits derived from its use, suggested its adoption for simple, as well as complicated, surgical problems.

In Japan, G-tube for gastrostomy is recognized in the insurance. But we have no problem in the insurance until October, 2012. The enteral route is considered more physiologic – the liver is not bypassed and the hepatic ability to take up, process, and store the various nutrients for subsequent release upon nervous or hormonal command, is maintained. It is often said that enteral nutrition is more safe and efficacious than the parenteral route (Sabiston Jr. *et al.*, 1997). The use of a jejunostomy tube was first described in 1891 by Witzel (Witzel., 1891). Liffman and Randall reported the jejunostomy placement of a small plastic catheter with a Witzel tunnel (Liffman & Randall, 1972). However, previous jejunostomy methods (Witzel., 1891; Kader.,1896 ; Stamm., 1894; Delany *et al.*, 1973)have utilized a long catheter out of the abdominal wall, which can be inconvenient in daily life. Some authors have reported methods of jejunostomy (Witzel., 1891; Kader., 1896 ; Stamm., 1894; Delany *et al.*, 1973). SLJT utilized the G-tube. Due to the technical steps required for the creation of a standard jejunostomy, most surgeons resist using this procedure as a routine adjunctive measure (Delany *et al.*, 1973). However, SLJT procedure requires less than five minutes for completion. It adds very little time or trauma to the surgical procedure, and intestinal manipulation is not required.

# 2   SLJT procedure

## 2.1   Jejunostomy techniques of using G-tube (20Fr)

A G-tube (20Fr) (Entristar; Tyco Healthcare, Mansfield, Mass) is used for the SLJT. The G-tube consisted of external and internal retention bolisters (Figure 1A, 1B, 1C and 1D).

During the procedure, the patient is placed in a supine position. The jejunostomy is performed during the abdominal procedure at the end of the esophageal cancer or gastric cancer operation. Nishi *et al.* reported jejunostomy placement from the Treitz ligament to about 20cm on the anal side (Nishi *et al.*, 1988). The G-tube is also inserted at the jejunostomy 20 cm from the Treitz ligament on the side opposing the jejunalmesenterium. A single purse string jejunostomy stitch is made using a 4-0 absorbable suture (Figure 1E). The stitch length is about 10mm and four stitches are performed in a square shape around the jejunostomy site.

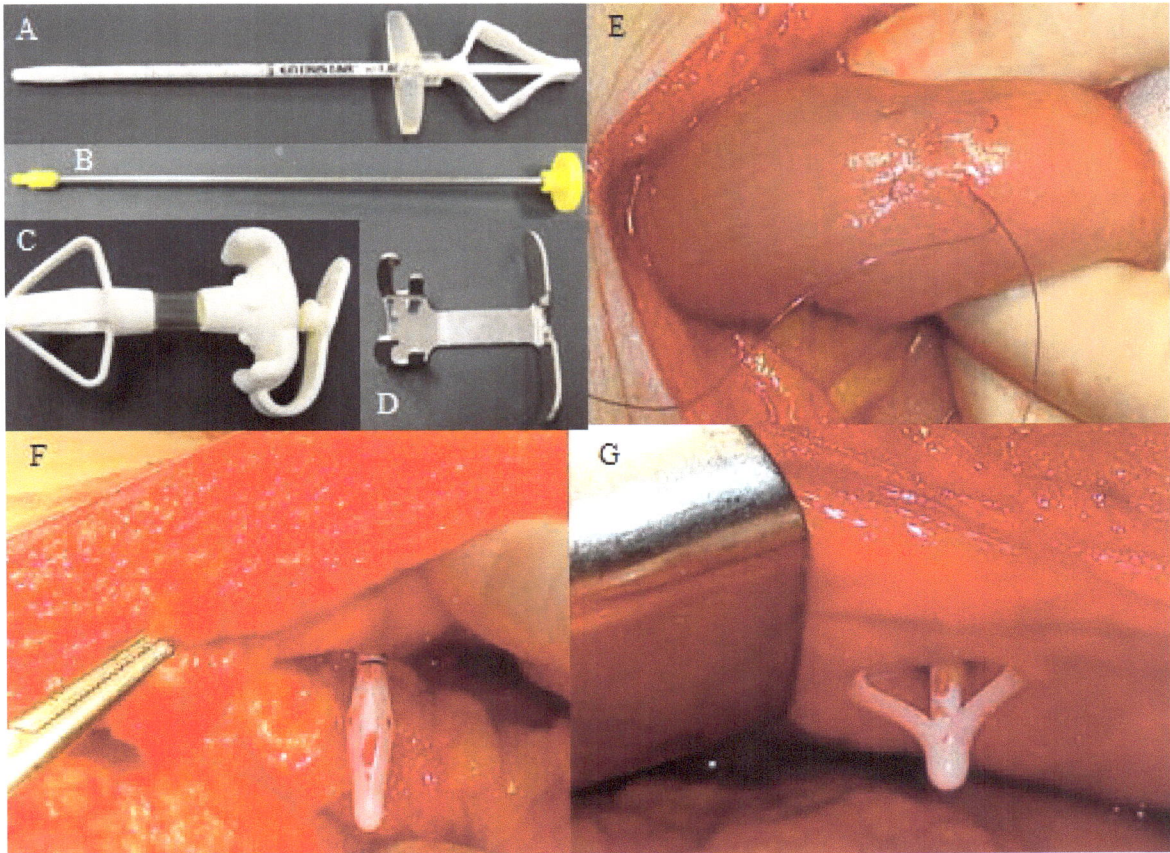

**Figure 1:** Skin-level gastrostomy tube (Entristar; Tyco Healthcare, Mansfield, Mass). **(A)** The Measuring device. **(B)** The Obturator. **(C)** Gastrostomytube comprised of external and internal retention bolisters. **(D)** The Gripstar.Jejunostomy technique: **(E)** A purse string suture of the jejunostomy tube using a 4-0 absorbable suture. **(F)** Insert the Stoma Measuring Device through the abdominal wall into the abdominal cavity. **(G)** Measure the abdominal wall thickness.

A skin incision, about 8mm in length, is made at the left upper quarter of the abdomen. Forceps are then used to pierce the abdominal wall and the Stoma Measuring Device is inserted through the abdominal wall into the abdominal cavity (Figure 1F). Based on the measurements obtained, a G-tube length is selected that allows for forward and backward-movement of the Entristar™ device (Figure 1G).

This could help reduce complications as a consequence of continual or excessive pressure to either the jejunal mucosa or the skin.

The surgeons open the G-tube tethered cap, load the GripStar Insertion/Removal Device by sliding the lower curved prongs of the GripStar device beneath the external retention portion of the G-Tube, and use the finger grips on the GripStar Device for retention during obturation and insertion (Figure 2A).

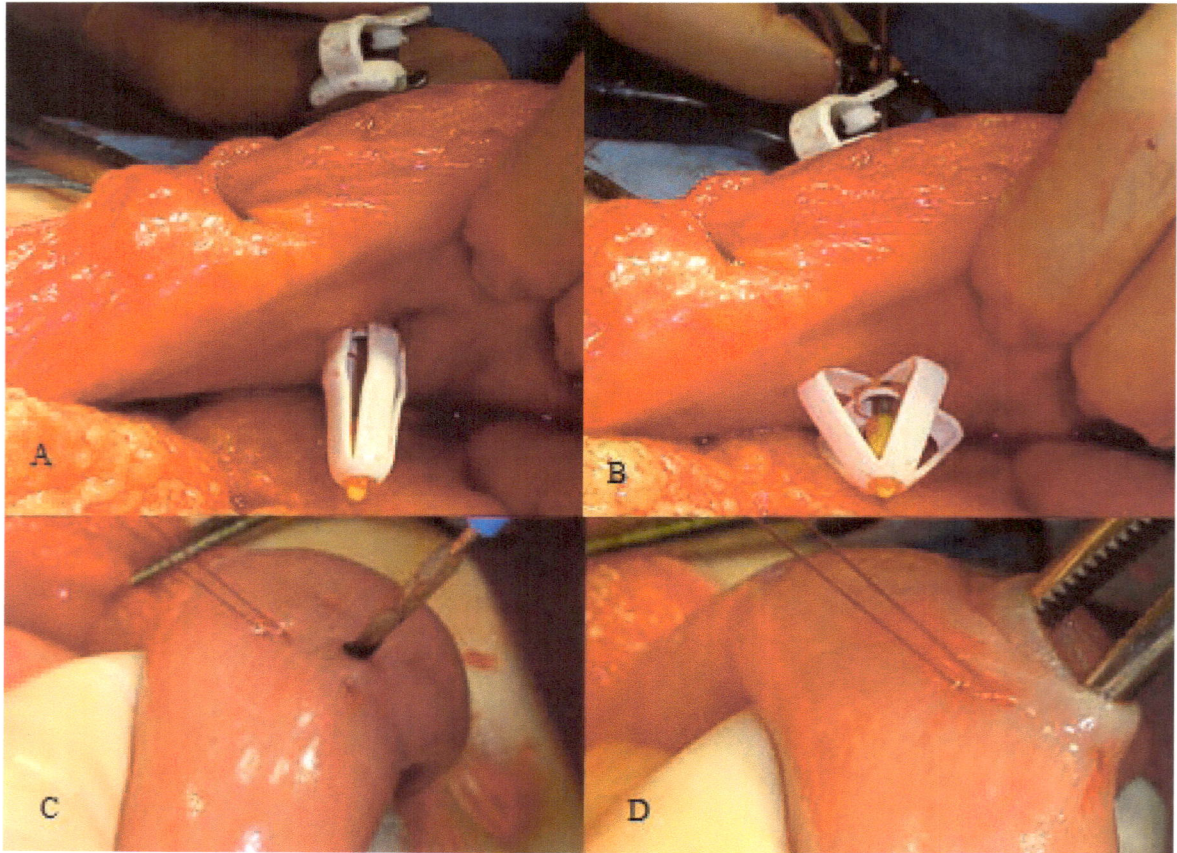

**Figure 2:** Jejunostomytechnique. **(A)** Use the finger grips on the GripStar Device for retention during obturation and insertion. **(B)** Insert the obturated G-Tube into the stoma tract until the internal retention portion can be seen perfectly in the abdominal cavity. **(C)** The center of the purse string suture of the jejunum is cut using an electronic knife. **(D)** Pierce using forceps.

The obturator is inserted into the G-tube without lubricating jelly. The surgeons obturate until moderate resistance is felt to reduce the diameter of the internal retention bolster. The obturated G-Tube is then inserted into the stoma tract until the internal retention portion can be seen perfectly in the abdominal cavity (Figure 2B). If excessive resistance is encountered during insertion, the procedure is stopped and the tract is dilated.

The center of the purse string suture of the jejunum is cut using an electronic knife (Figure 2C) and pierced using forceps (Figure 2D). The surgeons reduce the diameter of the internal retention bolster using the obturator and insert the internal retention bolster into the jejunal lumen via the small incision (Figure 3A). A purse string suture is tied tightly to the tube (Figure 3B). The intestine adjacent to tube is anchored to the peritoneum by a single stitch (Figure 3C).

Proper placement of the G-Tube (Figure 3D) should be confirmed through the injection of 20ml of air. Feedings should commence only after proper placement and patency have been confirmed.

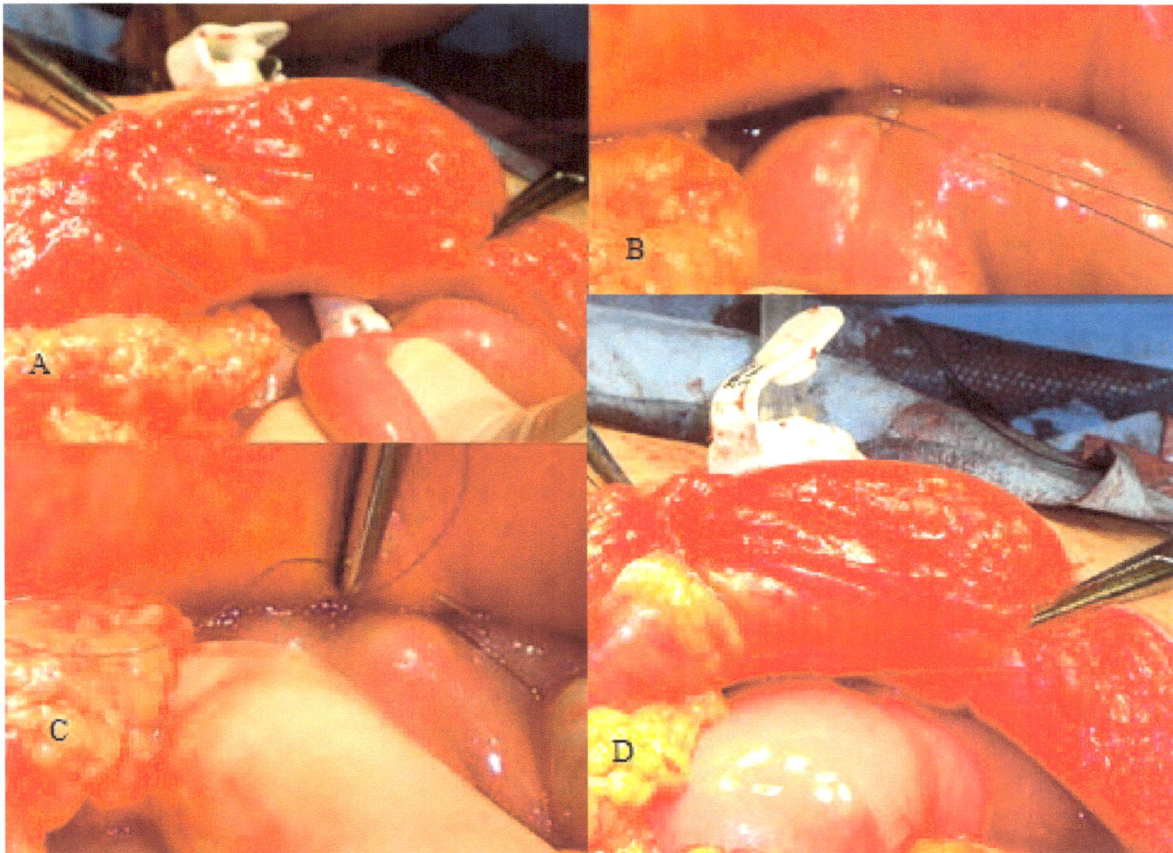

**Figure 3:** Jejunostomy technique. **(A)** Use obturator and insert the internal retention bolster into the jejunal lumen through the small incision. **(B)** Purse string suture thread is tied tightly to the tube. **(C)** The intestine adjacent to the tube is anchored to the peritoneum. **(D)** Proper placement of the G-Tube after operation.

A step-up spacer is placed beneath the external portion of the G-Tube. The entire procedure requires less than five minutes to perform, and it adds very little time or trauma to the overall surgical procedure nor does it require significant intestinal manipulation.

## 2.2   How to use SLJT

100ml liquefied standard diets and 50ml air is administered through the SLJT to confirm that there is no leakage or obstruction on the first day after the operation. Liquefied standard diets can be subsequently administered via the SLJT. The starting dose of the liquefied standard diet is 20 ml/hr and is increased in 10 ml/hr daily increments to a maximum dose of 60ml/hr.

## 2.3    Patient Follow-up and Complications

Complications were characterized and were recorded as early (those occurring < 24 hours after the procedure) or late (those occurring ≥ 24 hours after the procedure). Those complications arising after the procedure were further defined as minor (abdominal pain, wound infection, fever, peristomal leakage, dislocation, tract disruption, and catheter dislocation or fracture) or major (hemorrhage requiring blood transfusion, pneumoperitoneum, peritonitis, aspiration, and any complication of the tube insertion requiring radiologic intervention or surgery). Patient follow-up was assessed monthly, by the surgeons in all cases, to document subsequent complications. The occurrence of death was recorded and assessed to determine whether it had any relationship with the jejunostomy procedure.

The patients were followed up until removal of the G-tube for 19 – 906 days (median: 106 days) after tube insertion. The duration of administration of the liquefied diet was 7 – 905 days (median, 69 days) after tube insertion. In five out of 41 SLJT cases, the tubes were not removed. SLJT placement was performed successfully in all 41 patients. There were no procedural failures as a consequence of the tube insertion technique; all tubes were correctly positioned. Of the 41 patients, 20 (48.8%) used home enteral nutrition support through SLJT.

There were no early complications; i.e., no obstruction of the jejunal lumen and no tube failure as a result of tube fracture, displacement, or dislodgement. There were complications, including peristomal leakage, dermatitis, and ulceration, when the SLJT was used for more than three months. There were 6 cases of peristomal leakage (14.6%), 1 case of dermatitis and 1 case of peristomal ulceration as late complications in 6 patients. There are 4cases of peristomal granuloma (9.8%). No tube-related death or long-term major morbidity occurred as a consequence of the SLJT procedure.

This is the first study of jejunostomy using G-tube for esophageal cancer. There are no reports to compare with this study. Exchange of the G-tube under radiologic guidance was effective in patients with peristomal leakage. As a rule, the G-tube is generally removed after confirming the amount of postoperative oral meal intake and is performed postoperative removal of the G-tube one month later. Bleeding was observed after removal in some cases. However, the bleeding usually ceased within a short time. The fistula was generally closed within one or two days. But the tract was closed at about 3weeks after removal of the G-tube in only one case of 36 removed cases (2.8%).

## 3    Conclusion

This SLJ placement technique using the G-tube is a safe procedure in patients with EC that allows the creation of a long-term feeding jejunostomy.

## Reference

Delany HM, Carnevale NJ, Garvay JW. Jejunostomy by a needle catheter technique. Surgery, 1973, 73:786-790.

Derogar M, Orsini N, Sadr-Azodi O, Lagergren P: Influence of major postoperative complications on health-related quality of life among long-term survivors of esophageal cancer surgery. J Clin Oncol. 2012 May 10;30(14):1615-9.

Kader B. Zur Technik der Gastrostomie. Centralbl Chir, 1896, 23:-665-670.

Liffman KE, Randall HR. A modified technique for creating a jejunostomy.SurgGynecolObstet, 1972, 134: 663-664.

Nishi M, Kanemaki T, Imamura A, Hiramatsu Y, Hioki K, Yamamoto M. Postoperative enteral nutritional support by needle catheter feeding jejunostomy after esophagectomy and total gastrectomy. J JpnSurgAssoc, 1988, 49, 2237-2241.

Rino Y, Yukawa N, Murakami H, Sato T, Takata K, Hayashi T, Oshima T, Wada N, Masuda M, Imada T. Primary placement technique of jejunostomy using the entristarTM skin-level gastrectomy tube in patients with esophageal cancer. BMC Gastroenterol.2011 Jan 31;11:8.

Sabiston Jr., DC, Lyerly, HK. Textbook of Surgery.The biological basis of modern surgical practice. 15th ed. Philadelphia: W.B. Saunders Company, 1997: 147-148.

Saeki H, Rino Y, Cho H, Sato T, Kawamoto M, Takanashi Y, Yamada R, Oshima T, Hatori S, Imada T.: Evaluation of calorie intake according to age and sex in patients undergoing surgery for gastric cancer.Hepatogastroenterology. 55(82-83):795-8,2008.

Stamm M. Gastrostomy by a new method. Medical News, 1894, 65:324-326.

Witzel, O. ZurTechnik der Magenfistelanlegung. CentralblChir, 1891, 18: 601-604.

# Polyethylene Glycol: Re-establishing Gut-Barrier Function

Shruthi S Bharadwaj
*Biomedical Engineering*
*University of Florida, USA*

Sarah C Glover
*Department of Medicine*
*University of Florida, USA*

# 1    Introduction

Colon cancer remains one of the leading causes of mortality worldwide. A total of 1,638,910 new cancer cases and 577,190 deaths from cancer are projected to occur in the United States this year (Siegel *et al.*, 2012). Colon Cancers are unique since they arise in a microenvironment surrounded by bacteria. Under normal physiological circumstances, the skin, mouth, ileum, and colon encounter large numbers of bacteria. The colon, specifically, is continuously bathed in $10^{11}$ to $10^{12}$ cfu/ml of different kinds of both commensal as well as pathogenic bacteria(Gibson & Roberfroid, 1995). The relationship between some species of these bacteria and the epithelial cells lining the colon is symbiotic. This symbiotic relationship between the colonic cells and the surrounding bacteria is normally maintained by five major walls: the mucus layer atop the epithelial cells (Florey, 1955; Sheng *et al.*, 2012), the epithelia cells, a layer of sub-epithelial macrophages, dendritic cells, and lymph nodes as shown in Figure 1 (Macpherson *et al.*, 2009). This wall formed by layers of protective cells is what is known as gut barrier function. However, in the setting of diseases which lead to a loss of the protective mucosal layer such as inflammatory bowel disease or colon cancer, these commensal bacteria gain the ability to alter both the behavior of epithelial cells as well as the their surrounding extra cellular matrix (ECM) (Marteau & Chaput, 2011). Recent studies indicate that the invasion of bacteria though the barrier-function may in fact alter the surrounding ECM, especially tissue topography. There is also evidence that altered tissue topography may in fact induce abnormal cell behavior. This chapter focuses on PEGs role as a surrogate mucin in decreasing the pro-invasive effects of colon cancer cells as well as its role in re-establishing gut barrier function. Another goal of this chapter is to introduce PEG as a potential therapeutic agent in maintaining gut-barrier function.

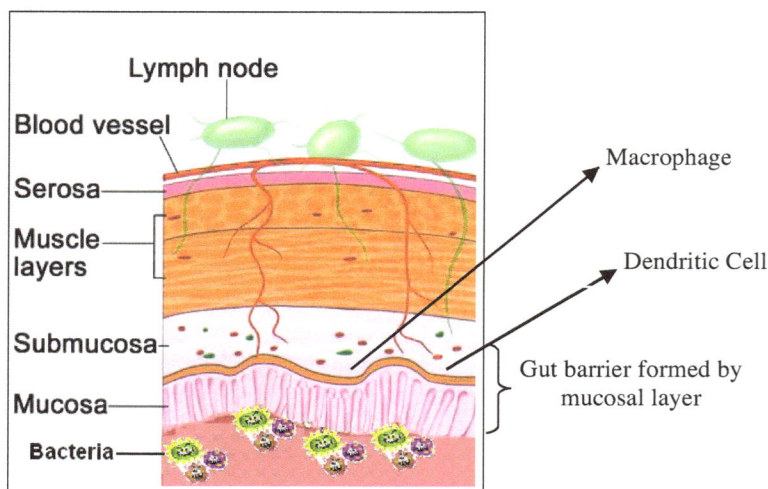

**Figure 1:** Schematic representation of the colonic intestinal wall with emphasis on the mucosal layer that forms the gut barrier function.

## 1.1    Commensal Bacteria

Colonic bacteria have both a positive and negative role in maintaining gut physiology. Bacteria, through the process of fermentation, produce several different compounds that affect the stability of colon. For example, colonic bacteria as shown in Figure 2 produce short-chain fatty acids from the metabolism of complex carbohydrates and proteins (Cummings, 1998; Cummings & Macfarlane, 1991; de Roos & Katan, 2000). Colonic bacteria, especially the pathogenic *E. Coli* has been known to cause diarrhea and several other digestive tract disorders (de Roos & Katan, 2000).

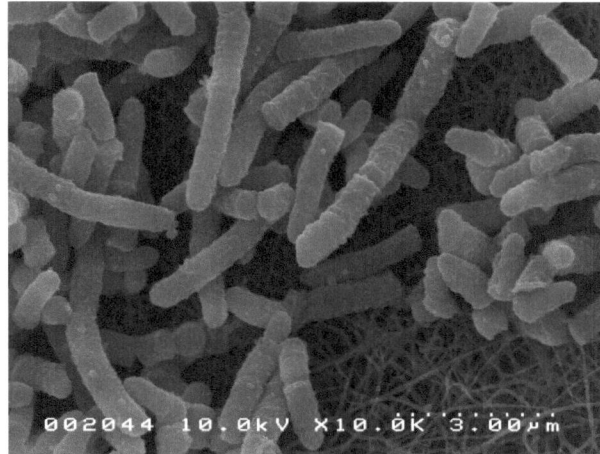

**Figure 2:** Commensal *E. coli* strain, 259, on collagen type I matrix. Scale bar = 3μm

The effect of bacterial strains on the onset of colon cancer is not clearly known. Several studies indicate that the presence of bacteria within the gut may influence cellular behavior and activate certain pathways that trigger carcinogenesis (de Roos & Katan, 2000). Although, the direct effect of a particular bacterial strain on cellular behavior is beyond the scope of this chapter, the effect that the bacteria have on the surrounding ECM will be emphasized in this chapter.

## 1.2  Commensal Bacteria Alter Topography

Bacteria differ from eukaryotic cells in several aspects. They have a cell wall, in addition to the phospholipid cell membrane found in eukaryotic cells, composed of peptidoglycans. Bacteria vary greatly in size, shape, and surface structures. They can be 1μm to several tens of microns, be spherical, rod-shaped, or twisted, and poses flagella, pili, or cilia, depending on the species and strain. However, in this chapter, we will focus primarily on commensal bacterial strains and one pathogenic *E. coli* strain. Both commensal bacterial strain and pathogenic *E. coli* strain discussed in this chapter are rod like bacteria that are similar in shape and size, approximately, 3 μm in length. These bacteria posses the ability to act independently of each other as a single cell organism, or form communities or colonies with a species and strain-specific extracellular polymeric substances called biofilms. These structural features of bacteria act through surface receptors, focal adhesions and either direct or indirect mechano-transduction pathways as well as alter the surrounding topography. Recent evidence suggests that commensal bacterial strains degrade and invade through collagen matrices as shown in Figure 3. Figure 3 shows commensal bacterial strain, 260, invading through a collagen type I matrix. Since, colonic tissue *in-vivo* primarily consists of type I collagen, it is evident that bacterial strains *in-vivo* invade through the colonic ECM. Although, further *in-vivo* studies are required to fully understand bacterial influencewithin the colon, this chapter introduces some of the major concerns associated with bacterial infection and the causal ECM degradation.

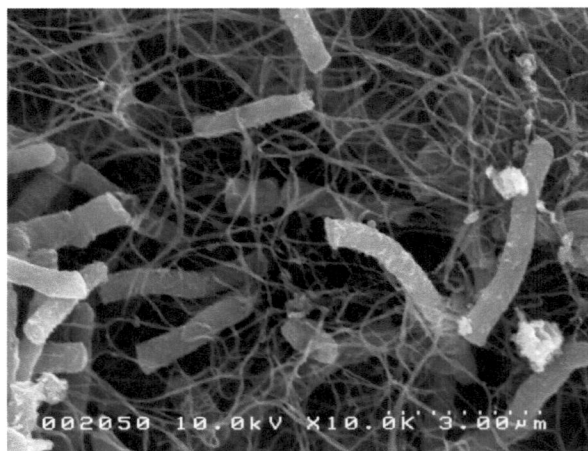

**Figure 3:** Scanning Electron Microscopy image of Commensal Bacterial strain, 260. Rod shaped commensal bacterial strain invades through the collagen type I matrix. Scale bar = 3 μm.

## 1.3    Topography Alters Cell Behavior

Several different mechanical cues play an important role in determining cell fate. It has been shown in literature that differentiation of stem cells in to endothelial lineage could be accomplished by inducing shear stress (Yamamoto *et al.*, 2005). Several studies have been conducted to measure the effect of topography on cellular function such as proliferation, differentiation and apoptosis supporting the hypothesis that mechanical features do influence cell fate (Figure 4). Another study states altering the dimensions of nanotubular-shaped titanium oxide surface structures independently allow either augmented human mesenchymal stem cell (hMSC) adhesion or a specific differentiation of hMSCs into osteoblasts by using only the geometric cues, absent of osteogenic inducing media (Oh *et al.*, 2009). Certain *in-vivo* studies conducted show the significance of tissue specific surface topography in determining the differentiation lineage of stem cells. Similarly, colon tissue *in-vivo* has distinct topographical features that influence the cellular function.

Since basement membranes of various tissues including the colon are composed of complex mixtures of nanoscale topography (5 – 200 nm) such as pits, pores, protrusions, striations, particulates, and fibers, nanotopography may be more significant in affecting cell behavior than the larger scale microtopography of underlining tissues (Lim & Donahue, 2007). In general, cell interaction with a nanotopographical surface is very much the same as interaction at any other scale; however, on a nanometer scale discrete attachment sites between the colonic tissue surface and the cell exist (Anselme, 2000). Although several different biological molecules are responsible for these discrete cell-to-surface attachments, the most common are integrins. Once the integrins attach to a surface, integrin receptors cluster togetherand recruit cytoplasmic proteins to form focal adhesions. The specific type of integrins recruited delegates on the structure and function of each focal adhesion and is dependent onthe environment outside the cell as well as the motifs programmed into the protein structure, the most common being the RGD peptide (Arginylglycylaspartic acid) motif. Although the majority of focal adhesions appear to be at a micrometer scale ranging from 1μm to 5 μm, integrins themselves are nanometer building blocks, about 8-12nm each, that arrange and rearrange together to form complete structures (Anselme *et al.*, 2010). In addition, surface chemistry on a nanometer scale plays a role in deciding which type of integrins are recruited and

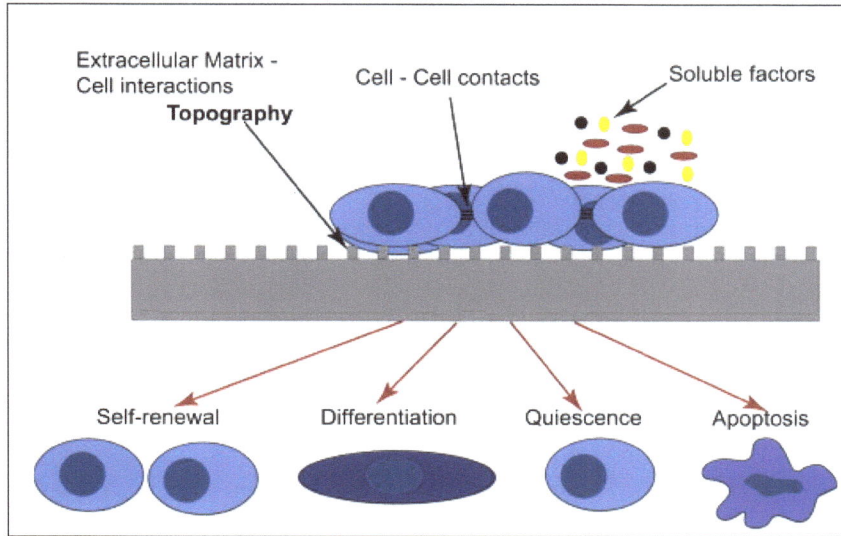

**Figure 4:** Schematic representing mechano-transduction. The figure represents cells exposed to three main factors that have been shown to influence cellular behavior (1) micron scaled topography (2) soluble factors and (3) cell-cell contact.

in turn also affects the function of the focal adhesion. For instance, self-assembled monolayers (SAMs) have been shown to increase $\alpha_5\beta_1$ integrin binding to fibronectin (FN) (Keselowsky *et al.*, 2003). Differences in FN structure have also been shown to alter integrin receptor binding, resulting in selective binding of $\alpha_5\beta_1$ on the COOH surface and poor binding of either integrin on the $CH_3$ SAM (Keselowsky *et al.* 2003; 2004). Upon adsorption to these surfaces, FN undergoes changes in structure, including alterations in the central cell-binding domain thus modulating functional activity and integrin binding. Focal adhesions are linked to the nucleus directly through cytoskeletal structures or indirectly through signal transduction pathways. These focal adhesions can have an influence on gene expression and thus alter cellular behavior.

Thus far, few studies have concentrated on the interaction between bacteria and nanotopographical surface features. Although one study has shown evidence that nanotopography plays a role in altering bacterial behavior through similar though far less known mechanisms as in eukaryotic cells, i.e. focal adhesions, mechano-receptors, and surface features such as flagella (Anselme *et al.*, 2010), less is known about how bacteria itself alters the nanotopography of the surface and by which mechanism it does so. Understanding the behavior of bacteria on nanostructured surfaces is essential for the design of surfaces that enhance or inhibit bacterial colonization and may potentially serve as a therapeutic measure for several disease conditions. However, it is just as important to study how bacteria alter the nanotopography of their surrounding environment primarily because these changes would also affect the behavior of the epithelial cells present there.

## 1.4    Polyethylene Glycol – What is it?

Polyethylene glycol (PEG) is used clinically to treat chronic constipation and to prep patients for colonoscopy examination and various other colon imaging procedures (Pampati & Fogel, 2004; Tran *et al.*,

2005). PEG has been used as drug delivery agent to successfully deliver chemotherapy in an *in-vitro* murine model of colon cancer (Chow *et al.*, 2009). Recently, it has been noted that PEG has profound chemo-preventive properties in both experimental models of colon carcinogenesis (Corpet & Parnaud, 1999) and in human population studies (Dorval, *et al.*). PEG's ability to act as a chemo-preventive agent is most likely due to its ability to induce apoptosis in damaged cells (Corpet & Parnaud, 1999; Corpet *et al.*, 2000; Roy, *et al.*, 2004). Furthermore, PEG has also been shown to reinforce epithelial barrier function in the colon in experimental models of colitis (Videla, *et al.*, 2007). PEG molecules have been known to adhere to proteins and surfactant phospholipids thereby forming barrier-like structures (Bedu-Addo *et al.*, 1996; Edwards *et al.*, 1997; Johnsson & Edwards, 2003).

While the most widely available form of PEG is the molecular weight of 3350, both high and low molecular weight forms of PEG have been shown to be of potential clinical importance. For example, PEG 15-20, a low molecular weight PEG, has been shown to protect against radiation-induced intestinal injury via its ability to bind lipid rafts and prevent their coalescence (Valuckaite *et al.*, 2009). Further, PEG 8000 has demonstrated functionality as a barrier inhibiting interactions between colonizing microbes and their epithelial cell targets, thereby forming a mucin-like layer (Wu *et al.*, 2004).

## 2     Effect of Commensal Bacterial Strains and PEG on Substrate Topography

The role bacteria play on substrate topography is a new paradigm that has several different implications. As mentioned previously, substrate topography is an essential parameter that provides insight to several disease states. Previously conducted studies provide evidence to suggest that commensal bacterial strains may in fact harm the surrounding extra-cellular matrix. Bacterial effects on scaffolds should be well understood before implanting an engineered tissue *in-vivo*. Bacteria native to the body may have a significant impact on scaffold integrity. Each commensal bacterial strain affects the surface topography of collagen substrates differently. The following section will focus on the role of bacterial strains in altering tissue integrity.

### 2.1     Commensal Bacterial Strains Alter Collagen Pore Size and Fiber Dimensions

It has been shown in literature that collagenases have the ability to degrade fibrillar collagen. The degradation caused by Collagenase activity decreases substrate integrity (Galis *et al.*, 1994; Varani *et al.*, 2001). Furthermore, low Collagenase activity has been associated with an increase in collagen turn-over (Shingleton *et al.* 1996).

It was previously shown in Bharadwaj *et al.* (2011) that commensal bacterial strain, especially 260, increased pore area although no Collagenase activity was detected (data not shown). Surprisingly, commensal bacterial strain HS4 did not alter pore size but had maximum Collagenase activity and in the case of substrates infected with 258 bacterial strain, a reduction in pore size and a slight increase in Collagenase activity were observed. Even though the pore size is increased, substrate integrity is maintained due to low Collagenase activity. In the case of HS4 infected substrates, the high Collagenase activity was compensated by keeping the pore size constant whereas in the case of 258 bacterial strains the pore size was reduced (Figure 5). This shows that bacterial strains, although in different ways, compensate for the disruption in the collagen matrix and maintain scaffold integrity.

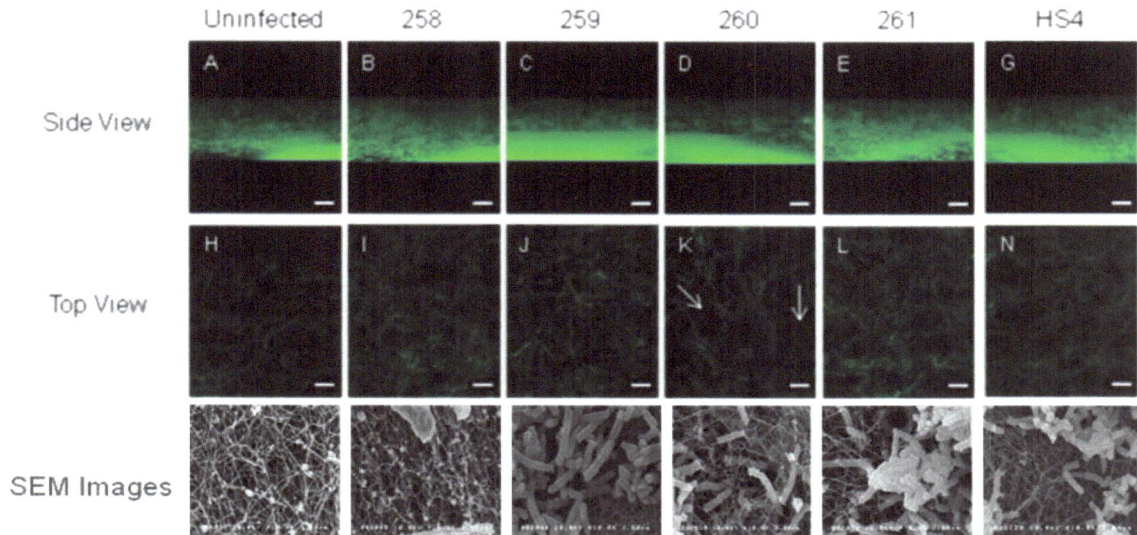

**Figure 5:** Samples infected with commensal *E. coli* strains affected collagen I substrate integrity by altering collagen fiber. The side view corresponds to substrate visualized in the Z-direction. No significant change was observed in collagen fiber integrity when treated with different commensal *E. coli* strains. Samples visualized from the top showed an increase in pore area especially in samples treated with commensal *E. coli* strain, 260 (indicated by arrow). Pore area decreased in samples treated with commensal *E. coli* strains 258 and 261. SEM images indicate change in fiber dimensions and an increase in pore size when infected with commensal bacterial strains 258, 260 and HS4. Image reproduced from Bharadwaj *et al.* (2011).

## 2.2   Commensal Bacterial Strains Alter Topographical Features

We have previously shown that bacterial infection degrades collagen matrices (Bharadwaj *et al.*, 2011). Collagen fibers are known to degrade over time regardless of bacterial influence. Previously published data indicate, samples infected with commensal *E. coli* strains 259, 260 and 261 do not degrade collagen excessively as determined by roughness profile analysis of SEM images shown in Figure 6. However, in substrates infected with commensal bacterial strains 258, 262 and HS4 an increase in overall roughness profile height is observed (data not shown). This shows that a few commensal bacterial strains, especially HS4, disrupt collagen matrix at nano-scale. Nano-scaled protrusions within the matrix have been shown to cause cellular apoptosis, differentiation and motility of cancerous cells in *in-vitro* models (Bettinger *et al.*, 2009; Biggs *et al.*, 2009; Hotary *et al.*, 2006). Also, epithelial cell morphology and cytokine production has been shown to be dependent on the underlying nano-topographical features *in vivo* (Andersson *et al.*, 2003). It is also shown in literature that in the event of inflammation, infection and malignant conditions of colon, the surrounding ECM is disrupted (Lo *et al.*, 2002; Vlodavsky & Friedmann, 2001). Although, probiotics have been known to have beneficial effect on the host organism and aid in digestion and overall health of the colon, in the event of colon cancer or other GI disorders, probiotics may, in fact, disrupt the collagen matrix further and worsen the already existing condition. Further studies, especially *in-vivo* experiments, are required in this area to confirm this hypothesis.

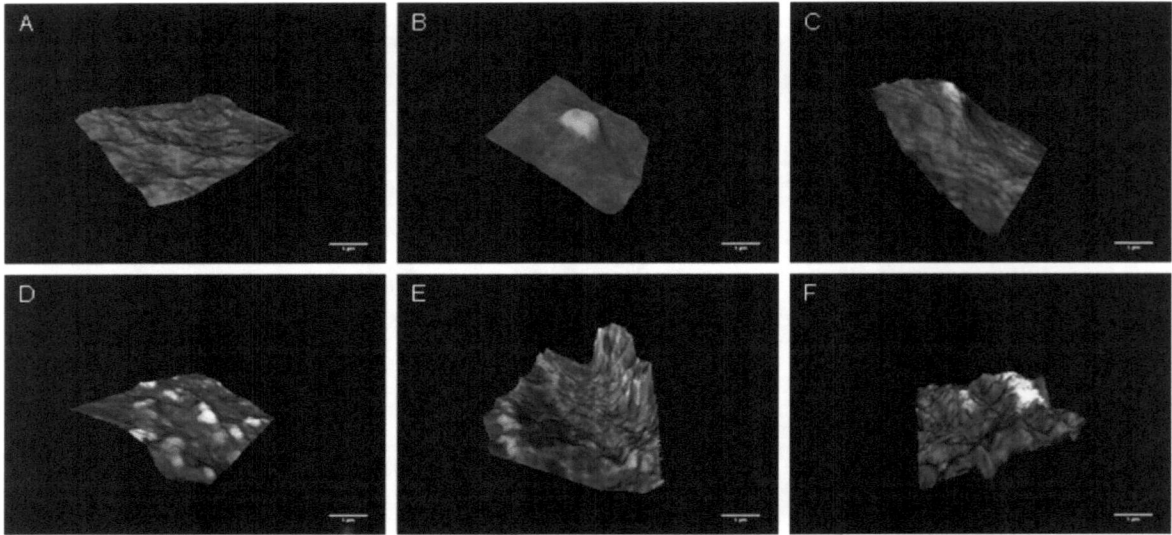

**Figure 6:** 3D Scaffold integrity stayed intact for the uninfected sample. (A) It is clear that the uninfected samples along with strains 259 (B) and 260 (C) have negligible collagen degradation while strain 261 (D) and 262 (E) have minimal degradation. Strain 161 or HS4 (F) exhibits significant collagen degradation. Bar length is 5 μm. Image reproduced from Bharadwaj *et al.* (2011).

## 2.3    Polyethylene Glycol Protects Against Bacterial Degradation and Acts a Surrogate Mucin

As mentioned previously in this chapter, bacterial degradation of collagen matrix is an important factor in determining the onset of several different disease states. Although commensal bacterial strains are known to be beneficial, previously published data suggest that these commensal strains may in fact degrade collagen matrices which in turn may induce the onset of several different diseases.

As seen in Figure 7, commensal bacterial strains degrade collagen matrix and invade through the collagen fibers. This invasion further disrupts the integrity of the tissue construct. Treatment with higher molecular weight PEG, especially PEG 8000, has been shown to reduce pro-invasiveness of aggressive cancer cells which will be further described in the next section. One of the reasons for this protective influence of PEG is that it directly influences and changes the collagen fiber dimension. PEG treated collagen tissue constructs have comparatively thicker and longer collagen fibers as compared to untreated collagen fibers. This change in dimensions further emphasizes PEGs role as a protective surrogate mucin that binds together collagen fibers creating a tightly knit barrier thus reducing bacterial invasion through the collagen tissue construct. Loss of mucin, in the event of colon cancer and other GI disorders enables gut flora to migrate through the epithelium. A protective layer atop the epithelial layer is required to maintain and segregate bacteria from the epithelial layer. PEG 8000, as shown in this chapter, creates a layer atop the collagen substrate thereby separating the bacteria and the collagen fibers.

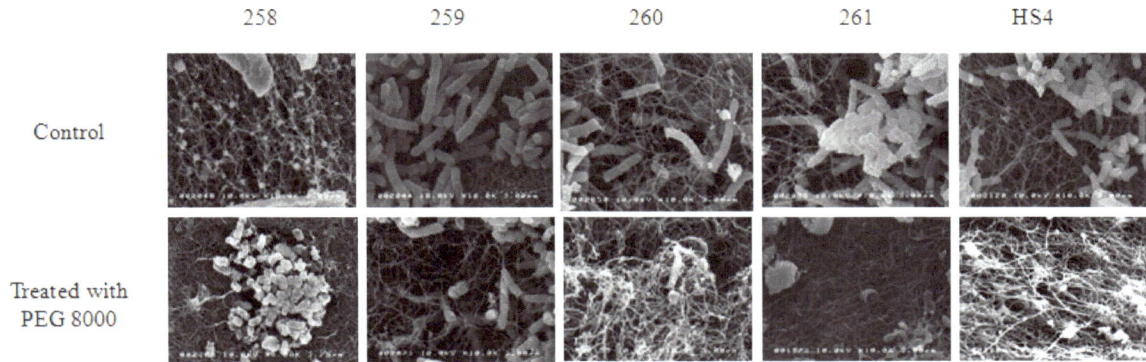

**Figure 7:** SEM images of collagen matrices infected with commensal *E. coli* strains alone and commensal *E. coli* strain infected collagen matrices treated with PEG 8000. PEG 8000 served as an adhesive that bound the collagen fibers together. The invasion of bacterial strains through the collagen matrix was drastically reduced in matrices treated with PEG 8000. This is especially seen in collagen matrix infected with bacterial strains 258, 260, 261 and HS4. Scale bar = 3 μm.

# 3    Effect of Polyethylene Glycol on Pro-invasive Effect of Colon Cancer Cells

So far we have discussed the role of bacterial strains on collagen substrates and how PEG might reduce the damage caused by these bacterial strains. This section will focus onPEGs role in decreasing the pro-invasive effects of cancerous cell line, Caco-2. Caco-2 cells are aggressive and invade through the extra-cellular matrix both *in-vitro* as well as *in-vivo*. As mentioned in the previous section, PEG has been shown to reduce the invasiveness of bacterial strains by increasing collagen substrate integrity. As previously shown, PEG acts as an adhesive to bind collagen fibers together. During the onset of cancer, cells are extremely aggressive and gain the ability to move through the extra-cellular matrix via several different enzymatic as well as non-enzymatic mechanisms. It is essential to control this motility of cells to avoid metastasis. The following sub-sections will emphasize PEGs role in controlling the proliferation, motility and invasion of cancerous Caco-2 cells.

## 3.1    Higher molecular weight PEGs increase Caco-2 cell proliferation

Previously published data indicate cellular proliferation increases in response to the two commensal *E. coli* strains, 261 and HS4. Specifically, proliferation increased 1.6 fold in response to treatment with strain 261 and 1.5 fold in response to treatment with HS4 (Bharadwaj, *et al.*, 2011). Although an increase in proliferation was observed when treated with PEG 8000, this increase is not statistically significant when treated with PEG 20,000 (Figure 8).

This indicates that it is not necessarily the molecular weight affecting the proliferation of cells but it is the structural property of the PEG that in turn increases the volume of macromolecules surrounding the cells. For example, Goverman *et al.* state that increasing the amount of macromolecules surrounding the cells aids in the formation of bundled F-actin(Goverman, Schick, & Newman). An early study conducted by Drenckahn *et al.*, also showed that the association rate constant of actin monomers to an actin filament increased in the presence of inert macromolecular 'crowders' (Drenckhahn & Pollard). Bundling

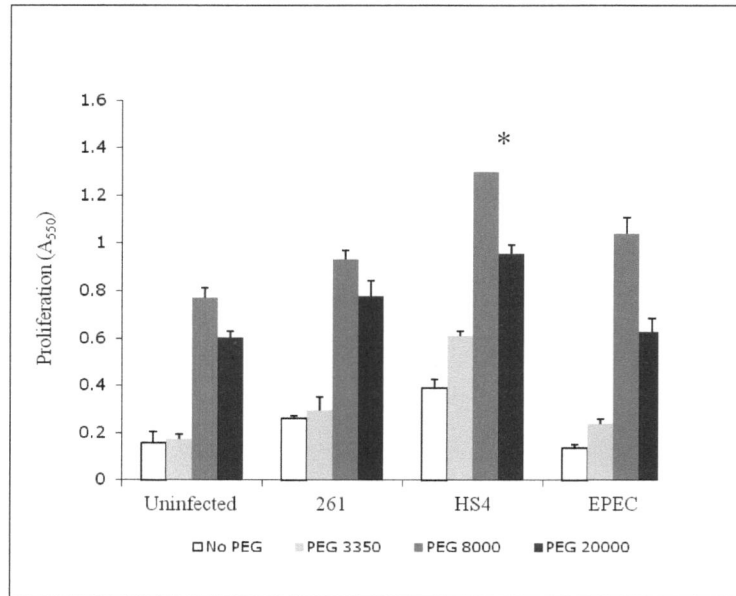

**Figure 8:** PEG 8000 increases proliferation of Caco-2. Caco-2 cells were plated on the surface of 400 um-thick collagen gels and allowed to remodel overnight. Proliferation of cells on the scaffold was observed using MTT proliferation assay. Scaffolds treated with PEG 8000 showed significant increase in proliferation. Standard student t-test was applied to the samples and $p < 0.05$ were obtained for samples treated with PEG 8000 and HS4 indicated by an asterisk (*). Image reproduced from Bharadwaj et al., 2011.

of actins has been shown to increase proliferation in colonic epithelial cells (Jawhari et al., 2003). Integrins induce polymerization and organization of actin through both physical protein-protein interactions that anchor actin filaments at sites of adhesion as well as through signaling pathways such as PtdLns(4,5)P$_2$ and Rho family GTPases. Therefore, actin bundling contributes to the integrin effects on cell cycle progression thereby inducing cell proliferation (Schoenwaelder & Burridge, 1999). Hence it is safe to assume that the overcrowding caused by PEG molecules aids in actin bundling which causes integrins to affect cell cycle progression resulting in an increases the proliferation rate of the cells. The proliferative response that was observed in Caco-2cells in response to the two commensal strains of E. coli and to EPEC is consistent with previously published results (Long et al., 2001). The reduction in proliferation in response to EPEC is also not surprising considering that EPEC is known to cause cellular apoptosis (Figueiredo et al., 2007; Shankar et al., 2009; Viswanathan et al., 2008). However, when treated with PEG 8000, the cell density increased most likely due to proliferation of cells. The dispersion of cells, especially when infected with HS4, may be caused by the increased proliferative response of cells when treated with PEG 8000 and infected with HS4.

## 3.2    PEG Decreases Pro-invasive Nature of Caco-2 cells

As shown in Bharadwaj et al. (2011), PEG binds the cells together reducing cluster thickness, however bacterial infection causes cells to pack less densely; Thus indicating that bacterial strains have a negative influence on PEGs binding properties. Caco-2 cells seeded on collagen I scaffolds were stained for phalloidin and DAPI to image the cytoskeleton and nucleus respectively as shown in Figure 9. The collagen scaffolds infected with bacterial strains showed that the cells were more spread out and were not as tightly packed as seen in control, especially in the case of samples infected with HS4.

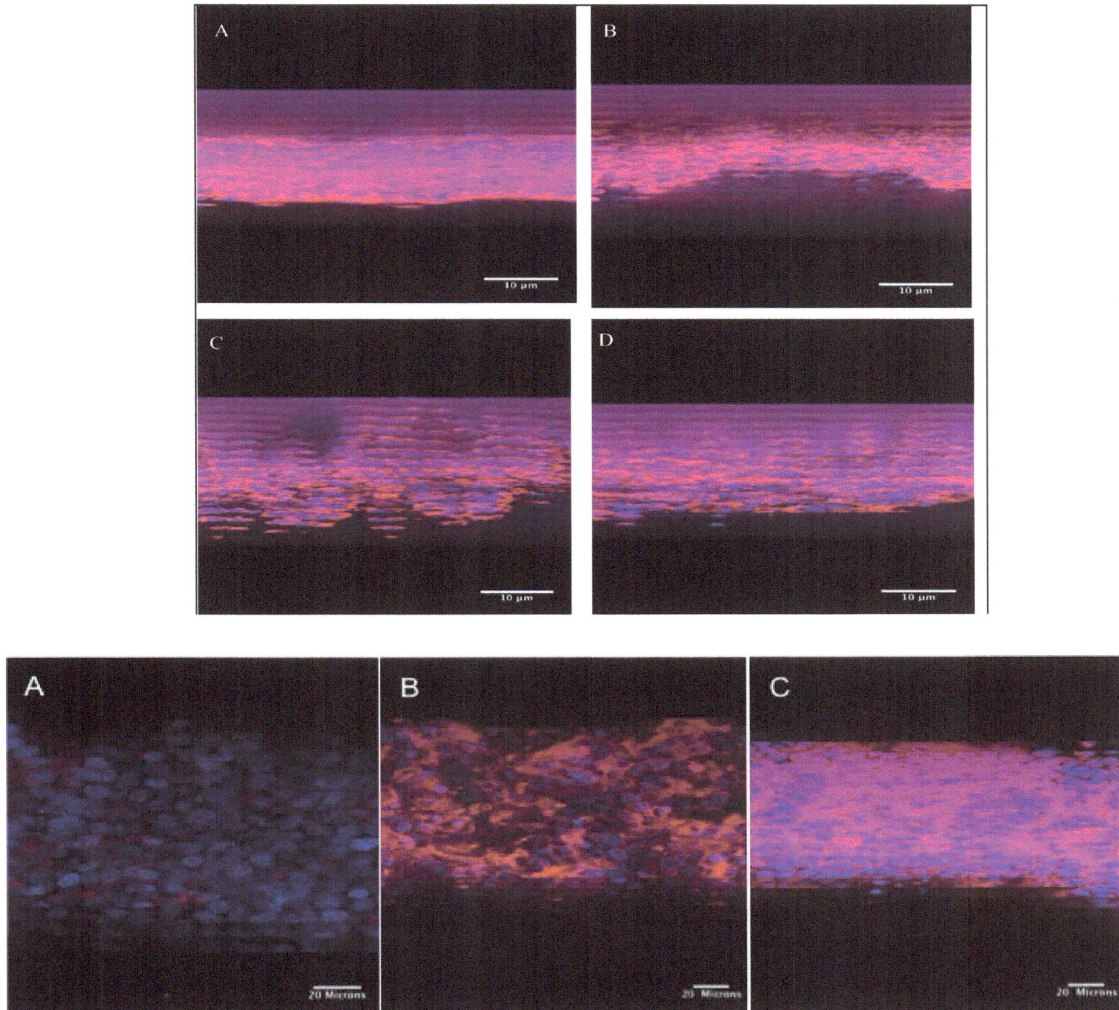

**Figure 9:** Multiphoton Images of Caco-2 cells treated with various molecular weight PEG (A) Untreated cells served as control in both pictures above. In the picture on top, (B, C) Caco-2 cells were infected with commensal strains 261, HS4 (D) and EPEC. Depth of invasion increased in response to bacterial infection. The maximum depth of invasion was seen in scaffolds infected with HS4. PEG had no significant effect on the depth of invasion. PEG prevented the pro-invasive effects of the bacterial strains, but increased Caco-2 proliferation. Each stack is approximately 5μm thick. The overall thickness of the scaffold was approximately 400 μm and the penetration depth was approximately 80 μm. The actin filaments are shown in red and the DAPI staining of nuclei are shown in blue. Bar length=10 μm. In the picture below, (B, C) Caco-2 cells were treated with PEG 3350 and PEG 8000 respectively. Cluster thickness decreased when treated with higher molecular weight PEG. The cluster thickness when treated with PEG 8000 was approximately 50 μm. The actin filaments are shown in red and DAPI staining of nuclei is in blue. Bar length=20 μm.

Cancer cell cluster thickness was similar to the control for samples treated with PEG 3350; However, higher molecular weight PEGs (8,000 and 20,000), reduced cluster thickness as shown in Figure 9. Since higher molecular PEG, especially PEG 8000, increased cell proliferation, the reduction of cell cluster thickness when treated with PEG 8000 indicates that higher molecular weight PEG may cause the cells to pack more tightly, with a higher cell-cell contact.

The quantification of depth of invasion is essential in determining the role each of the variables, PEG and bacterial strains respectively, in terms of pro-invasive effect they have on the cancerous Caco-2 cells. As seen in Figure 9 and Figure 10, Caco-2 cells are highly aggressive when treated with higher molecular weight PEG and infected with HS4. Since proliferation increased with higher molecular weight PEG, it is essential to see if the invasiveness of Caco-2 cells were affected as well.

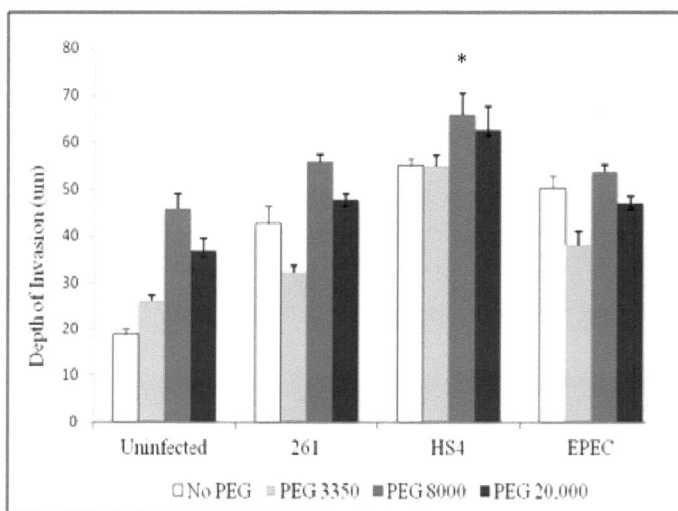

**Figure 10:** Quantitative Analysis of Depth of Invasion. Cell cluster thickness is decreased by PEG Quantitative analysis of depth of invasion of Caco-2 cells in 1.2 mg/mL collagen type I substrate. The images in Figure.3 were analyzed using commercially bought software. The depth of invasion in seen in Figure 9 was determined by measuring the distance travelled by the cells in micrometers. Standard student t-test was applied to the samples and the $p < 0.05$ were obtained for samples treated with PEG 8000 and HS4 indicated by an asterisk (*). Image reproduced from Bharadwaj *et al.*, 2011.

As described in Bharadwaj *et al.* (2011) the depth of invasion can be quantified by measuring the distance that Caco-2 cells invaded within the 3D collagen matrix. As shown in Figure 10, the depth of invasion was significantly higher when Caco-2 cells were treated with PEG 8000 and infected with HS4 bacterial strain, with a penetrationdepth of approximately 65 μm. PEG 8000 alone also significantly increased penetration depth of Caco-2 cells to approximately 45 μm when compared to a control sample with a depth of invasion of 15 μm. The combination of higher molecular weight PEG and commensal bacterial strain, especially HS4, significantly increases the pro-invasiveness of Caco-2 cancer cells.

Although both proliferation and depth of invasion are increased when treated with higher molecular weight PEG, the data in Figure 9 and Figure 10 suggest that cell density may not be a major factor in increasing cellular invasion. The cells when infected with bacterial strains are loosely packed, establishing fewer cell-cell contact; thus indicating that invasion of Caco-2 cells through the 3D collagen matrix is not due to the force generated by cell-cell contact.

## 3.3 PEG Decreases MMP Activity

Matrix metalloproteinase (MMP) activity *in-vivo* plays an important role in tissue remodeling. Most MMPs are involved in breaking down the proteins that form tissues, especially collagen. MMPs are secreted by cells to aid in motility and/or invasion through the matrices. This is most commonly seen in the event of cancer, where cells invade through the matrix towards the blood stream during metastasis. MMPs are activated stepwise via a cyteine-switch mechanism either proteolytically or chemically (Springman *et al*, 1990; Van Wart & Birkedal-Hansen, 1990). A zymogen, which is an inactive enzyme precursor, is often activated prior to MMP activation. We speculate that PEG, especially PEG 8000 may inhibit the activation of precursor zymogens thereby reducing MMP-1 activity. Another speculation is that Tissue Inhibitors of Metalloproteinases (TIMPs) may have been up-regulated which in turn suppressed MMP-1 activity. Since higher molecular weight PEG affects proliferation and depth of invasion of Caco-2 cells, it is no surprise that MMP activity is also affected by PEG. Interstitial collagenase (MMP-1) is involved in the initial breakdown of collagen during tumor growth and invasion (Figueiredo *et al.*, 2007). With the increased invasion of Caco-2 cells as shown in Figure 11, it is expected to see an increase in collagenase activity. However, as shown previously, MMP-1 activity for Caco-2 cells significantly decreased when treated with various molecular weight PEG, especially PEG 8000.

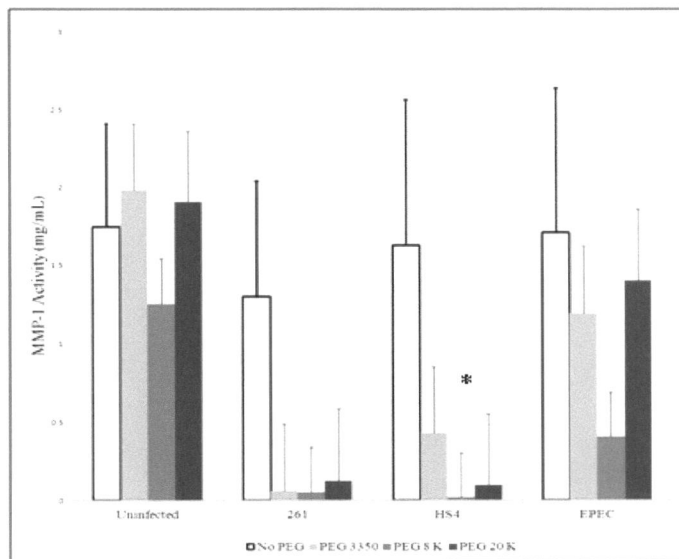

**Figure 11:** MMP-1 activity in the commensal strains was comparatively lower than when infected with pathogenic (EPEC). PEG significantly reduced the MMP-1 activity when infected with bacteria (both commensal and pathogenic). A 5-fold decrease in MMP-1 activity was noted in samples treated with PEG 8000 and infected with commensal bacteria. Standard student t-test was applied to the samples and the $p < 0.05$ were obtained for samples treated with PEG 8000 and HS4 indicated by an asterisk (*). Image reproduced from Bharadwaj *et al.*, 2011.

The pathogenic strain (EPEC) also decreased MMP-1 activity when treated with PEG 8000 as shown in Figure 11. Infecting with bacterial strains alone did not significantly reduce MMP-1 activity. Treatment with PEG 8000 decreased MMP-1 activity from 1.7 mg/mL (control) to 1.3 mg/ml. Although there was a reduction in MMP-1 activity, the decrease was not significant when treated with PEG alone. However, combining PEG with bacterial strains reduced MMP-1 activity drastically. As shown in Figure 11, MMP-1 activity of samples treated with PEG 8000 and infected with HS4 decreased from 1.4 mg/mL (treated with PEG 8000 alone) to 0.1 mg/mL (Bharadwaj et al., 2011). This indicates that neither PEG nor bacterial strains have an effect on MMP-1 activity by themselves, although combining PEG with bacterial strains reduces the pro-invasiveness of Caco-2 cells by significantly reducing MMP-1 activity. Collagenase-3 (MMP-13) plays a crucial role in the modulation of extracellular matrix degradation and cell-matrix interactions involved in metastasis (Toriseva et al., 2012) . Due to its ability to degrade an exceptionally wide range of ECM components such as type I, II, II and IV collagen, the physiologic expression of MMP-13 is seen in situations in which rapid and effective remodeling of collagenous ECM is required, especially in a tumor (Noel et al., 2012; Shah et al., 2012). MMP-13 activity was determined for Caco-2 cells when infected with EPEC and commensal strains of E. Coli under different PEG conditions. No significant change in MMP-13 activity was observed when infected with commensal and pathogenic E. Coli strains.

Although higher molecular weight PEG showed higher MMP-13 activity when compared to lower molecular weight PEG, the bacterial strains do not contribute significantly to MMP-13 expression. An increase inMMP-13 due to treatment with PEG indicates PEGs role as a surrogate mucin and aiding in tissue remodeling.

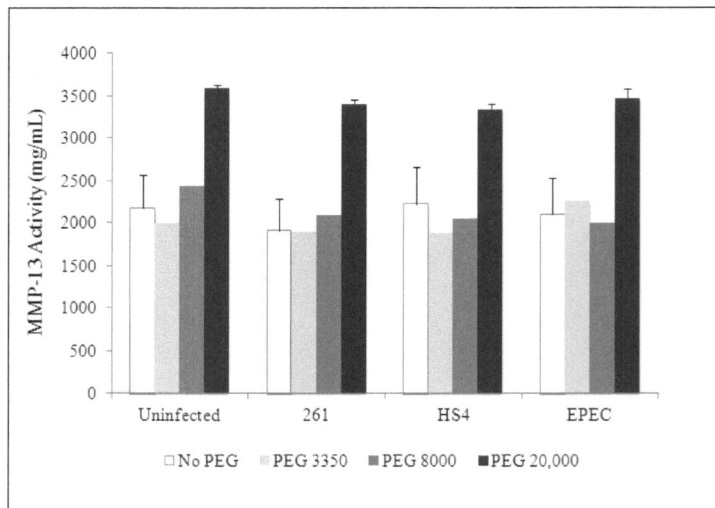

**Figure 12**: MMP-13 activity for the samples treated with DMEM/F12 (No PEG), PEG 3350 and PEG 8000 showed no significant change. The bacterial strains, especially the commensal bacteria, slightly decreased the MMP-13 activity. Image reproduced from Bharadwaj et al., 2011.

## 4   Implications of PEG as a therapeutic agent

The data presented in this chapter suggest that commensal bacterial strains disrupt collagen matrix, thereby degrading the tissue construct. This degradation of matrix causes the gut barrier function to be disrupted and commensal bacterial strains gain the ability to invade through the extra-cellular matrix or the tissue construct. We also emphasize in this chapter that colonic bacterial strains have the ability to alter epithelial cell behavior and several studies have confirmed bacterial influence on the onset of colitis-like disease states. Thus, using probiotics in the event of GI disorders may have a negative impact. Although, probiotics have been known to have beneficial effect on the host organism and aid in digestion and overall health of the colon, in the event of colon cancer or other GI disorders, probiotics may, in fact, disrupt the collagen matrix further and worsen an already existing condition. Similarly, we speculate that antibiotics may also have an effect on tissue integrity. Further studies are definitely in need to support this.

PEGs role as a surrogate mucin becomes extremely important in subjugating the bacterial influence on the tissue. Since, PEG is widely used as a laxative, especially PEG 3350, it is deemed safe to be used in human populations. During the onset of colon cancer and several other GI disorders, the gut barrier function is disrupted. Ideally, a layer of mucin protects the epithelial lining from bacterial influence. We propose in this chapter, that PEG 8000 may in fact act as a surrogate mucin based on the fact that PEG 8000 serves as an adhesive and binds the collagen fibers together forming a thick-knit mesh like framework. PEG 3350 has been proven safe to be administered orally. Similarly, administering PEG 8000 orally could be an effective way of re-establishing the lost barrier function. Further studies, especially in an animal model, are required to fully understand the implications of using PEG as a surrogate mucin.

The data presented in this chapter also suggest that PEG directly influences and decreases the invasiveness of cancer cells by forming a close knit mesh-work of collagen fibers. PEGs influence on cancer cell proliferation further enhances its role as a potential therapeutic agent that can be used in conjunction with an anti-cancer drug to successfully re-create gut barrier function and potentially reduce risk of metastasis. Chemo-therapeutic agents utilize the fact that cancer cells are fast proliferating and target these cells accordingly. Our data as shown in this chapter indicate that PEG, especially PEG 8000, increases cellular proliferation. This increase in cell proliferation may in fact be of therapeutic use since this will enhance the potency of chemotherapeutic agents in targeting fast proliferating cells.

# References

Andersson, A. S., Backhed, F., von Euler, A., Richter-Dahlfors, A., Sutherland, D., & Kasemo, B. (2003). Nanoscale features influence epithelial cell morphology and cytokine production. Biomaterials, 24(20), 3427-3436.

Anselme, K. (2000). Osteoblast adhesion on biomaterials. Biomaterials, 21(7), 667-681.

Anselme, K., Davidson, P., Popa, A. M., Giazzon, M., Liley, M., & Ploux, L. (2010). The interaction of cells and bacteria with surfaces structured at the nanometre scale. Acta Biomater, 6(10), 3824-3846.

Bedu-Addo, F. K., Tang, P., Xu, Y., & Huang, L. (1996). Effects of polyethyleneglycol chain length and phospholipid acyl chain composition on the interaction of polyethyleneglycol-phospholipid conjugates with phospholipid: implications in liposomal drug delivery. Pharm Res, 13(5), 710-717.

Bettinger, C. J., Langer, R., & Borenstein, J. T. (2009). Engineering substrate topography at the micro- and nanoscale to control cell function. Angew Chem Int Ed Engl, 48(30), 5406-5415.

Bharadwaj, S., Nekrasov, V., Vishnubhotla, R., Foster, C., & Glover, S. C. (2012). Commensal *E. coli* Strains Uniquely Alter the ECM Topography Independent of Colonic Epithelial Cells. Journal of Biomaterials and Nanobiotechnology, 3, 70-78.

Bharadwaj, S., Vishnubhotla, R., Shan, S., Chauhan, C., Cho, M., & Glover, S. C. Higher molecular weight polyethylene glycol increases cell proliferation while improving barrier function in an in vitro colon cancer model. J Biomed Biotechnol, 2011, 587470.

Biggs, M. J., Richards, R. G., Gadegaard, N., McMurray, R. J., Affrossman, S., Wilkinson, C. D., *et al.* (2009). Interactions with nanoscale topography: adhesion quantification and signal transduction in cells of osteogenic and multipotent lineage. J Biomed Mater Res A, 91(1), 195-208.

Chow, T. H., Lin, Y. Y., Hwang, J. J., Wang, H. E., Tseng, Y. L., Pang, V. F., *et al.* (2009). Therapeutic efficacy evaluation of 111In-labeled PEGylated liposomal vinorelbine in murine colon carcinoma with multimodalities of molecular imaging. J Nucl Med, 50(12), 2073-2081.

Corpet, D. E., & Parnaud, G. (1999). Polyethylene-glycol, a potent suppressor of azoxymethane-induced colonic aberrant crypt foci in rats. Carcinogenesis, 20(5), 915-918.

Corpet, D. E., Parnaud, G., Delverdier, M., Peiffer, G., & Tache, S. (2000). Consistent and fast inhibition of colon carcinogenesis by polyethylene glycol in mice and rats given various carcinogens. Cancer Res, 60(12), 3160-3164.

Cummings, J. H. (1998). Dietary carbohydrates and the colonic microflora. Curr Opin Clin Nutr Metab Care, 1(5), 409-414.

Cummings, J. H., & Macfarlane, G. T. (1991). The control and consequences of bacterial fermentation in the human colon. J Appl Bacteriol, 70(6), 443-459.

de Roos, N. M., & Katan, M. B. (2000). Effects of probiotic bacteria on diarrhea, lipid metabolism, and carcinogenesis: a review of papers published between 1988 and 1998. Am J Clin Nutr, 71(2), 405-411.

Dorval, E., Jankowski, J. M., Barbieux, J. P., Viguier, J., Bertrand, P., Brondin, B., *et al.* (2006). Polyethylene glycol and prevalence of colorectal adenomas. Gastroenterol Clin Biol, 30(10), 1196-1199.

Drenckhahn, D., & Pollard, T. D. (1986). Elongation of actin filaments is a diffusion-limited reaction at the barbed end and is accelerated by inert macromolecules. J Biol Chem, 261(27), 12754-12758.

Edwards, K., Johnsson, M., Karlsson, G., & Silvander, M. (1997). Effect of polyethyleneglycol-phospholipids on aggregate structure in preparations of small unilamellar liposomes. Biophys J, 73(1), 258-266.

Figueiredo, P. M., Furumura, M. T., Aidar-Ugrinovich, L., Pestana de Castro, A. F., Pereira, F. G., Metze, I. L., *et al.* (2007). Induction of apoptosis in Caco-2 and HT-29 human intestinal epithelial cells by enterohemolysin produced by classic enteropathogenic *Escherichia coli*. Lett Appl Microbiol, 45(4), 358-363.

Florey, H. (1955). Mucin and the protection of the body. Proc R Soc Lond B Biol Sci, 143(911), 147-158.

Galis, Z. S., Sukhova, G. K., Lark, M. W., & Libby, P. (1994). Increased expression of matrix metalloproteinases and matrix degrading activity in vulnerable regions of human atherosclerotic plaques. J Clin Invest, 94(6), 2493-2503.

Gibson, G. R., & Roberfroid, M. B. (1995). Dietary modulation of the human colonic microbiota: introducing the concept of prebiotics. J Nutr, 125(6), 1401-1412.

Goverman, J., Schick, L. A., & Newman, J. (1996). The bundling of actin with polyethylene glycol 8000 in the presence and absence of gelsolin. Biophys J, 71(3), 1485-1492.

Hotary, K., Li, X. Y., Allen, E., Stevens, S. L., & Weiss, S. J. (2006). A cancer cell metalloprotease triad regulates the basement membrane transmigration program. Genes Dev, 20(19), 2673-2686.

Jawhari, A. U., Buda, A., Jenkins, M., Shehzad, K., Sarraf, C., Noda, M., *et al.* (2003). Fascin, an actin-bundling protein, modulates colonic epithelial cell invasiveness and differentiation in vitro. Am J Pathol, 162(1), 69-80.

Johnsson, M., & Edwards, K. (2003). Liposomes, disks, and spherical micelles: aggregate structure in mixtures of gel phase phosphatidylcholines and poly(ethylene glycol)-phospholipids. Biophys J, 85(6), 3839-3847.

Keselowsky, B. G., Collard, D. M., & Garcia, A. J. (2003). Surface chemistry modulates fibronectin conformation and directs integrin binding and specificity to control cell adhesion. J Biomed Mater Res A, 66(2), 247-259.

Keselowsky, B. G., Collard, D. M., & Garcia, A. J. (2004). Surface chemistry modulates focal adhesion composition and signaling through changes in integrin binding. Biomaterials, 25(28), 5947-5954.

Lim, J. Y., & Donahue, H. J. (2007). Cell sensing and response to micro- and nanostructured surfaces produced by chemical and topographic patterning. Tissue Eng, 13(8), 1879-1891.

Lo, E. H., Wang, X., & Cuzner, M. L. (2002). Extracellular proteolysis in brain injury and inflammation: role for plasminogen activators and matrix metalloproteinases. J Neurosci Res, 69(1), 1-9.

Long, E., Capuco, A. V., Wood, D. L., Sonstegard, T., Tomita, G., Paape, M. J., et al. (2001). Escherichia coli induces apoptosis and proliferation of mammary cells. Cell Death Differ, 8(8), 808-816.

Macpherson, A. J., Slack, E., Geuking, M. B., & McCoy, K. D. (2009). The mucosal firewalls against commensal intestinal microbes. Semin Immunopathol, 31(2), 145-149.

Marteau, P., & Chaput, U. (2011). Bacteria as trigger for chronic gastrointestinal disorders. Dig Dis, 29(2), 166-171.

Noel, A., Gutierrez-Fernandez, A., Sounni, N. E., Behrendt, N., Maquoi, E., Lund, I. K., et al. (2012). New and paradoxical roles of matrix metalloproteinases in the tumor microenvironment. Front Pharmacol, 3, 140.

Oh, S., Brammer, K. S., Li, Y. S., Teng, D., Engler, A. J., Chien, S., et al. (2009). Stem cell fate dictated solely by altered nanotube dimension. Proc Natl Acad Sci U S A, 106(7), 2130-2135.

Pampati, V., & Fogel, R. (2004). Treatment Options for Primary Constipation. Curr Treat Options Gastroenterol, 7(3), 225-233.

Roy, H. K., Gulizia, J., DiBaise, J. K., Karolski, W. J., Ansari, S., Madugula, M., et al. (2004). Polyethylene glycol inhibits intestinal neoplasia and induces epithelial apoptosis in Apc(min) mice. Cancer Lett, 215(1), 35-42.

Schoenwaelder, S. M., & Burridge, K. (1999). Bidirectional signaling between the cytoskeleton and integrins. Curr Opin Cell Biol, 11(2), 274-286.

Shah, M., Huang, D., Blick, T., Connor, A., Reiter, L. A., Hardink, J. R., et al. (2012). An MMP13-selective inhibitor delays primary tumor growth and the onset of tumor-associated osteolytic lesions in experimental models of breast cancer. PLoS One, 7(1), e29615.

Shankar, B., Krishnan, S., Malladi, V., Balakrishnan, A., & Williams, P. H. (2009). Outer membrane proteins of wild-type and intimin-deficient enteropathogenic Escherichia coli induce Hep-2 cell death through intrinsic and extrinsic pathways of apoptosis. Int J Med Microbiol, 299(2), 121-132.

Sheng, Y. H., Hasnain, S. Z., Florin, T. H., & McGuckin, M. A. (2012). Mucins in inflammatory bowel diseases and colorectal cancer. J Gastroenterol Hepatol, 27(1), 28-38.

Shingleton, W. D., Hodges, D. J., Brick, P., & Cawston, T. E. (1996). Collagenase: a key enzyme in collagen turnover. Biochem Cell Biol, 74(6), 759-775.

Siegel, R., Naishadham, D., & Jemal, A. (2012). Cancer statistics, 2012. CA Cancer J Clin, 62(1), 10-29.

Springman, E. B., Angleton, E. L., Birkedal-Hansen, H., & Van Wart, H. E. (1990). Multiple modes of activation of latent human fibroblast collagenase: evidence for the role of a Cys73 active-site zinc complex in latency and a "cysteine switch" mechanism for activation. Proc Natl Acad Sci U S A, 87(1), 364-368.

Toriseva, M., Laato, M., Carpen, O., Ruohonen, S. T., Savontaus, E., Inada, M., et al. (2012). MMP-13 Regulates Growth of Wound Granulation Tissue and Modulates Gene Expression Signatures Involved in Inflammation, Proteolysis, and Cell Viability. PLoS One, 7(8), e42596.

Tran, L. C., & Di Palma, J. A. (2005). Lack of lasting effectiveness of PEG 3350 laxative treatment of constipation. J Clin Gastroenterol, 39(7), 600-602.

Valuckaite, V., Zaborina, O., Long, J., Hauer-Jensen, M., Wang, J., Holbrook, C., et al. (2009). Oral PEG 15-20 protects the intestine against radiation: role of lipid rafts. Am J Physiol Gastrointest Liver Physiol, 297(6), G1041-1052.

Van Wart, H. E., & Birkedal-Hansen, H. (1990). The cysteine switch: a principle of regulation of metalloproteinase activity with potential applicability to the entire matrix metalloproteinase gene family. Proc Natl Acad Sci U S A, 87(14), 5578-5582.

Varani, J., Spearman, D., Perone, P., Fligiel, S. E., Datta, S. C., Wang, Z. Q., *et al.* (2001). Inhibition of type I procollagen synthesis by damaged collagen in photoaged skin and by collagenase-degraded collagen in vitro. Am J Pathol, 158(3), 931-942.

Videla, S., Lugea, A., Vilaseca, J., Guarner, F., Treserra, F., Salas, A., *et al.* (2007). Polyethylene glycol enhances colonic barrier function and ameliorates experimental colitis in rats. Int J Colorectal Dis, 22(6), 571-580.

Viswanathan, V. K., Weflen, A., Koutsouris, A., Roxas, J. L., & Hecht, G. (2008). Enteropathogenic *E. coli*-induced barrier function alteration is not a consequence of host cell apoptosis. Am J Physiol Gastrointest Liver Physiol, 294(5), G1165-1170.

Vlodavsky, I., & Friedmann, Y. (2001). Molecular properties and involvement of heparanase in cancer metastasis and angiogenesis. J Clin Invest, 108(3), 341-347.

Wu, L., Zaborina, O., Zaborin, A., Chang, E. B., Musch, M., Holbrook, C., *et al.* (2004). High-molecular-weight polyethylene glycol prevents lethal sepsis due to intestinal Pseudomonas aeruginosa. Gastroenterology, 126(2), 488-498.

Yamamoto, K., Sokabe, T., Watabe, T., Miyazono, K., Yamashita, J. K., Obi, S., *et al.* (2005). Fluid shear stress induces differentiation of Flk-1-positive embryonic stem cells into vascular endothelial cells in vitro. Am J Physiol Heart Circ Physiol, 288(4), H1915-1924.

# Small Bowel Adenocarcinoma

Nishant Poddar, Arsh Singh, Bhawna Sharma
RishitaSolanki Singh, Shahzad Raza, Hemant Singh Sindhu
Madhumati Kalavar
*Division of Hematology/Oncology*
*Brookdale University Hospital Medical Center, New York, USA*

# 1    Introduction

Cancer of the small bowel is an uncommon tumor accounting for only 0.1% – 0.3% of all malignancies and 1% – 2 % of primary gastrointestinal tract malignancies (Lowenfels, 1973; Chow *et al.*, 1996). As a result of its relative rarity, data accumulation regarding its natural history has been limiting both the clinical and molecular understanding of this cancer. Furthermore, presence of different histological subtypes has complicated its typical disease expression characteristics. Adenocarcinomas, one of the most common occurring histological subtypes, represent about 40% of all malignant small bowel tumors. Other subtypes include malignant carcinoids tumors (~50%), lymphomas (15%), and sarcomas (GIST) (Chow *et al.*, 1996). Even though historically, adenocarcinoma has been the most common histological subtype, the steady rise of incidence of carcinoid tumor over the past few decades make them the most common subtype (Bilimoria *et al.*, 2009). According to the recent data analysis from cancer registries participating in Surveillance, Epidemiology, and End Results (SEER) program, an estimated 8,070 persons (4,380 men and 3,690 women) will be diagnosed with and 1,150 men and women will die of cancer of the small intestine in 2012 (Howlader *et al.*, 2009).

Due to the rare nature of small bowel adenocarcinoma and paucity of information available, there is a poor understanding of its pathogenesis leading to delay in diagnosis and unclear standard guidelines for appropriate therapeutic options.

# 2    Histopathology

About 40 different histological subtypes have been reported in literature. The four most common types are adenocarcinoma (Figure 1), carcinoid, lymphomas, and sarcomas (Sai & Howard, 2011).

Though adenocarcinoma comprises about 30% – 50% of small intestinal malignancies, its percentage is much lower than the proportion in the colon where the overwhelming majority is adenocarcinoma. The majority of the tumorsare located in the duodenum and duodenal-jejunal junction (50 – 70%) followed by jejunum (16%), ileum (13%), and the remainder 'not identified' (Sai & Howard, 2011; Schottenfeld *et al.*, 2009; Sperenza *et al.*, 2010). Some of these studies have also included adenocarcinoma of the ampulla of vater and periampullary region as a part of small bowel adenocarcinoma.

Neuroendocrine cancers of the small intestine are almost always carcinoid tumors with most of them originating from ileum and rarely in duodenum (Hamilton & Aaltonen, 2000). Over the past several decades four-fold increase has been noted in the incidence of carcinoid tumors with less dramatic rise in adenocarcinomas and lymphomas.

Lymphoma comprises about 15% of small intestinal malignancies. Ileum and jejunum are the most commonly affected sites with MALT being the most common type. Other primary lymphomas seen include large B-cell lymphoma, mantle cell lymphoma, burkitt lymphoma, and enteropathy associated T-cell lymphoma (Nakamura *et al.*, 2000).

A very small percentage of small intestinal malignancies constitute sarcomas (10%) (Sai & Howard, 2001; Howe *et al.*, 2001). GIST, being the most common type, represents over 90% of all small intestinal sarcomas (Howe *et al.*, 2001; Katz & DeMatteo, 2008). Lipoma, leiomyomas, leiomyosarcomas, angiosarcoma, and Kaposi's sarcoma are the other subtypes.

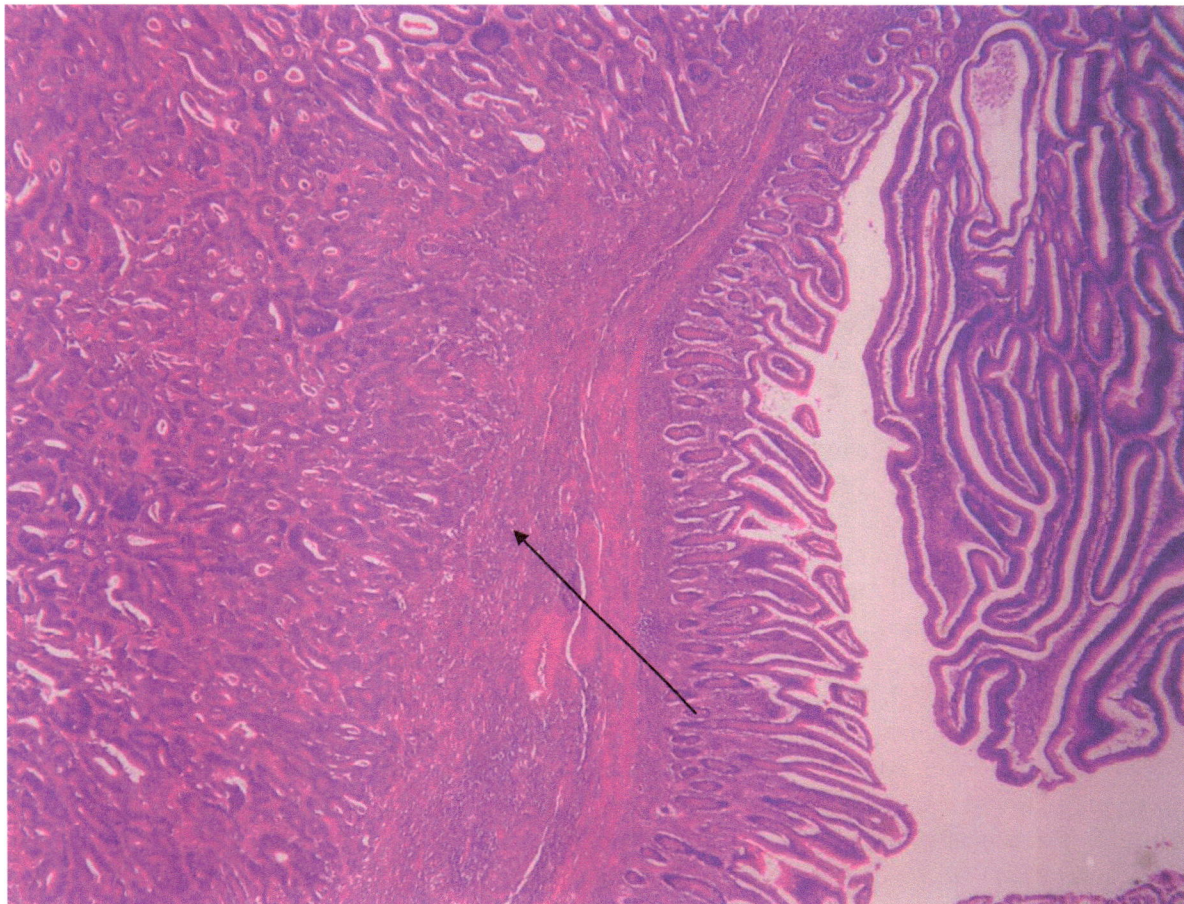

**Figure 1**: Hematoxylin-eosin stain at 100× showing infiltrative small bowel adenocarcinoma withadjacent villous adenoma.

## 3   Etiology

Given the rarity of this disease little is known regarding its molecular etiology. Despite the fact that small intestines represent majority of the length of our alimentary tract (about 75% of length with approximately 90% of surface area) a striking contrast is seen between the incidence rate of adenocarcinoma of the large intestine and small intestine with latter being about 40 to 50 fold less common (Neuget & Santos, 1993; Cross *et al.*, 2008, Perzin & Bridge, 1981).

Patients with adenocarcinoma of small or large bowel are at a higher risk of second malignancy at either intestinal site (Neuget & Santos, 1993; Cross *et al.*, 2008, Perzin & Bridge, 1981). Hereditary genetic syndromes such as HNPCC and FAP result in increased risk of not only colon cancer but small bowel adenocarcinoma as well (Schulmann *et al.*, 2005). An increased risk has also been noted for individuals with crohn's disease, celiac disease, adenoma, and peutz-jeghers syndrome (Sai & Howard, 2001). A similar process of carcinogenesis has been suggested at both sites given the similarities found in environmental and genetic factors between the two. The dietary correlates of adenocarcinoma of the small bowel have been found to be very similar to those of colon cancer, or at the least of the same magnitude. As is the case with colon cancer, increased risk of small bowel cancer is correlated with diet high in red or smoked meat, saturated fat, bread, pasta whereas an inverse relation is seen with intake of fiber from grains, whole grain foods, and vegetables conferring a protective effect (Cross *et al.*, 2008, Negri *et al.*, 1999).

Akin to colorectal cancer, the adenoma-carcinoma transformation sequence in the small bowel is postulated to be of similar significance (Howe *et al.*, 1999). In contrast to colon, small bowel adenomas are much rarer and on average, occur a decade earlier than carcinomas. However, the distribution of adenomas in the small bowel is quite similar to that of carcinomas (Sellner *et al.*, 1984). Similar to colon cancer, molecular analysis shows a good subset of small intestinal cancer result from inherited mismatch repair (MMR) gene mutation. The frequency of MSI in adenocarcinomas of the small intestine equals that of colon cancer (Planck *et al.*, 2003). Variable incidence of MMR gene abnormalities has been reported in literature so far, ranging anywhere from 5% – 45% by microsatellite testing and 0% – 26% by immunohistochemical testing (Planck *et al.*, 2003; Hibi *et al.*, 1995; Rashid A & Hamilton SR, 1997; Bläker *et al.*, 2002; Brueckl *et al.*, 2004; Zhang *et al.*, 2006). Overman *et al.* recently reported an incidence of 35% in a study of 54 patients confirmed by MSI PCR (Overman *et al.*, 2010). As is the case with colorectal cancer, patients with MSI tend to be younger and have earlier stage disease. However, in contrast to colorectal cancer, no evidence of improved prognosis was seen in this subset of patients.

A major role in the progression of carcinoma of the small bowel is played by p53 as well with its expression more frequently associated with poorly differentiated carcinoma (Nishiyama *et al.*, 2002). K-ras mutation is common as well and its incidence is considered to be comparable to that in colon cancer (Overman *et al.*, 2010; Younes *et al.*, 1997). A recent attempt at characterizing the tumor genetics and epigenetics showed that chromosomal instable tumor was associated with high frequency of K-ras mutation (55%) as compared to microsatellite and chromosomally stable tumor (10%). This inverse relationship between K-ras mutation and microsatellite instability is similar to that seen in colon cancer (Wade *et al.*, 2001). Mutation in APC has also been demonstrated but unlike colon cancer, these are uncommon in small bowel adenocarcinoma.

Though the exact reason behind such discrepancies between small and large bowel cancer incidence remains unclear, a number of possible theories have been entertained. It is thought that the rapid turnover time of cells in small intestine results in shedding of cells prior to accumulation of genetic damage conferring a relative protection to the small bowel from development of cancer (Michael, 2009). In a study carried out by Gao and Wang, a significantly higher level of enterocyte apoptosis was noted for normal small intestine tissue as compared to normal colonic tissue and small intestinal adenocarcinoma tissue. The median apoptotic index for each of the three was 15.2%, 1.6% and 0.1% respectively. In their study, a similar pattern was also observed for the expression level of pro-apoptotic molecule BAX (77.5% v/s 53.3% and 28.6% respectively). For the expression level of BCL-2, an anti-apoptotic molecule, no difference was observed (Chun & Ai-Ying, 2009). Also if one takes into account the physiologic characteristic of the small intestine, its dilute alkaline environment, lack of bacterial degradation activity, and rapid transit time, the actual exposure time to carcinogens present in the diet is relatively very limited compared to colon. It is considered that a changed micro-ecology of colon is responsible for an enhanced metabolic activation of ingested as well as endogenously formed pro-carcinogenic substrates. It is also hypothesized that small intestinal enterocytes may have inherent resistance to the development of APC mutation leading to subsequently low rate of adenoma formation (Michael, 2009; Miyaki *et al.*, 1994).

Regardless, understanding the pathogenesis of this rare tumor requires further insight into its molecular abnormalities and carcinogenesis. This is of utmost importance especially given its poor prognosis. Recently with improved imaging modalities and a trend towards newer chemotherapeutic agents, the management of small bowel adenocarcinoma has changed.

# 4  Epidemiology

Demographic and geographic patterns of small bowel adenocarcinoma show a correlation between the incidence rates of small bowel and colon cancer, suggesting that the two cancers share some common risk factors (Haselkorn *et al.*, 2005; Sai & Howard, 2001).

Small bowel cancer incidence in the U.S. and Western Europe is higher compared to Asia as per international data (Curado *et al.*, 2007). One of the highest age-adjusted incidences of small bowel tumor worldwide is seen in U.S (Haselkorn *et al.*, 2005). A rise in the incidence rate is seen after the age of 40 with peaks noted in the seventh and eighth decades. Mean age of presentation is 65 years (Haselkorn *et al.*, 2005; Sai & Howard, 2001). Patients with predisposing conditions such as inflammatory bowel disease, HNPCC, FAP or celiac disease tend to present earlier. Incidence rate is higher among men than women. Higher incidence and mortality rate is also seen among U.S. black population in both men and women as compared to the Whites. The reason for differences in survival between U.S. black and white populations is largely unexplained.

# 5  Presentation and Diagnosis

In early stages of the disease, patients are usually asymptomatic or present with very nonspecific symptoms which are often overlooked by not only the patient but by the physician as well. Diagnostic delay has been noted in many studies ranging from months to years with an average delay of approximately 6 – 8 months (Michael, 2009; Zollinger *et al.*, 1986; Bauer *et al.*, 1994; Holzheimer & Mannick, 2001). The most common presenting symptom of vague abdominal pain is often misdiagnosed as neurotic or having irritable bowel syndrome (Holzheimer & Mannick, 2001). Hence, a high index of suspicion is required for diagnosis given its nonspecific presenting symptoms.

Ninety percent of patients become symptomatic after the seventh decade of life. A retrospective case series of 129 patients by Talamonti *et al* showed abdominal pain as the most common symptom followed by vomiting, weight loss and Gastro intestinal tract bleeding (Talamonti *et al.*, 2002). This distribution however included subtypes of adenocarcinoma, carcinoid, lymphoma, and sarcoma. (Table1).

Metastasis to the small bowel is also seen and mainly originates from ovary, colon, lung, and kidney malignancies. Metastatic spread is via intraperitoneal and hematogenous routes.

One of the main reasons behind the delay in diagnosis is inaccessibility of the small bowel to endoscopic examination especially distal to duodenum. Examination of the entire small bowel has always remained a challenge. Plain radiographs do not detect these tumors clearly unless an obstruction is present. Small bowel barium follow-through series was somewhat considered to be the radiographic gold standard with few retrospective studies showing a sensitivity of approximately 60% in diagnosis of advanced stage disease with majority being duodenal tumor. For jejunal and ileal lesions,the sensitivity drops down to 20% – 30% (Michael J, 2009; Bauer *et al.*, 1994; Bessette *et al.*, 1989). However, the sen-

| Symptom/signs | All patients (%) |
|---|---|
| Abdominal pain | 81 |
| Vomiting | 62 |
| Weight Loss | 57 |
| GI Bleed | 30 |
| Diarrhea | 26 |
| Mass | 36 |
| Acute abdomen | 28 |
| Carcinoid syndrome | 9 |

**Table 1**: Common Symptoms/ Signs of Small Bowel Cancer

sitivity of barium small bowel series is increased by enteroclysis, which involves infusion of contrast enema directly in the small intestine via a nasogastric tube, followed by compression radiographs of each segment (Maglinte *et al*., 1984).

Computerized Tomography (CT) and Magnetic Resonance Imaging (MRI) are mainly useful as adjunct studies and are more helpful in assessing the extent of loco-regional nodal spread and metastatic disease. Their role in identifying primary lesions is limited with some retrospective studies showing an overall staging accuracy of 45% when compared to surgical intra-operative reports; sensitivity ranges from 0% to 58% for stage 1 to stage 4 respectively (Bucklet *et al*., 1997; Laurent *et al*., 1995). Their diagnostic yield is further increased by contrast enterography where instead of a naso-enteric tube, a high volume of neutral oral contrast is ingested. An added advantage of CT/MRI imaging compared to other modalities is the detection of extra-intestinal abnormalities (Figure 2 and Figure 3).

As mentioned earlier, small bowel cancer distal to duodenum is relatively inaccessible to an endoscopic exam unlike gastric and colon cancer, which are amenable to endoscopic biopsy. The length of small bowel can measure up to 575 cm and along with its tortuous anatomy, multiple complex loop configurations, continues to be a considerable challenge for an endoscopic exam. Push enteroscopy examines the small bowel with a long enteroscope and is generally only capable of visualizing proximal small bowel, mainly jejunum to a level of 40 – 100 cm past ligament of treitz (Sturniolo *et al*., 2005; Lida *et al*., 1986). Newer techniques, such as double balloon endoscopy and wireless capsule endoscopy, have considerably improved visualization of the small bowel in the last decade.

Double balloon endoscopy involves an endoscope and an over tube, (a tube that fits over the endoscope) with balloon attached to both. Using a push and pull technique, the small intestine is pleated onto the over tube allowing insertion of the endoscope deep into the intestine. An advantage of double balloon endoscopy over capsule endoscopy is that it offers the possibility of biopsy and polyp resection. However it is time consuming and is only available at specialized centers (May *et al*., 2003).

Capsule endoscopy is a procedure which can be done as an outpatient over a period of approximately 8 hours. It requires the ingestion of a pill that contains a tiny camera and is capable of acquiring approximately 50,000 images. These images are then collected on a digital recording device. The wireless capsule endoscopy is simple and a non-invasive procedure that has allowed clinicians to visualize the entire small bowel and detect its pathology. Its role has primarily been in obscure GI bleeding evaluation. In a retrospective analysis of 562 patients conducted at New York's Mt Sinai Hospital, who underwent capsule endoscopy for various reasons (bleeding, abnormal imaging, etc), 50 patients (8.9%) were diagnosed with small bowel cancer. The rate rose to 13% for patients under 50 years of age (Cobrin *et al*.,

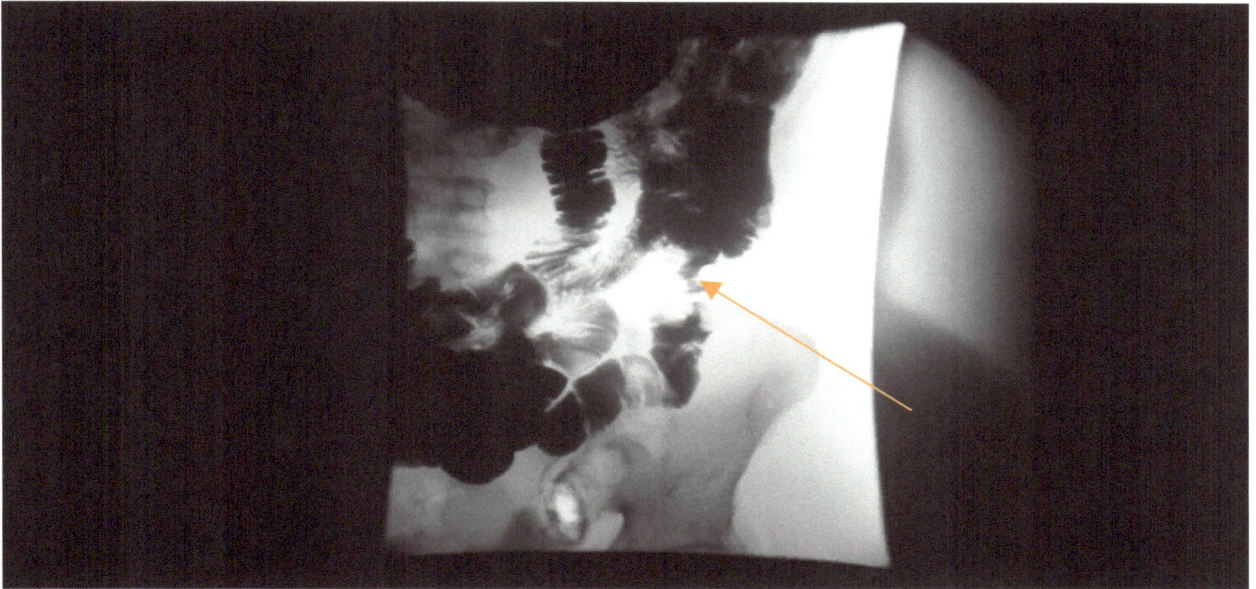

**Figure 2:** CT Scan with oral contrast showing irregular filling defect of the Jujenum secondary to Small Bowel Adenocarcinoma (Arrowindicating filling defect).

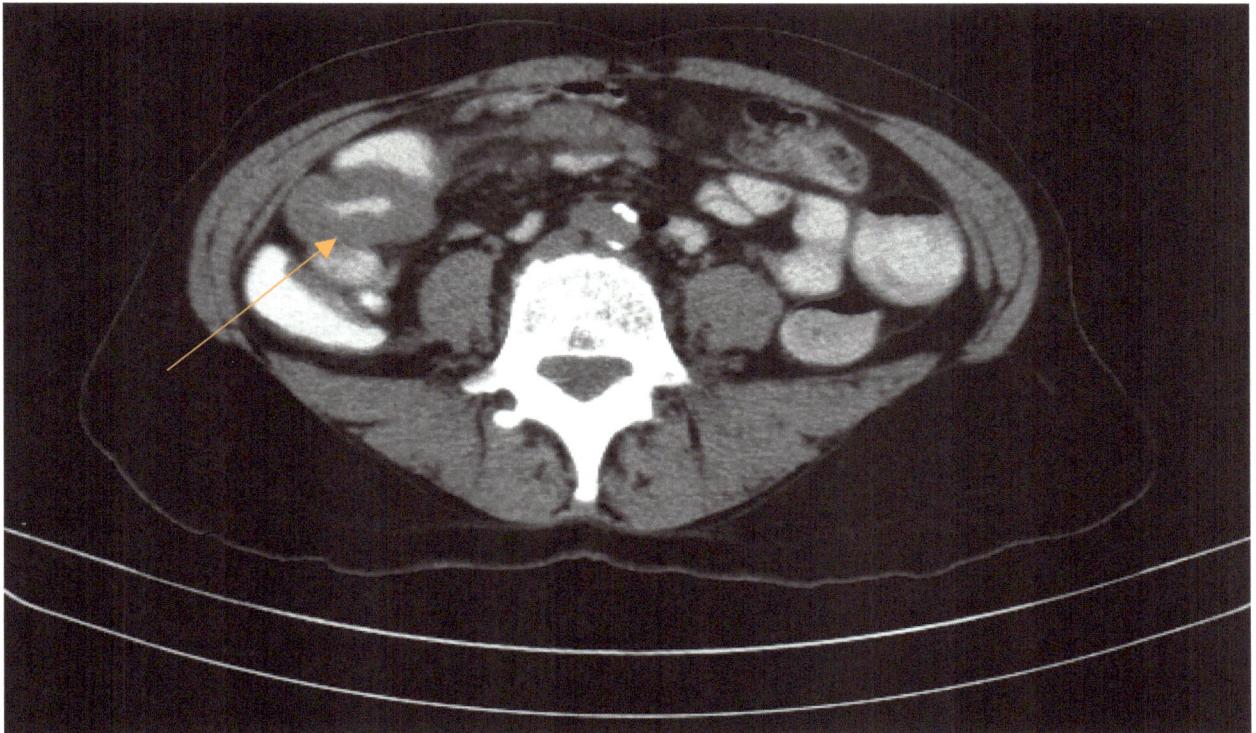

**Figure 3:** Small Bowel thickening suspicious of Small Bowel Cancer, later confirmed on biopsy (Indicated by arrow).

2006). In a review of prospectively collected data of 416 capsule endoscopies from three Australian centers, prior radiological exam had identified only 6.3% of the 27 tumors picked up by capsule endoscopy (Bailey *et al.*, 2006). Another study involving capsule endoscopy evaluation in patients with suspected small bowel cancer and without any gastrointestinal bleeding showed a diagnostic yield of about 62%(Sturniolo *et al.*, 2005). One of the complications of this procedure is retention of the capsule which can occur at the pathologic site. Capsule endoscopy can miss small lesions due to improper bowel preparation, presence of blood in the lumen, or rapidity of transit time. Both double balloon and capsule endoscopy have their unique advantages and should be used in a complementary manner.

Endoscopic ultrasound (EUS) has not been directly studied, but it can be very useful in assessing the nodal status and depth of invasion of the tumor especially in the cases of duodenal adenocarcinomas (Michael JO, 2009; Oh *et al.*, 2005). Though, with the advent of these newer techniques the work up for small bowel cancer has changed, the algorithm used in clinical practice depends largely on the availability of these modalities at individual institutions.

# 6   Staging

The staging system for small bowel cancer is mainly from American Joint Committee on Cancer (AJCC) utilizing TNM staging system (Table 2). These cancers are typically advanced at the time of diagnosis. The grading system includes grade I (well differentiated ~ 0% – 42%) grade II (moderately differentiated 24% – 45%) and grade III (poorly differentiated 34% – 42%) (Howe *et al.*, 1999; Wade *et al.*, 2001).

According to the National Cancer Data Base, the distribution of presenting stage is 12% in stage I, 30% in stage II, 26% in stage III, and 32% in stage IV (Bilimoria *et al.*, 2009).

# 7   Treatment

The only hope of cure for patients with this disease is with surgical intervention. One of the most important prognostic factors for survival is the ability to completely resect the disease. In most studies, surgical intervention provides a curative resection in 40% – 65% of patients with a 5 year survival rate of 40% – 60% for resected tumor as compared to only 15% – 30% for non-resected tumor. In a retrospective study conducted at M.D. Anderson institute of 217 patients, 146 patients underwent cancer directed surgery (including whipple procedure) as their primary definitive surgery. In a multivariate analysis of the study, surgical resection and lymph node involvement ratio (percentage of total lymph nodes removed with cancer involvement) were the only independent predictors of overall survival (OS) (Dabaja *et al.*, 2004). 5 year overall survival for stage IV disease was significantly shorter compared to stage I-III disease (5% vs. 36%). Also the 5 year OS was significantly shorter for LN involvement ratio of greater than75% as compared to those with less than 75% (12% vs. 51%).

Another study of 80 patients from Taiwan reported a similar experience. Out of 60 patients who underwent surgical resection, 45 had resection with curative intent. The cumulative 1, 3, and 5 year survival rates for all patients compared to those who underwent resection with curative intent (43.6% vs. 54.9%, 22.8% vs. 30.5%, and 17.5% vs. 27.4% respectively) again demonstrated earlier tumor stage and curative resection as two independent factors favoring overall survival. In patients who underwent resec-

| TNM staging for adenocarcinoma of the small intestine | | | |
|---|---|---|---|
| **Primary tumor (T)** | | | |
| TX | Primary tumor cannot be assessed | | |
| T0 | No evidence of primary tumor | | |
| Tis | Carcinoma in situ | | |
| T1 | Tumor invades lamina propria or submucosa | | |
| T2 | Tumor invades muscularispropria | | |
| T3 | Tumor invades through muscularispropria into the subserosa or into the nonperitonealizedperimuscular tissue (mesentery or retroperitoneum) with extension 2 cm or less* | | |
| T4 | Tumor perforates the visceral peritoneum or directly invades other organs or structures (includes other loops of small intestine, mesentery, or retroperitoneum more than 2 cm, and abdominal wall by way of serosa; for duodenum only, invasion of pancreas) | | |
| **Regional lymph nodes** | | | |
| NX | Regional lymph nodes cannot be assessed | | |
| N0 | No regional lymph node metastasis | | |
| N1 | Regional lymph node metastasis | | |
| **Distant metastasis** | | | |
| MX | Distant metastasis cannot be assessed | | |
| M0 | No distant metastasis | | |
| M1 | Distant metastasis | | |
| **Stage grouping** | | | |
| Stage 0 | Tis | N0 | M0 |
| Stage I | T1 | N0 | M0 |
| | T2 | N0 | M0 |
| Stage II | T3 | N0 | M0 |
| | T4 | N0 | M0 |
| Stage III | Any T | N1 | M1 |
| Stage IV | Any T | Any N | M1 |

*The peritonealizedperimuscular tissue is for the jejunum and ileum, part of the mesentery; and for duodenum in areas where serosa is lacking, part of the retroperitoneum

**Table 2:** TNM Staging (adapted from AJCC Cancer Staging Manual, Sixth Edition).

tion with curative intent, lymph node involvement was the only predictive factor of poor disease free survival (Wu *et al.*, 2006).

Analysis of Surveillance Epidemiology and End Results (SEER) database on the impact of lymph nodes evaluation on the survival of patients with small bowel adenocarcinoma who undergo curative resection was presented in 2009. The database identified patient's aged 18 – 90 years with small intestinal adenocarcinoma from 1988 to 2005. The total number of lymph nodes assessed considerably influenced survival of stage I, II, III adenocarcinoma. The survival of patients with stage I/II disease (*n* = 1,216 from a total of 1991) was dependent upon the total number of lymph nodes assessed. Stage II 5-year disease specific survival was 66%, 82%, and 88% for 1 – 8, 9 – 12, and more than 12 lymph nodes examined, respectively. For stage III disease (n=775), the optimal cut point of positive lymph nodes was 3. The 5 year disease specific survival for < 3 compared to > 3 positive lymph nodes was 58% vs. 37% (Overman *et al.*, 2009).

The primary modality of treatment is also significantly influenced by primary tumor site. Tumors in distally located adenocarcinoma (jejunum, ileum) are more amenable to surgical resection than duodenal adenocarcinoma (83% vs. 57%) (Bailey *et al.*, 2006). Presence of extensive local disease or metastases to multiple regional/distant lymph nodes and/or other organs/peritoneum renders them surgically unresectable. These surgeries include whipple procedure and wide local excision (WLE) with lymphadenectomy for tumors of jejunum and proximal ileum. Ileocolectomy may be required for distal ileal lesions (Bauer *et al.*, 1994; Frost *et al.*, 1994; Dabaja *et al.*, 2004).

Compared to jejunum and ileum adenocarcinoma, duodenal adenocarcinoma has a higher loco-regional failure rate. One study reported a loco-regional failure rate of 39% with positive margin status as a strong predictor of recurrence (Kelsey *et al.*, 2007; Overman, 2009).

# 8   Adjuvant Therapy

Due to the rarity of this disease, large case studies and randomized trials are very difficult to perform and frankly not feasible. Most of the data available are in the form of retrospective studies mainly from single institution reports and hence subject to selection bias.

At present, data on adjuvant chemotherapy is limited and unconvincing. Due to the similarities and multiple parallels recognized by clinicians, epidemiologists, and geneticists between large and small bowel cancer (as mentioned earlier) similar adjuvant therapeutic approach has been adopted for small bowel cancer by clinicians in current practice. Among the majority of the studies reported to date, 5-FU is the most commonly used agent and remains the mainstay of treatment. Newer agents such as irinotecan (CPT-11), used as second line treatment for colon cancer, are also considered for refractory cases of small bowel adenocarcinoma.

Despite the lack of randomized trials to clearly demonstrate the supporting role of adjuvant chemotherapy, its use has only increased as projected by National Cancer Data Base (8.1% to 23.8% from 1985 to 2005) (Bilimoria *et al.*, 2009). It is likely that the clinical decision-making by the physician for patients with small bowel adenocarcinoma is influenced by the proven benefit of adjuvant chemotherapy in colorectal cancer. Patients with positive lymph node involvement after curative resection for small bowel adenocarcinoma exhibit a higher risk of recurrence with 5 years survival rate of only 22% – 27% (Oh *et al.*, 2005; Talamonti *et al.*, 2002) clearly emphasizing the role of adjuvant chemotherapy in these patients. Moreover, despite the lack of clear-cut evidence, the primarily distant failure pattern of small bowel adenocarcinoma further strengthens the argument for use of chemotherapy in adjuvant settings especially given the marked improvement in the activity seen with the combination of oxaliplatin with 5-FU in colon cancer.

Dabaja *et al.* (2004) conducted a retrospective study of 217 patients at M.D. Anderson Institute. Out of 217 patients with small bowel adenocarcinoma (registered between 1978 and 1998), adjuvant chemotherapy was administered to only 59 (27%) patients as compared to 62 patients who did not receive chemotherapy post resection. In a multivariate analysis of the study, patients receiving chemotherapy had no survival benefit. However this study did not describe the type of chemotherapy given.

Another retrospective study of 113 patients from Princess Margaret Hospital also was inconclusive regarding the role of adjuvant chemotherapy. However, it was noted by authors that chemotherapy was more likely to be offered to patients with worse prognostic factors (Fishman *et al.*, 2006).

Small bowel cancer is generally considered to be resistant to radiotherapy. However role of radiation, as an adjuvant therapy was evaluated in a limited way by European Organization for Research and Treatment of Cancer (EORTC). In this prospective phase III study, concurrent radiation with 5-FU as an adjuvant therapy was evaluated in patients with pancreatic and periampullary carcinoma (which included adenocarcinoma of the bile duct, duodenum, and ampulla of vater). There was no difference in the 5-year survival rate when compared to observation alone group (Klinkenbijl *et al.*, 1999).

Duke University investigators reported a study of 32 patients (between 1975 to 2005) undergoing potentially curative treatment for duodenal adenocarcinoma. Surgery alone was compared with surgery and concurrent chemotherapy with radiation (either pre-operatively or post-operatively). Chemotherapy was mainly with 5-FU. Five-year survival did not differ between the two groups (57% for chemo-radiation versus 44% for surgery, $p = 0.42$). However in patients with margin negative resection (R0), chemo-radiation appeared to improve five year overall survival (83% vs. 53%, $p = 0.07$). Two of the eleven patients (18%) who received pre-operative chemo-radiation had complete pathologic response (Kelsey *et al.*, 2007). A smaller study at Fox Chase Cancer Center evaluating the role of chemo-radiation (5-FU and mitomycin-C) in pancreatic and duodenal cancer also reported a complete pathologic response in four out of five patients with duodenal adenocarcinoma (Yeung *et al.*, 1993). In both studies, no lymph node involvement was seen at the time of surgical resection. However pretreatment radiographic description of the disease was not defined either.

As mentioned earlier, despite the lack of any concrete evidence, the use of adjuvant chemotherapy has increased in the last few decades and is likely to continue to rise given the current clinical practice trends, the pattern of distant disease recurrence and the adverse prognostic effect of lymph node involvement. Again, the rarity of the disease precludes the possibility of conducting a prospective randomized trial. However, more studies with larger data sets should be generated from multi- institutional collaboration in an attempt to characterize the role of adjuvant therapy and guide the treatment.

## 9    Palliative Chemotherapy

Though there are a number of retrospective analyses from various single-institution reports exhibiting a survival benefit with palliative chemotherapy (Dabaja *et al.*, 2004; Halfdanarson *et al.*, 2006; Fishman *et al.*, 2006), its role compared to best supportive care has not been evaluated in any randomized prospective trial. The majority of small bowel adenocarcinoma chemotherapy experience has been with 5-FU-based regimens. Newer agents evaluated thus far include irinotecan, platinum agents, and gemcitabine.

In one of the largest series reported by Fishman *et al.* from Princess Margaret Hospital, 44 patients who received palliative chemotherapy showed an overall response rate of 36% (9% complete response and 27% partial response) during first or second line regimen. Various chemotherapy regimens were used including irinotecan, gemcitabine, capecitabine, platinum agents, and 5-FU. Retrospective analysis showed a survival benefit in patients who received palliative chemotherapy compared to those who did not (18.6 mo vs. 13.4 mo) (Fishman *et al.*, 2006). Interestingly, it was noted that regimens including irinotecan, gemcitabine, or platinum agents had higher response rates compared to older fluorouracil regimen (42 – 50% vs. 0 – 13%).

In another retrospective study of 80 patients at MD Anderson Cancer Center (MDACC) conducted by Overman *et al.*, the combination of 5-FU with platinum agents (29 patients) was compared with 5-FU without a platinum compound (41 patients) and non 5-FU-based treatment (10 patients). Treatment with

5-FU and platinum agents resulted in a higher response rate compared to other regimens (41% vs. 16%) and a longer median progression free survival (8.7 months vs. 3.9 months) (Overman *et al.*, 2008).

To date, only two prospective studies have been conducted on this relatively rare tumor. One of the two prospective studies conducted on this tumor evaluated CAPOX in patients with advanced adenocarcinoma of small bowel or ampullary origin. Overman *et al.* conducted a single institution phase II study at MDACC in an attempt to evaluate capecitabine in combination with oxaliplatin (CAPOX) in patients with locally advanced or metastatic adenocarcinoma of small bowel or ampullary origin. The primary end point of the study was overall response rate as assessed by the RECIST criteria. Out of 30 patients who received study treatment, overall response rate (ORR) was confirmed in 50% of patients with median time to progression of 11.4 months and median overall survival of 20.4 months. A durable complete response rate of 10% was also observed. The median time to progression and overall survival in patients with metastatic disease (n=25) was 9.4 months and 15.5 months respectively. Patients with small bowel adenocarcinoma only (n=18) had a response rate of 61% (Overman *et al.*, 2009). This study showed a superior outcome with CAPOX compared to other regimens in literature.

The second study was a multicenter study conducted by ECOG in patients with adenocarcinoma of small bowel or ampulla of vater. Between 1983 and 1985, 39 patients with advanced and recurrent disease were enrolled. Chemotherapy with combination of 5-FU, doxorubicin, and mitomycin C (FAM) was administered. An overall response rate of 18.4% with median overall survival of 8 months was observed (Gibson *et al.*, 2005).

Irinotecan, which is used as a second line in colon cancer, has also shown efficacy in case series as a salvage therapy in patients refractory to 5-FU (Polyzos *et al.*, 2003). A recent case report showed a complete response to FOLFIRI regimen in a patient with FOLFOX refractory metastatic duodenal adenocarcinoma (Catania *et al.*, 2010). Data collected at a single institute over a 9 year period was reviewed to assess the efficacy of 5-FU and either platinum compound or irinotecan. The overall response rate with 5-FU combined with carboplatin, cisplatin or oxaliplatin was 21% with median progression free and overall survival of 8 and 14 months respectively. 5-FU with irinotecan used as second line chemotherapy in patients who progressed on 5-FU and a platinum agent resulted in disease stablization in 4 of 8 patients (50%) with median progression free survival of 5 months (Locher *et al.*, 2005). Another retrospective study reported response in 5 of 12 patients with irinotecan-based therapy such as FOLFIRI, XELIRI, or single agent irinotecan. Gemcitabine is another chemotherapy agent to have demonstrated some activity in this tumor. Response was seen in 4 of 8 patients (50%) with the combination of gemcitabine and 5-FU (Fishman *et al.*, 2006) and one of two patients with single agent gemcitabine in the refractory setting (Overman *et al.*, 2008).

Locally advanced, inoperable or metastatic small bowel adenocarcinoma shows survival benefit with systemic chemotherapy unlike the unproven role in adjuvant setting. Response rates and median survival have ranged from 6-61% and 14 to 20 months respectively (Overman *et al.*, 2008; Overman *et al.*, 2009; Locher *et al.*, 2005; Zaanan *et al.*, 2009; Ono *et al.*, 2008).

The role of targeted therapies such as anti-vascular endothelial growth factor receptor (VEGFR) and anti-epidermal growth factor receptor (EGFR) has not been studied so far in small bowel adenocarcinoma. In an attempt to better understand the molecular abnormalities, Overman *et al.* conducted one of the largest clinico pathologicstudies of small bowel adenocarcinoma, providing a robust immunophenotypic characterization and molecular expression of various oncogenic pathways in 54 patients. Loss of mismatch repair protein (MMR) was seen in 35% of patients, confirmed with MSI PCR in all tested cases. EGFR expression was present in 71% of cases, similar to the rate of expression seen in colorectal cancer. VEGF expression was also seen in 91% of patients (Overman *et al.*, 2010). This high rate of expression of EGFR and VEGFR in patients with small bowel adenocarcinoma provides strong support to the idea of further clinical investigations into the therapies particularly targeted at these oncogenic pathways.

Few case series reported to date have shown benefit of anti-EGFR therapy in patients with small bowel adenocarcinoma, especially those harboring the K-ras wild type. In one case report, disease stabilization with clinical benefits was achieved with addition of cetuximab to irinotecan as a third line regimen (De Dosso *et al.*, 2010). Similar benefit has been reported in case studies by other institutions as well (Santini *et al.*, 2010; Poddar *et al.*, 2011). Unlike anti-EGFR therapy, anti-VEGF agents have not been studied in this rare tumor. Bevacizumab is a humanized monoclonal antibody targeted against VEGF and is routinely used in colorectal cancer. A recent single case report showed impressive palliation result achieved in a patient with advanced small bowel adenocarcinoma treated with bevacizumab in conjunction with gemcitabine and oxaliplatin and then maintained on bevacizumab and capecitabine (Tsang *et al.*, 2008).

# 10    Follow up and Recurrence

There are no standard guidelines for follow up schedule in small bowel adenocarcinoma. Plans are usually devised based on the individual situation. Recurrence rates are as high as 39% even after curative resection, thus emphasizing the importance of close follow-up (Tomoki *et al*, 2010). Follow-up visits generally are scheduled 3 months or less initially. Routine blood work such as CBC and chemistry including liver function tests are obtained along with history and physical on every visit. Tumor marker carcinoembryonic antigen (CEA) is also followed serially depending on patient's symptoms. Imaging and procedures such as CT and endoscopy are done if there is suspicion of recurrence.Fordistant recurrence, treatment options are usually based on clinical experience from colon cancer and include chemotherapy or biologic agents in combination with chemotherapy as reported in few case reports. For locally recurrent small bowel adenocarcinoma, treatment options may include surgery, radiation and chemotherapy.

# 11    Prognosis

The overall 5-year survival rate for adenocarcinoma of the small bowel ranges from 15 – 30%. For surgically resectable cancer studies have shown 5-year survival rate of 40 – 60%. Prognosis is dismal in cases of unresectable tumor. 5 year disease specific survival by stage as reported by National Cancer Data Base (from 1985 – 1995) was 65% for stage I, 48%stage II, 35% for stage III and 4% for stage IV (Overman, 2009; Wu *et al.*, 2006).

Factors associated with poor prognosis are advanced disease stage, elderly age, poor histological differentiation, positive margins and duodenal primary (Overman, 2009). Duodenal adenocarcinoma is associated with higher loco-regional failure rate. Median OS is shorter for patients with duodenal adenocarcinoma when compared with jejunum and ileum tumor (18 monthsvs. 26 months) (Dabaja *et al.*, 2004). The reason for poorer outcome for patients with duodenal adenocarcinoma is unclear. Whether it is related to its complex retroperitoneal anatomy or different intrinsic tumor biology is not known. Predisposing conditions such as crohn's disease and pathologic evidence of vascular invasion is also associated with worse outcomes.

The primary pattern of failure in small bowel adenocarcinoma is predominantly systemic. Among patients with Stage IV, liver is the most common site of metastasis (59%) followed by carcinomatosis (25%), pelvis (9%) and lungs (4%). Metastasis to brain is infrequent (Dabaja *et al.*, 2004).

## 12   Summary

The small bowel comprises most of the length of the entire alimentary tract (approximately 75%). However, the incidence of small bowel adenocarcinoma is about 50-fold less than that of colon adenocarcinoma. The specific reason behind this disparity remains unclear though many theories are entertained regarding its distinct physiology.

Though newer techniques such as double balloon enteroscopy and wireless capsule endoscopy have facilitated the diagnostic work-up for small bowel pathology, examination of the entire length of small intestine remains a considerable challenge. Both clinicians and patients often overlook its vague and non-specific symptoms, leading to delays in diagnosis.

Curative resection remains the only hope for long-term survival in these patients. Lymphovascular invasion and a positive surgical margin are predictors of loco-regional recurrence and poor outcome.

Due to the lack of randomized prospective trials, the role of adjuvant therapy has not been clearly outlined. Multiple single institutional analyses have suggested a role of 5-FU-based therapy. Most of the decisions in clinical practice are influenced by the proven benefit of adjuvant therapy in colorectal cancer.

Encouraging median survival data are seen with palliative chemotherapy for patients with advanced disease. 5FU infusional and capecitabine combination regimen appears to be the most active in this disease and should be considered as first line therapy. Other agents such as irinotecan and gemcitabine have been tried as salvage therapy.

Targeted therapy has not been evaluated in small bowel adenocarcinoma. Randomized prospective controlled trials are warranted to ascertain the role of biological agents in patients with this rare tumor.

## References

Bailey, A.A., Debinski, H.S., Appleyard, M.N., Remedios, M.L., Hooper, J.E., Walsh, A.J.&Selby, W.S. Diagnosis and outcome of small bowel tumors found by capsule endoscopy: a three-center Australian experience.Am J Gastroenterol. 2006 Oct;101(10):2237-43.

Bauer, R. L., Palmer, M. L., Bauer, A. M., Nava, H. R. & Douglass, H. O. Adenocarcinoma of the small intestine: 21-year review of diagnosis, treatment, and prognosis. Ann SurgOncol. (1994);1(3):183–188.

Bessette, J.R., Maglinte, D.D., Kelvin, F.M.&Chernish, S.M. Primary malignant tumors in the small bowel: a comparison of the small-bowel enema and conventional follow-through examination. AJR Am J Roentgenol. 1989 Oct;153(4):741-4.

Bilimoria, K.Y., Bentrem, D.J., Wayne J.D., Ko, C.Y., Bennett, C.L.&Talamonti, M.S.Small bowel cancer in the United States: changes in epidemiology, treatment, and survival over the last 20 years. Ann Surg. 2009 Jan; 249(1):63-71.

Bläker, H., Von, H. A., Penzel, R., Gross, S.&Otto, H.F.Genetics of adenocarcinomas of the small intestine: frequent deletions at chromosome 18q and mutations of the SMAD4 gene.Oncogene. 2002 Jan 3;21(1):158-64.

Brueckl, W.M., Heinze, E., Milsmann, C., Wein, A., Koebnick, C., Jung, A., Croner, R.S., Brabletz, T., Günther, K., Kirchner, T., Hahn, E.G., Hohenberger, W., Becker, H.&Reingruber, B. Prognostic significance of microsatellite instability in curatively resected adenocarcinoma of the small intestine.Cancer Lett. 2004 Jan 20;203(2):181-90.

Buckley, J. A., Siegelman, S. S., Jones, B. & Fishman, E. K. The accuracy of CT staging of small bowel adenocarcinoma: CT/Pathologic correlation. J Comp Ass Tomo. (1997);21:986–991.

Catania, C., Pelosi, G., Fazio, N., Biffi, R., Spitaleri, G., Noberasco, C., Zampino, M.G., Maggioni, A., Trifirò, G., Toffalorio, F., Vigna, PD., De Braud, F.&De Pas, T. A FOLFIRI-induced complete tumor response in a patient with FOLFOX-refractory metastatic duodenal adenocarcinoma.ActaOncol. 2010;49(1):120-1.

Chow, J.S., Chen, C.C., Ahsan, H. &Neugut, A.I. A population-based study of the incidence of malignant small bowel tumours: SEER, 1973–1990. Int J Epidemiol 1996;25:722-8.

Cobrin, G.M., Pittman, R.H.&Lewis, B.S. Increased diagnostic yield of small bowel tumors with capsule endoscopy.Cancer. 2006 Jul 1;107(1):22-7.

Cross, A.J., Leitzmann, M.F., Subar, A.F.,et al.A prospective study of meat and fat intake in relation to small intestinal cancer.Cancer Res. 2008;68:9274–9279.

Curado, M.P., Edwards, B., Shin, H.R., Storm, H., Ferlay, J., Heanue, M. & Boyle, P.Cancer Incidence in Five Continents Vol. IX. Lyon: IARC, IARC Scientific Publication, No. 160; 2007.

Dabaja, B.S., Suki, D., Pro, B., Bonnen, M.&Ajani, J. Adenocarcinoma of the small bowel: presentation, prognostic factors, and outcome of 217 patients.Cancer. 2004 Aug 1;101(3):518-26.

De Dosso, S., Molinari, F., Martin, V., Frattini, M.&Saletti, P. Molecular characterisation and cetuximab-based treatment in a patient with refractory small bowel adenocarcinoma.Gut. 2010 Nov;59(11):1587-8.

DeSesso, J.M. & Jacobson, C.F. (2001).Anatomical and physiological parameters affecting gastrointestinal physiological parameters affecting gastrointestinal absorption in humans and rats.Food ChemToxicol39:209–228.

Fishman, P. N., Pond, G.R., Moore, M.J., et al. (2006). Natural history and chemotherapy effectiveness for advanced adenocarcinoma of the small bowel: a retrospective review of 113 cases. Am J ClinOncol29:225–231.

Frequent genetic instability in small intestinal carcinomas.Jpn J Cancer Res. 1995 Apr;86(4):357-60.

Frost, D. B., Mercado, P. D. & Tyrell, J. S. Small bowel cancer: a 30-year review. Ann SurgOncol. (1994);1(4):290–295.

Gao, C. & Wang, Ai-Ying.,Significance of Increased Apoptosis and Bax Expression in Human Small Intestinal Adenocarcinoma.J HistochemCytochem. 2009 December; 57(12): 1139–1148.

Gibson, M.K., Holcroft, C.A., Kvols, L.K., et al. Phase II study of 5-fluorouracil, doxorubicin, and mitomycin C for metastatic small bowel adenocarcinoma.Oncologist. 2005;10:132–137.

Halfdanarson, T., Quevedo, F. & McWilliams, R.R. Small bowel adenocarcinoma: A review of 491 cases. J ClinOncol. 2006;24:209. (abstr 4127)

Halfdanarson, T., Quevedo, F., McWilliams, R.R., et al. (2006): Small bowel adenocarcinoma: A review of 491cases. J ClinOncol24:209, (abstr 4127).

Hamilton, S.R. &Aaltonen, L.A. World Health Organization Classification of Tumours.Pathology and Genetics of Tumours of the Digestive System. Chapter 4; Lyon: IARC Press; 2000. pp. 69–92.

Haselkorn, T., Whittemore, A.S. &Lilienfeld, D.E.(2005). Incidence of small bowel cancer in the United States and worldwide: geographic, temporal, and racial differences. Cancer Causes Control;16:781–787.

Hibi, K., Kondo, K., Akiyama, S., Ito, K.&Takagi, H.

Holzheimer, R.G., &Mannick, J.A., editors.Surgical Treatment: Evidence-Based and Problem-Oriented. Part III Adenocarcinoma of the small bowel. Alfred I Neugut, M.D., Michael R Marvin, Ph.D., M.D., and John A Chabot, M.D.Munich: Zuckschwerdt; 2001.

Howe, J.R., Karnell, L.H. & Scott-Conner, C. Small bowel sarcoma: analysis of survival from the National Cancer Data Base. Ann SurgOncol. 2001;8:496–508.

Howe, J.R., Karnell, L.H., Menck, H.R.,et al. The American College of Surgeons Commission on Cancer and the American Cancer Society. Adenocarcinoma of the small bowel: review of the National Cancer Data Base, 1985–1995. Cancer. 1999;86:2693–2706.

Howlader, N., Noone, A.M., Krapcho, M., Neyman, N., Aminou, R., Altekruse, S.F., Kosary, C.L., Ruhl, J., Tatalovich, Z., Cho, H., Mariotto, A., Eisner, M.P., Lewis, D.R., Chen, H.S., Feuer, E.J. & Cronin, K.A. (eds). SEER Cancer Statistics Review, 1975-2009 (Vintage 2009 Populations), National Cancer Institute. Bethesda, MD.

Katz, S.C. &DeMatteo, R.P. Gastrointestinal stromal tumors and leiomyosarcomas.J SurgOncol. 2008;97:350–359.

Kelsey, C.R., Nelson, J.W., Willett, C.G., Chino, J.P., Clough, R.W., Bendell, J.C., Tyler, D.S., Hurwitz, H.I., Morse, M.A., Clary, B.M., Pappas, T.N.&Czito, B.G. Duodenal adenocarcinoma: patterns of failure after resection and the role of chemoradiotherapy.Int J RadiatOncolBiol Phys. 2007 Dec 1;69(5):1436-41.

Klinkenbijl, J.H., Jeekel, J., Sahmoud, T., Van Pel, R., Couvreur, M.L., Veenhof, C.H., Arnaud, J.P., Gonzalez, D.G., de Wit, L.T., Hennipman, A.&Wils, J. Adjuvant radiotherapy and 5-fluorouracil after curative resection of cancer of the pancreas and periampullary region: phase III trial of the EORTC gastrointestinal tract cancer cooperative group. Ann Surg. 1999 Dec;230(6):776-82; discussion 782-4.

Laurent, F., Drouillard, J., Lecesne, R. &Bruneton, J. CT of small-bowel neoplasms.Semin Ultrasound, CT MRI. (1995);16(2):102–111.

Lida, M., Yamamoto, T., Yao, T., Fuchigami, T. &Fujishima, M. Jejunal endoscopy using a long duodenofiberscope.GastrointestEndosc. (1986);32:233–236.

Locher, C., Malka, D., Boige, V., et al. Combination chemotherapy in advanced small bowel adenocarcinoma. Oncology. 2005;69:290–294.

Lowenfels AB. Why are small-bowel tumours so rare? Lancet 1973; 1:24-6.

Maglinte, D. T., Hall, R., Miller, R. E., Chernish, S. M., Rosenak, B., Elmore, M. & Burney, B. T. Detection of surgical lesions of the small bowel by enteroclysis. Am J Surg. (1984);147:225–229.

May, A., Nachbar, L., Wardak, A., Yamamoto, H., &Ell, C. Double-balloon enteroscopy: preliminary experience in patients with obscure gastrointestinal bleeding or chronic abdominal pain.Endoscopy. 2003 Dec;35(12):985-91.

Miyaki, M., Konishi, M., Kikuchi-Yanoshita, R., Enomoto, M., Igari, T., Tanaka, K., Muraoka, M., Takahashi, H., Amada, Y., Fukayama, M., et al. Characteristics of somatic mutation of the adenomatous polyposis coli gene in colorectal tumors. Cancer Res. 1994 Jun 1;54(11):3011-20.

Nakamura, S., Matsumoto, T., Takeshita, M., Kurahara, K., Yao, T., Tsuneyoshi, M., Iida, M. &Fujishima, M. A. Clinicopathologic study of primary small intestine lymphoma: prognostic significance of mucosa-associated lymphoid tissue-derived lymphoma. Cancer. 2000;88:286–294.

Negri, E., Bosetti, C., La, V. C.,et al. Risk factors for adenocarcinoma of the small intestine. Int J Cancer. 1999;82:171–174.

Neugut, A.I.&Santos, J. Cancer Epidemiol Biomarkers Prev.The association between cancers of the small and large bowel.1993; Nov-Dec; 2(6):551-3.

Nishiyama, K., Yao, T., Yonemasu, H., Yamaguchi, K., Tanaka, M.&Tsuneyoshi, M.

Oh, Y.S., Early, D.S. &Azar, R.R. Clinical applications of endoscopic ultrasound to oncology.Oncology. 2005;68(4-6):526-37.

Ono, M., Shirao, K., Takashima, A., Morizane, C., Okita, N., Takahari, D., Hirashima, Y., Eguchi-Nakajima, T., Kato, K., Hamaguchi, T., Yamada, Y.&Shimada, Y. Combination chemotherapy with cisplatin and irinotecan in patients with adenocarcinoma of the small intestine.Gastric Cancer. 2008;11(4):201-5.

Ouriel, K. &Adams, J.T. (1984).Adenocarcinoma of the small intestine. Am J Surg; 147:66–71.

Overexpression of p53 protein and point mutation of K-ras genes in primary carcinoma of the small intestine.Oncol Rep. 2002 Mar-Apr;9(2):293-300.

Overman, M. J. Recent Advances in the Management of Adenocarcinoma of the Small Intestine.Gastrointest Cancer Res. 2009 May-Jun; 3(3): 90–96.

Overman, M. J., Hu, C., Wolff, R. A. & Chang G. J.; University of Texas M. D. Anderson Cancer Center, Houston, TX. 2009 ASCO Annual Meeting.Impact of lymph node evaluation on survival for small bowel adenocaricnoma: Analysis of the Surveillance, Epidemiology and End Results (SEER) database. J ClinOncol27:15s, 2009 (suppl; abstr 4596)

Overman, M.J., Kopetz, S., Wen S, et al. Chemotherapy with 5-fluorouracil and a platinum compound improves outcomes in metastatic small bowel adenocarcinoma. Cancer. 2008;113:2038– 2045.

Overman, M.J., Kopetz, S., Wen, S., et al. (2008). Chemotherapy with 5-fluorouracil and a platinum compound improves outcomes in metastatic small bowel adenocarcinoma. Cancer 113:2038-2045.

Overman, M.J., Pozadzides, J., Kopetz, S., Wen, S., Abbruzzese, J.L., Wolff, R.A.&Wang, H. Immunophenotype and molecular characterisation of adenocarcinoma of the small intestine.Br J Cancer. 2010 Jan 5;102(1):144-50.

Overman, M.J., Varadhachary, G.R., Kopetz, S., et al. Phase II study of capecitabine and oxaliplatin for advanced adenocarcinoma of the small bowel and ampulla of Vater.J ClinOncol. 2009

Perzin, K.H. &Bridge, M.F. Adenomas of the small intestine: a clinicopathologic review of 51 cases and a study of their relationship to carcinoma. 1981 Aug 1;48(3):799-819.

Planck, M., Ericson, K., Piotrowska, Z., Halvarsson, B., Rambech, E.&Nilbert, M. Department of Oncology, University Hospital, Lund, Sweden.Microsatellite instability and expression of MLH1 and MSH2 in carcinomas of the small intestine.Cancer. 2003 Mar 15;97(6):1551-7.

Poddar , N. , Raza, S., Sharma, B., Liu, M., Gohari, A.&Kalavar, M. Small Bowel Adenocarcinoma Presenting with Refractory Iron Deficiency Anemia – Case Report and Review of Literature. Case Rep Oncol. 2011 Sep-Dec; 4(3): 458–463.

Polyzos, A., Kouraklis, G., Giannopoulos, A., Bramis, J., Delladetsima, J.K.&Sfikakis PP.Irinotecan as salvage chemotherapy for advanced small bowel adenocarcinoma: a series of three patients.J Chemother. 2003 Oct;15(5):503-6.

Rashid, A., &Hamilton, S.R.Genetic alterations in sporadic and Crohn's-associated adenocarcinomas of the small intestine.Gastroenterology. 1997 Jul;113(1):127-35.

Sai, Y. P. &Howard, M. Epidemiology of cancer of the small intestine.World J GastrointestOncol. 2011 March 15; 3(3): 33–42.

Santini, D., Fratto, M. E., Spoto, C., Russo, A., Galluzzo, S., Zoccoli, A., Vincenzi, B.&Tonini, G. Cetuximab in small bowel adenocarcinoma: a new friend?Br J Cancer. 2010 October 12; 103(8): 1305.

Schottenfeld, D., Beebe-Dimmer, J.L.&Vigneau, F.D. The epidemiology and pathogenesis of neoplasia in the small intestine. Ann Epidemiol. 2009 Jan;19(1):58-69.

Schulmann, K., Brasch, F.E., Kunstmann, E., Engel, C., Pagenstecher, C., Vogelsang, H., Krüger, S., Vogel, T., Knaebel, H.P., Rüschoff, J., Hahn, S.A., Knebel-Doeberitz, M.V., Moeslein, G., Meltzer, S.J., Schackert, H.K., Tympner, C., Mangold, E.&Schmiegel, W.; German HNPCC Consortium.HNPCC-associated small bowel cancer: clinical and molecular characteristics.Gastroenterology. 2005 Mar;128(3):590-9.

Sellner, F. &Dtsch, Z. V. S.Adenomas and carcinomas of the small intestine in familial polyposis and Gardner syndrome--analysis of a literature survey. 1986;46(5):287-93.

Abrahams, N.A., Halverson, A., Fazio, V.W., et al. (2002). Adenocarcinoma of the small bowel: a study of 37 cases with emphasis on histologic prognostic factors. Dis Colon Rectum 45:1496–1502.

Speranza, G., Doroshow, J.H. &Kummar, S. Adenocarcinoma of the small bowel: changes in the landscape? CurrOpinOncol. 2010 Jul;22(4):387-93 Gastrointestinal tract: Edited by Alain Hendlisz July 2010 - Volume 22 - Issue 4 - p 387–393.

Sturniolo, G.C., Di Leo, V., Vettorato, M.G., et al. (2005). Clinical relevance of small-bowel findings detected by wireless capsule endoscopy.ScandJGastroenterol40:725–733.

Sturniolo, G.C., Di Leo, V., Vettorato, M.G.&D'Inca, R. Clinical relevance of small-bowel findings detected by wireless capsule endoscopy.Scand J Gastroenterol. 2005 Jun;40(6):725-33.

Talamonti, M.S., Goetz, L.H., Rao, S., et al. (2002). Primary cancers of the small bowel: analysis of prognostic factors and results of surgical management Arch Surg137:564–571.

Talamonti, M.S., Goetz, L.H., Rao, S.& Joehl, R.J. Primary cancers of the small bowel: analysis of prognostic factors and results of surgical management. Arch Surg. 2002 May;137(5):564-70; discussion 570-1

The presence of K-12 ras mutations in duodenal adenocarcinomas and the absence of ras mutations in other small bowel adenocarcinomas and carcinoid tumors.Cancer1997 May 1;79(9):1804-8.

Tomoki, Y., Eiichi, M., Isao, A., Toshiaki, T., &Katsuyuki, A. Successful treatment of recurrent small bowel adenocarcinoma by cytoreductive surgery and chemotherapy: a case report and review of the literature. J Med Case Reports.2010; 4: 213.

Tsang, H., Yau, T., Khong, P.L.&Epstein, R.J. Bevacizumab-based therapy for advanced small bowel adenocarcinoma.Gut. 2008 Nov;57(11):1631-2.

Wade, S., Samowitz, J. A., Holden, K. C., Sandra, L. E., Adrianne R. W., Heather A. L., Margaret A. R., Melanie. F. N., Kristin M. G., Beverly J. L., Mark F. L., and Martha L. S. Inverse Relationship between Microsatellite Instability and K-ras and p53 Gene Alterations in Colon Cancer.Am J Pathol. 2001 April; 158(4): 1517–1524.

Wu, T.J., Yeh, C.N., Chao, T.C., Jan, Y.Y.&Chen, M.F. Prognostic factors of primary small bowel adenocarcinoma: univariate and multivariate analysis. World J Surg. 2006 Mar; 30(3): 391-8; discussion 399.

Yeung, R.S., Weese, J.L., Hoffman, J.P., Solin, L.J., Paul, A.R., Engstrom, P.F., Litwin, S., Kowalyshyn, M.J.&Eisenberg, B.L.Neoadjuvantchemoradiation in pancreatic and duodenal carcinoma.A Phase II Study.Cancer. 1993 Oct 1;72(7):2124-33

Younes, N., Fulton, N., Tanaka, R., Wayne, J., Straus, F.H. 2nd. &Kaplan, E.L.

Zaanan, A., Costes, L., Liegard, M., et al. Final analysis of the multicentric retrospective AGEO study on 99 advanced small bowel adenocarcinomas. Presented at the ASCO GI Symposium 2009; San Francisio, CA. January 15–17, 2009; (abstr 238)

Zhang, M.Q., Chen, Z.M.&Wang, H.L. Immunohistochemical investigation of tumorigenic pathways in small intestinal adenocarcinoma: a comparison with colorectal adenocarcinoma. Mod Pathol. 2006 Apr;19(4):573-80.

Zollinger, R. M., Sternfeld, W. & Schreiber, H. Primary neoplasms of the small intestine. Am J Surg. (1986);151:654–658.

# The Search for a Non-Invasive Test for Colon Cancer and other Gastrointenstinal Disorders

Andrew P. Smith

*California Pacific Medical Center Research Institute, San Francisco, USA*

Nancy M. Lee

*California Pacific Medical Center Research Institute, San Francisco, USA*

## 1   Introduction

Colorectal cancer is the third most common cancer in the US and continues to be the second leading cause of cancer deaths. Each year, about 150,000 new cases will be diagnosed and 50,000 patients will die of this disease. Most colon cancers begin as an adenomatous polyp (Day & Morson, 1978), so the use of colonoscopy to detect and remove polyps can in principle prevent most colon cancers. In practice, however, colonoscopy has fallen well short of this goal. A major problem is that it is expensive, invasive, and inconvenient, requiring prior bowel preparation in addition to the procedure itself, performed in a hospital or clinic. Compliance is thus relatively low, 40-50%, as compared to over 80% for breast, cervix and prostate cancer screening. Moreover, if all recommended individuals, including not only those with a family history of cancer, but everyone over 50 years of age, were to seek a colonoscopy, it would seriously strain if not exceed the capacity of this country's estimated ten thousand qualified endoscopists to perform the necessary procedures.

For these and other reasons, colonoscopy is currently only one of several recommended screening options. The fecal occult blood test, carried out annually, is non-invasive and much less expensive than colonoscopy. Flexible sigmoidoscopy, recommended every five years, is also less expensive. The capsule camera approach, while relatively expensive and also requiring a colon prep, is another less invasive alternative to colonoscopy (Sieg, 2011). While all of these approaches show some promise, none of them to date has achieved a degree of sensitivity or specificity equal to that of colonoscopy (Ransohoff, 2005).

It has long been recognized that we need a non-invasive test of sufficiently high sensitivity and specificity that it could identify individuals likely to have polyps or cancers, and therefore recommend them for colonoscopy, while sparing the large majority of clean individuals from this procedure. A non-invasive test will almost certainly make use of biological markers for colon cancer, alterations in certain molecules that can be reliably used to indicate presence of the cancer or of polyps (Alhquist, 2010). Several possible alternatives are currently being researched, including stool tests for DNA mutations associated with colon cancer (Imperiale *et al.*, 2004; Ahlquist *et al.*, 2008) and various types of blood tests for colon cancer markers (Hundt *et al.*, 2007). We will briefly review recent progress in developing these tests here, and then discuss our own studies aimed at developing a screening test for colon cancer based on rectal swabs, and its possible application to other disorders of the gastrointestinal tract.

## 2   Biomarkers for Colon Cancer and Risk of Colon Cancer

Biomarkers indicative of colon cancer or colon cancer risk might in principle be found in colon tissue itself or in the circulation. One would expect that molecular changes that could serve as biomarkers would be easiest to detect at the source of the cancer itself, in the colon. Biomarkers in the blood will be present only to the extent that certain molecules find their way from the colon to the circulation, which means there is probably a smaller pool of potential candidates. Nevertheless, a great deal of effort is being made to find such markers in blood, since it would make it possible to add a colon cancer test to other tests that are already routinely applied to patient blood samples.

### 2.1   Colon Cancer Biomarkers in Blood

A large number of studies have evaluated plasma substances, including soluble proteins, mRNA and DNA, and cytological assays, as markers for colon cancer (Leung *et al.*, 2005; Wang *et al.*, 2006; Hundt *et al.*, 2007; Leman *et al.*, 2007, 2008; Cordero *et al.*, 2011). Sensitivities and specificities reported by these investigators were generally in the range of 60-80%, in a few cases higher. However, in most of these studies, sensitivity for polyp detection, if it was even examined, was much lower. In fact, many blood-based tests are likely to be relatively insensitive to polyps, unless they are fairly advanced, since these tests generally depend on the presence of cells, or portions of them, from the site of the tumor breaking off and entering the circulation. Another downside of blood tests is that the markers used are frequently relatively nonspecific, indicative of cancers other than those in the colon.

In a study of a little more than one hundred individuals, however, Leman *et al.* (2008), reported that a colon cancer-specific antigen (CCSA) – 2, was able to detect cancers and advanced adenomas with close to 100% sensitivity, and smaller adenomas with about 50% sensitivity. This antigen is a nuclear protein thought to be released during changes in nuclear structure during carcinogenesis. Levels of this protein also had a specificity of nearly 100% when cancer patients were compared with respect to individuals with normal colons or hyperplastic polyps, as well as individuals with other types of cancers. Moreover, there appeared to be a correlation between the antigen level and the size/advancement of the adenoma, so that the test might distinguish different stages of progression. However, in this preliminary study, the authors selected an arbitrary level of the protein, one high enough to eliminate all controls, yet low enough to include all cancers and most adenomas. If this test were to be used for screening, it would be necessary to define a non-arbitrary control value, based on a large population of subjects, which could be used confidently for an unknown group of individuals.

Another promising antigen is sCD26, a constitutively expressed protease thought to be involved in processing of certain regulatory peptides (Cordero *et al.*, 2011). In an initial study of 175 individuals, an immunoassay for this antigen showed 90% sensitivity and 90% specificity in detecting colon cancers (Cordero *et al.*, 2000). In a larger follow-up study of more than 2500 individuals (DiChiara *et al.*, 2009), this antigen was able to identify the two cases of colon cancer, and a number of individuals with polyps, but there was a large proportion of false positives, with an overall positive predictive value (PPV) of about 40%. A third study of about 300 cohorts found a lower sensitivity for colon cancer and still lower for adenomas, with again, a relatively low PPV (DiChiara *et al.*, 2010).

Another potential blood-borne marker for colon and other types of cancer is methylated DNA (Kim *et al.*, 2010). DNA activity is regulated in an epigenetic fashion by alterations of methylation patterns, and aberrant patterns have specifically been shown to be associated with certain cancers (Laird & Jaenisch 1994; Jones, 1996; Lengauer *et al.*, 1997; Kondo *et al.*, 2004). Several studies have evaluated methylation patterns in certain genes found in either serum or in immune cells as biomarkers for colon cancer (Lofton-Day *et al.*, 2008; Payne, 2010; Woo & Kim, 2010; Herbst *et al.*, 2011). Most of these studies have failed to identify a large fraction of colon cancers. Warren *et al.* (2011) reported a sensitivity and specificity of about 90% for detection of colon cancers, analyzing methylated DNA of the septin9 gene. However, detection of adenomas was far lower, on the order of 10%.

## 2.2   Detection of DNA Mutations in Stool

While the search for blood-borne biomarkers of colon cancer continues, a logically more fruitful place to investigate is in colon tissue itself. Since carcinogenesis in the colon is known to involve accumulation of genetic mutations and other abnormalities of the genome (Kinzler & Vogelstein, 1996; Beerenwinkel *et al.*, 2007), many studies have attempted to identify such pathologies in stool. This contains colon mucosa cells, the DNA of which can be isolated and analyzed (Itzkowitz, 2009). Biomarkers examined include mutations in genes such as adenomatous polyposis coli (APC), p53, b-catenin, and k-ras, as well as markers of microsatellite instability and as in blood plasma, gene methylation. Many of these changes occur with high frequency not only in colon cancers but in adenomatous polyps, suggesting that they may be an early, precancerous indicator of the disease (Powell *et al.*, 1992; Pretlow *et al.*, 1993; Sparks *et al.*, 1998; Ieda *et al.*, 1996; Mosnier *et al.*, 1996; Iino *et al.*, 1999; Jass, 2000; Osborn & Ahlquist, 2005; Zhang *et al.*, 2007; Chien *et al.*, 2007; Mixich *et al.*,, 2007; Ausch *et al.*, 2009; Kim *et al.*, 2009; Hellebrekers et al., 2009; Mori *et al.*, 2011; Lind *et al.*, 2011).

Several laboratories initially reported that the presence of such changes, identified by analysis of DNA present in stool, correlates with a fairly high degree of both specificity and sensitivity (70-90%) to the presence of colon cancer (Ahlquist *et al.*, 2000; Dong *et al.*, 2001; Koshiji *et al.*, 2002; Traverso *et al.*, 2002; Berger *et al.*, 2003; Calistri *et al.*, 2003; Tagore *et al.*, 2003). However, most of these studies failed to detect a large fraction of advanced adenomas (50% or greater), with smaller polyps usually not studied. Moreover, most studies analyzed a small and unrepresentative subject pool.

One of the first multicenter studies to examine a large population, by Imperiale *et al.* (2004), detected only about 50% of colon cancers, though this was substantially better than the fecal occult blood test. More recently, another multicenter study compared two fecal occult blood tests with two DNA tests (Ahlquist *et al.*, 2008). One of the DNA tests actually detected fewer cancers than either of the fecal occult blood tests used. The second DNA test was somewhat better, but still detected only about 60% of cancers, and less than 50% of large adenomas (as determined by colonoscopy). Moreover, the false positive rate for both DNA tests was significantly greater than that for the occult blood tests. As a result, the investigators concluded that the DNA tests did not provide significant improvement in screening over the occult blood tests.

The following year, in a smaller study, the same investigators reported an improved assay that was able to detect a larger proportion of both cancers and adenomas (Zou *et al.*, 2009). Some DNA tests are currently on the market, and the prospects for continued improvement are good (Kiesel & Ahlquist, 2011). However, at this time there is still no test based on DNA nor any other biomarker that has been shown capable of detecting cancers and adenomas as reliably as colonoscopy. Another significant issue is that the DNA test, while cheaper than colonoscopy, is considerably more expensive than the fecal occult blood test. Since either test is more likely to detect cancers or adenomas if used annually, a less reliable but cheaper test might be just as effective.

## 2.3   Detecting Colon Cancer and Colon Cancer Risk by Gene Expression Analysis

Because of the current limitations in DNA tests, we are interested in an alternative approach, involving identification of changes in the expression of certain genes. It is now well recognized that a wide variety of cancers are accompanied by such changes in gene expression (Giordano *et al.*, 2001; Baron *et al.*, 2001; Hsu *et al.*, 2007; Jurik *et al.*, 2007). Many studies have revealed changes in expression of a large and diverse group of genes in both adenomatous polyps and colon cancers (Bartman *et al.*, 1999; Buckhaults *et al.*, 2001; Notterman *et al.*, 2001; Chen *et al.*, 2004; Sugiyama *et al.*, 2005; Ahmed *et al.*, 2007; Yang *et al.*, 2011; Loboda *et al.*, 2011; Nastase *et al.*, 2011), as well as in circulating tumor cells (Bustin *et al.*, 1999; Hundt *et al.*, 2007; Bukurova *et al.*, 2011). Gene expression can be determined using either microarrays, which are suitable for analysis of very large numbers of genes, and thus for screening for candidate biomarkers; or real time quantitative PCR (RT-PCR), which focuses on a smaller number targets, and may be more appropriate if the most likely targets have been identified.

A major advantage of gene expression analysis, as shown in some studies that will be discussed below, is that some of these changes occur very early in the process of carcinogenesis, prior to any morphological alterations, and in some cases even prior to the appearance of major genetic mutations. The regulation of most genes is highly controlled in the normal cell, and only slight alterations in this regulation may result in detectable changes in expression level. Hence expression analysis is a highly sensitive indicator of metabolic events that may long precede the extensive genetic and morphological derangements that are typical of cancer. This is crucially important in screening, as the goal is not to detect cancers that have already begun to develop, but to identify individuals who may be at risk for cancer, so that the disease can be prevented entirely.

In initial studies with a mouse model of colon cancer, we found changes in gene expression in both adenomatous polyps, and in normal appearing colon mucosa distant from the polyps (Chen *et al.*, 2004). For these studies, we employed a panel of fifteen or sixteen genes that studies by other groups had shown to be involved in cancer. We found these same gene expression changes also were present in normal appearing colon mucosa tissue in human cancer patients (Chen *et al.*, 2004). That is, these genes exhibited changes in expression relative to levels in normal mucosa of individuals with no cancer or polyps. Moreover, these changes were found not simply close to the cancer or polyps, but throughout the colon. This finding demonstrated that molecular changes occur not only in polyps or cancer, but in normal tissue of individuals with cancer, and suggested that these changes might serve as biomarkers for colon cancer.

In support of this, Polley *et al.* (2004) reported changes in protein expression in normal appearing mucosa of colon cancer patients. This is an extremely important finding, as it not only supports the conclusion that changes in gene expression may occur prior to any morphological alterations, but that these changes may be detected throughout the colon. This makes screening methods simpler, as it becomes possible to sample tissue anywhere in the colon, rather than being dependent on obtaining material from a localized polyp or other morphological abnormality.

Based on this finding, we subsequently asked whether such changes in gene expression could also be found in individuals without colon cancer, but at significant risk for colon cancer. For this study, we used subjects with either adenomatous polyps or with a personal or family history of cancer. These individuals submitted to colonoscopy, during which we removed biopsies of normal appearing colon mucosa. Using the same panel employed in our earlier studies, we again found significant changes in expression in individuals with either polyps or history, compared to controls with no polyps or history (Hao *et al.*, 2005a,b). We subsequently confirmed these results using rectal swabs, a less invasive procedure that requires no colonoscopy nor colon preparation (Smith *et al.*, 2012).

Ahmed *et al* (2007) also reported changes in expression, in some cases detectable using a single gene, in individuals with cancer or polyps, using material isolated from stool samples. While these results using RT-PCR have been quite promising, to obtain the full benefit of gene expression analysis, it will be important to identify other candidate genes, using procedures capable of greater screening, such as microarrays. In addition to making it possible to increase the sensitivity and selectivity of the panel, by addition of new genes, this work may identify genes capable of serving as biomarkers for other disorders of the colon or the gastrointestinal tract.

## 2.4   Microarray Analysis of Colon Mucosa from Individuals with Colon Cancer or Risk for Colon Cancer

Our initial studies were carried out with unamplified RNA, obtained from biopsies of nine subjects (three controls, three polyps, three histories). After extraction, RNA samples were sent to the Microarray Facility at Berkeley National Laboratory, where they were analyzed on an oligo chip containing 45,000 probes representing 39,000 transcripts from approximately 33,000 genes. Because of the difficulty in obtaining enough RNA for analysis, subsequent studies employed amplified DNA obtained from this RNA. These studies used biopsies from a total of forty subjects: seven individuals with personal or family history of cancer, ten individuals with polyps, nine individuals with colon cancer, and fourteen controls, who had no polyps, cancer or personal/family history of cancer. This RNA was subjected to microarray analysis at Phalanx Biotech (Palo Alto, CA), using a total of 30,968 probes.

Our preliminary microarray studies have identified several hundred candidate genes, which have higher expression values in individuals with colon cancer or at risk for colon cancer than controls. We selected five of these genes to add to our original panel, and were able to improve sensitivity and specificity of detection of individuals with colon cancer risk (manuscript in preparation). Further work will be required to validate other genes, perhaps replacing some currently on the panel, but based on our preliminary results, we believe this approach has great promise to improve our colon cancer screening procedure.

## 3    Barrett's Esophagus

We also want to assess the possibility of extending gene expression analysis to screening for other disorders of the gastrointestinal tract. As a preliminary step in this direction, we conducted a small study on individuals with Barrett's esophagus (BE). BE is a pre-malignant condition that is associated with a greatly increased risk of esophageal adenocarcinoma (EAC) (Lagergren *et al.*, 1999), which is the seventh leading cause of cancer deaths (Jemal *et al.*, 2006). The excess risk of developing EAC in BE relative to the general population ranges between 30- and 60-fold (Cameron *et al.*, 1985; Hage *et al.*, 2004; Spechler *et al.*, 2000). In most Western countries, the incidence of EAC has increased rapidly over the past two decades and at present comprises at least 60 % of all esophageal cancer cases (Blot *et al.*, 1991; Bytzer *et al.*, 1999; Bollschweiler *et al.*, 2001; Van Soest *et al.*, 2005). The condition develops when gastroesophageal reflux disease damages the squamous esophageal mucosa and the injury heals through a metaplasia process in which columnar cells replace squamous ones. The abnormal columnar epithelium that characterizes BE is an incomplete form of intestinal metaplasia that predisposes patients to adenocarcinoma.

The problem of identifying patients with Barrett's dysplasia is substantial. Many patients with BE have few symptoms, while many reflux patients do not have BE. At present this necessitates use of a very large number of endoscopy procedures to screen for BE, with many missed cases. The incidence of BE is not well established, because it is frequently asymptomatic and difficult to detect, but it is present in at least 10% of patients with gastroesophageal reflux disease who submit to endoscopy (Haggitt, 1994; Lagergren *et al.*. 1999), and about 10% of patients with BE have EA at time of diagnosis.

Early treatment of BE is possible if the disease is detected or diagnosed. Treatment involves therapy with drugs to suppress acid reflux, while in more advanced cases esophagectomy may be recommended (Haggitt, 1994). However, the diagnosis of BE is based on endoscopic findings of columnar epithelium lining the distal esophagus. Like colonoscopy, endoscopy is a relatively expensive procedure, and currently, the general population is not routinely screened for BE by endoscopy. So diagnosis of BE, like that of colon cancer, would benefit greatly from a cheaper, non-invasive test. Our preliminary study was designed to determine if BE could be identified by expression of the same genes that we have shown are altered in individuals with colon cancer or risk of colon cancer.

Our preliminary study of Barrett's patients was limited by the small number of patients (8). Furthermore, all but two of these patients exhibited either polyps or history of cancer, and so would be expected to show significant changes in our gene expression panel on this basis, above and beyond any correlation with Barrett's. It is relevant in this light to note a study reporting that Barrett's patients are at increased risk for colorectal cancer (Van Soest *et al.*, 2005). With those caveats in mind, each of the eight Barrett's patients exhibited expression values significantly different from controls using two different tests of multivariate analysis (manuscript in preparation).

However, it remains to be determined whether these two diseases can be distinguished by gene expression values alone. Large scales studies of individuals with BE but no GI abnormalities will be necessary to address this issue. Another factor we intend to test is whether tissue samples can be obtained by buccal or cheek swabs. This would be an even simpler and less invasive approach than that offered by rectal swabs.

# 4    Conclusions

The use of biomarkers to detect certain diseases or enhanced risk for developing these diseases has several important advantages, including cost, ease of administering, and availability. Both colonoscopy and endoscopy generally cost several thousand dollars, with prices varying considerably in different hospitals and clinics across the U.S. In contrast, the gene expression analysis approach we have described here, properly developed, could be carried out for a few hundred dollars, with this cost also less subject to regional variation. Rectal swabs could be submitted during a routine visit to any physician, which are then sent to a laboratory for analysis. These advantages in cost and ease are likely to improve compliance substantially among those at risk, which include everyone over fifty years of age.

In the case of colonscopy, another factor often not appreciated is that there are not enough practitioners of the process to provide colonoscopy to all individuals at risk who should be screened. This state of affairs exists despite the fact that more than half of those at risk may have no polyps, and only about 10% exhibit a large (> 1 cm diameter) adenoma (Imperiale *et al.*, 2004). Moreover, the great majority of even large polyps are thought not to develop to cancer. An benefit of screening with biomarkers, therefore, would be to reduce the work load of colonoscopists. Screening cqn identify those who actually have polyps that need to be removed, freeing colonoscopists from what has proven to be a very large number of unnecessary procedures. Ultimately, it may even be possible using screening to determine which polyps are potentially harmful, and which are not and do not need to be removed.

While several different approaches are being applied to identifying biomarkers for colon cancer, the use of gene expression analysis has several advantages. First, as our studies and those of Polley *et al.* (2006) and Ahmed *et al.* (2007) show, changes in expression may signal not simply the presence of cancer, or even some morphological abnormality, such as an adenomatous polyps, that could develop into cancer, but molecular abnormalities that would not be detectable by any procedure focused on morphology. Individuals in this state could be closely monitored for the first sign of a morphological abnormality that might require removal. A similar situation may exist with respect to upper gastrointestinal diseases such as BE.

Moreover, the approach lends itself to an endless amount of modification, by altering the composition of the panel of genes. This would be obviously necessary to extend the procedure to different diseases, such as colon cancer or BE, but it may also prove helpful in screening for different types of the same general disease, and perhaps also for different stages of a particular disease. With respect to the latter, Ahmed *et al.* (2007) have reported some success in distinguishing individuals with polyps from those with colon cancer. As our preliminary studies with microarrays show, candidate genes—those that exhibit altered expression in individuals with colon cancer or polyps—can be added to the pre-existing panel to see if they improve sensitivity and/or specificity for detection of any particular disease. The data obtained from such studies are also likely to be useful in understanding the underlying mechanisms of the disease. The screening process therefore should not be thought of as a fixed method, but as one evolving over time.

# References

Ahlquist, D.A., Skoletsky, J.E., Boynton, K.A., Harrington, J.J., Mahoney, D.W., Pierceall, W.E., Thibodeau, S.N. & Shuber, A.P. (2000). Colorectal cancer screening by detection of altered human DNA in stool: feasibility of a multitarget assay panel, Gastroenterology, 119,1219-1227.

hlquist, D.A., Sargent, D.J., Loprinzi, C.L., Levin, T.R., Rex, D.K., Ahnen, D.J., Knigge, K., Lance, M.P., Burgart, L.J., Hamilton, S.R., Allison, J.E, Lawson, M.J., Devens, M.E., Harrington, J.J., & Hillman, S.L. (2008). Stool DNA and occult blood testing for screen detection of colorectal neoplasia, Annals of Internal Medicine, 149(7), 441–450.

Ahlquist, DA. (2010). Molecular detection of colorectal neoplasia.Gastroenterology,138(6), 2127-2139.

Ahmed, F.E., Vos, P., James, S., Lysle, D.T., Allison, R.R., Flake, G., Sinar, D.R., Naziri, W., Marcuard, S.P., & Pennington, R. (2007). Transcriptomic molecular markers for screening human colon cancer in stool and tissue. Proteomics, 4(1), 1-20

Ausch, C., Buxhofer-Ausch, V., Oberkanins, C., Holzer, B., Minai-Pour, M., Jahn, S., Dandachi, N., Zeillinger, R., & Kriegshäuser, G. (2009). Sensitive detection of KRAS mutations in archived formalin-fixed paraffin-embedded tissue using mutant-enriched PCR and reverse- hybridization.Journal of Molecular Diagnosis, 11(6), 508-13.

Baron, A., Moore, P.S., & Scarpa, A. (2001). DNA array/microarrays in oncological research with focus on pancreatic cancer, Advances in Clinical Pathology, 5(4),115-120

Bartman, A.E., Sanderson, S.J., Ewing, S.L., Niehans, G.A., Wiehr, C.L., Evans, M.K., & Ho, S.B. (1999). Aberrant expression of MUC5AC and MUC6 gastric mucin genes in colorectal polyps, International Journal of Cancer, 80(2), 210-218.

Beerenwinkel, N., Antal, T., Dingli, D., Traulsen, A., Kinzler, K.W., Velculescu, V.E., Vogelstein, B., & Nowak, M.A. (2007). Genetic progression and the waiting time to cancer. PLoS, Computational Biology, 3(11), e225.

Berger, B.M., Vucson, B.M., & Diteberg, J.S. (2003). Gene mutations in advanced colonic polyps: potential marker selection for stool-based mutated human DNA assays for colon cancer screening, Clinical Colorectal Cancer 3(3), 180-185

Blot, W.J., Devesa, S.S., Kneller, R.W., &Fraumeni, J.F. Jr. (1991). Rising incidence of adenocarcinoma of the esophagus and gastric cardia. Journal of the American Medical Association, 265(10), 1287-1289.

Bollschweiler, E., Wolfgarten, E., Gutschow, C., &Hölscher, A.H. (2001). Demographic variations in the rising incidence of esophageal adenocarcinoma in white males, Cancer, 92(3), 549-555.

Bresalier R.S. (2009). Barrett's Esophagus and esophageal adenocarcinoma, Annual Review of Medicine, 60, 221-231.

Buckhaults, P., Rago, C., St. Croix, B., Saha, S., Zhang, L., Vogelstein, B., Kinzler, K.W. (2001). Secreted and cell surface genes expressed in benign and malignant colorectal tumors, Cancer Research, 61(19), 6996-7001

Bukurova, Iu.A., Nikitina, S.L., Khankin, S.L., Krasnov, G.S., Lisitsin, N.A., Karpov, V.L., & Beresten,' S.F. (2011). Identification of protein markers for serum diagnosis of cancer based on microRNA expression profiling.Molecular Biology (Mosk), 45(2),376-81

Bustin, S.A., Gyselman, V.G., Williams, N.S., & Dorudi, S. (1999). Detection of cytokeratins 19/20 and guanylyl cyclase C in peripheral blood of colorectal cancer patients, British Journal of Cancer, 79(11-12),1813–1820

Bytzer P, Christensen PB, Damkier P., Vinding, K., & Seersholm, N. (1999). Adenocarcinoma of the esophagus and Barrett's esophagus: a population-based study, American Journal of Gastroenterology, 94(1), 86-91.

Calistri, D., Rengucci, C., Bocchini, R., Saragoni, L., Zoli, W., & Amadori D. (2003). Fecal multiple molecular tests to detect colorectal cancer in stool, Clinical Gastroenterology and Hepatology, 1(5), 377-83

Cameron, A.J., Ott, B.J., Payne, W.S. (1985). The incidence of adenocarcinoma in columnar-lined (Barrett's) esophagus, New England Journal of Medicine, 313, 857-859.

Chen, L.-C., Hao, C.Y., Chiu, Y.S.Y., Wong, P., Melnick, J.S., Brotman, M., Moetto, J., Mendes, F., Smith, A.P., Bennington, J.L., Moore, D., & Lee, NM (2004). Alteration of gene expression in normal-appearing colon mucosa of APCMin mice and human cancer patients, Cancer Research 64(10), 3694-3700.

Chien, C.C., Chen, S.H., Liu. C,C., Lee, C.L., Yang, R.N., Yang, S.H., & Huang, C.J. (2007). Correlation of K-ras codon 12 mutations in human feces and ages of patients with colorectal cancer (CRC), Translation Research, 149(2), 96-102.

Cordero, O.J., Imbernon, M., Chiara, L.D., Martinez-Zorzano, V.S., Ayude, D., de la Cadena, M.P., & Rodriguez-Berrocal, F.J. (2011). Potential of soluble CD26 as a serum marker for colorectal cancer detection, World Journal of Clinical Oncology, 2(6), 245-61.

Cordero, O.J., Ayude, D., Nogueira, M., Rodriguez-Berrocal, F.J., & de la Cadena, M.P. (2000). Preoperative serum CD26 levels: diagnostic efficiency and predictive value for colorectal cancer, British Journal of Cancer, 83(9), 1139–1146.

Day, D.W. & Morson, B.C. (1978). The adenoma-carcinoma sequence, Major Problems in Pathology, 10 58-71.

De Chiara, L., Rodríguez-Piñeiro, A.M., Rodríguez-Berrocal, F.J., Cordero, O.J., Martínez-Ares, D. & Páez de la Cadena, M. (2010). Serum CD26 is related to histopathological polyp traits and behaves as a marker for colorectal cancer and advanced adenomas, BMC Cancer, 10, 333.

De Chiara, L., Rodríguez-Piñeiro, A.M., Cordero, O.J., Rodríguez-Berrocal, F.J., Ayude, D., Rivas-Hervada, F.J. & de la Cadena, M.P. (2009). Soluble CD26 levels and its association to epidemiologic parameters in a sample population, Disease Markers, 27(6), 311–316.

Dong, S.M., Traverso, G., Johnson, C., Geng, L., Favis, R., Boynton, K., Hibi, K., Goodman, S.N,, D'Allessio, M., Paty, P., Hamilton, S.R., Sidransky, D., Barany, F., Levin, B., Shuber, A., Kinzler, K.W., Vogelstein, B., &Jen, J. (2001). Detecting colorectal cancer in stool with the use of multiple genetic targets, Journal of the National Cancer Institute, 93(11), 858-865.

Giordano, T.J., Shedden, K.A,, Schwartz, D.R., Kuick, R., Taylor, J.M.G., Lee, N., Misek, D.E., Greenson, J.K., Kardia, S.L.R., Beer, D.G., Rennert, G., Cho, K.R., Gruber, S.B., Fearon, E.R., & Hanash, S. (2001). Organ-specific molecular classification of primary lung, colon, and ovarian adenocarcinomas using gene expression profiles, American Journal of Pathology 159 (4), 1231-1238.

Hage M, Siersema PD, van Dekken, H., Steyerberg, E.W. & Dees, J., Kuipers, E.J. (2004). Oesophageal cancer incidence and mortality in patients with long-segment Barrett's oesophagus after a mean follow-up of 12.7 years, Scandinavian Journal of Gastroenterology 39(12), 1175-1179.

Haggitt, R.C. (1994). Barrett's esophagus, dysplasia, and adenocarcinoma, Human Pathologies 25(10), 982-993.

Hao, C.Y., Moore, D., Chiu, Y.S.Y., Wong, P., Bennington, J.L., Smith, A.P., Chen, L.-C., & Lee, NM (2005a). Altered gene expression in normal colonic mucosa of individuals with polyps of the colon, Diseases of the Colon and Rectum 48(12), 2329-2335.

Hao, C.Y., Moore, D., Wong, P., Bennington, J.L., Smith, A.P., Lee, N.M. & Chen, L.-C. (2005b). Alteration of Gene Expression in Macroscopically Normal Colonic Mucosa from Individuals with a Family History of Sporadic Colon

Cancer. Clin. Cancer Res. 11, 1400-1407.

Hellebrekers, D.M., Lentjes, M.H., van den Bosch S.M., Melotte, V,, Wouters, K.A., Daenen, K.L., Smits, K.M., Akiyama, Y., Yuasa, Y,. Sanduleanu, S., Khalid-de Bakker, C.A., Jonkers, D., Weijenberg, M.P., Louwagie, J., van Criekinge, W., Carvalho, B., Meijer, G.A., Baylin, S.B., Herman, J.G., de Bruïne, A.P., & van Engeland, M. (2009). GATA4 and GATA5 are potential tumor suppressors and biomarkers in colorectal cancer.Clinical Cancer Research, 15(12), 3990-7.

Herbst, A., Rahmig, K., Stieber, P., Philipp, A., Jung, A., Ofner, A., Crispin, A., Neumann, J., Lamerz, R., &Kolligs, F.T. (2011). Methylation of NEUROG1 in serum is a sensitive marker for the detection of early colorectal cancer, American Journal of Gastroenterology, 106(6),1110-8. E

Hsu, C.N., Lai, J.M., Liu, C.H., Tseng, H.H., Lin, C.Y., Lin, K.T., Yeh, H.H., Sung, T.Y., Hsu, W.L., Su, L.J., Lee, S.A., Chen, C.H., Lee, G.C, Lee, D.T., Shiue, Y.L., Yeh, C.W., Chang, C.H., Kao, C.Y., & Huang, C.Y. (2007). Detection of the inferred interaction network in hepatocellular carcinoma from EHCO (Encyclopedia of Hepatocellular Carcinoma genes Online), BMC Bioinformatics 8, 66.

Hundt, S., Haug, U., & Brenner, H. (2007). Blood markers for early detection of colorectal cancer: a systematic review, Cancer Epidemiology Biomarkers and Prevention, 16(10), 1935–1953.

Imperiale, T.F., Ransohoff, D.F., Itzkowitz, S.H., Turnbull, B.A., & Ross, M.E. (2004). Fecal DNA versus fecal occult blood for colorectal-cancer screening in an average-risk population, New England Journal of Medicine, 351(26), 2704–2714.

Itzkowitz, S.H. (2009). Incremental advances in excremental cancer detection tests,Journal of the National Cancer Institute101(18),1225-1227.

Jemal, A, Siegel, R, & Ward E., Murray, T., Xu, J., Smigal, C., Thun, M.J.(2006). Cancer statistics, 2006, CA Cancer Journal of Clinicians, 56(2),106-30.

Jones, P.A. (1996). DNA methylation errors and cancer, Cancer Research, 56(11), 2463–2467.

Juric, D, Lacayo, N.J., Ramsey, M.C., Racevskis, J., Wiernik, P.H., Rowe, J.M., Goldstone, A.H., O'Dwyer, P.J., Paietta, E., & Sikic, B.I. (2007). Differential gene expression patterns and interaction networks in BCR-ABL-positive and -negative adult acute lymphoblastic leukemias. Journal of Clinical Oncology 25(11), 1341-1349.

Kisiel, J.B., &Ahlquist, D.A. (2011). Stool DNA screening for colorectal cancer: opportunities to improve value with next generation tests.Journal of Clinical Gastroenterology, 45(4), 301-8.

Kim, M.S., Louwagie, J., Carvalho, B., Terhaar Sive Droste, J.S., Park, H.L., Chae, Y.K., Yamashita, K., Liu, J., Ostrow, K.L., Ling, S., Guerrero-Preston, R., Demokan, S., Yalniz, Z., Dalay, N., Meijer, G.A., Van Criekinge, W,, & Sidransky, D. (2009). Promoter DNA methylation of oncostatin m receptor-beta as a novel diagnostic and therapeutic marker in colon cancer.PLoS One, 4(8), e6555.

Kim, M.S., Lee, J., &Sidransky, D. (2010). DNA methylation markers in colorectal cancer, Cancer Metastasis Review, 29(1), 181-206.

Kinzler, K.W, & Vogelstein, B. (1996). Lessons from hereditary colorectal cancer, Cell 87(2), 159-170.

Kondo, Y., & Issa, J.P.J. (2004). Epigenetic changes in colorectal cancer, Cancer Metastasis Review, 23(1-2), 29–39.

Koshiji, M,, Yonekura, Y., Saito, T., & Yoshioka, K. (2002). Microsatellite analysis of fecal DNA for colorectal cancer detection, Journal of Surgical Oncology, 80(1), 34-40.

Lagergren J, Bergstrom R, Lindgren A,& Nyren, O. (1999). Symptomatic gastroesophageal reflux as a risk factor for esophageal adenocarcinoma, New England Journal of Medicine, 340(11), 825-31.

Laird, P.W., & Jaenisch, R. (1994). DNA methylation and cancer, Human Molecular Genetics, 3, 1487–1496.

Leman, E.S., Schoen, R.E., Weissfeld, JL, Cannon, G.W., Sokoll, L.J., Chan, D.W., & Getzenberg, R.H. (2007). Initial analyses of colon cancer-specific antigen (CCSA)-3 and CCSA-4 as colorectal cancer-associated serum markers, Cancer Research, 67(12), 5600–5605.

Leman, E.S., Schoen, R.E., Magheli, A., Sokoll, L.J., Chan, D.W., & Getzenberg, R.H.(2008) Evaluation of colon cancer-specific antigen 2 as a potential serum marker for colorectal cancer, Clinical Cancer Research,14(5), 1349–1354.

Lengauer, C., Kinzler, K., & Vogelstein, B. (1997). Genetic instability in colorectal cancers, Nature, 386(6712), 623–627.

Leung, W.K., To, K.F., Man, E.P., Chan, M.W., Bai, A.H., Hui, A.J., Chan, F.K., & Sung, J.J. (2005). Quantitative detection of promoter hypermethylation in multiple genes in the serum of patients with colorectal cancer, American Journal of Gasteroenterology, 100(10), 2274–2279.

Lind, G.E., Danielsen, S.A., Ahlquist, T., Merok, M.A., Andresen, K., Skotheim, R.I., Hektoen, M., Rognum, T.O., Meling, G.I., Hoff, G., Bretthauer, M., Thiis-Evensen, E., Nesbakken, A., & Lothe, R,A. (2011). Identification of an epigenetic biomarker panel with high sensitivity and specificity for colorectal cancer and adenomas, Molecular Cancer, 10(1), 85.

Loboda, A., Nebozhyn, M.V., Watters, J.W., Buser, C.A., Shaw, P.M., Huang, P.S., Van't Veer, L., Tollenaar, R.A., Jackson, D.B., Agrawal, D., Dai, H., & Yeatman, T.J. (2011). EMT is the dominant program in human colon cancer.BMC Medical Genomics, 20, 4-9.

Lofton-Day, C., Model, F., Devos, T., Tetzner, R., Distler, J., Schuster, M., Song, X., Lesche, R., Liebenberg, V., Ebert, M., Molnar, B., Grützmann, R., Pilarsky. C,, &Sledziewski, A. (2008). A DNA methylation biomarkers for blood-based colorectal cancer screening, Clinical Chemistry, 54(2), 414-23.

Lu, S., Chiu, Y.S., Smith, A.P., Moore, D., &Lee, N.M. (2009). Biomarkers correlate with colon cancer and risks: a preliminary study.Diseases of the Colon and Rectum, 52(4), 715-24.

Mahalanobis, P.C. (1936). On the generalized distance in statistics, Proceedings of the National Institute of India, 12, 49-55.

Mixich, F., Ioana, M., Voinea, F., Săftoiu, A., & Ciurea, T. (2007). Noninvasive detection through REMS-PCR technique of K-ras mutations in stool DNA of patients with colorectal cancer.Journal of Gastrointestinal and Liver Disease, 16(1), 5-10.

Mori, Y., Olaru, A.V., Cheng, Y., Agarwal, R., Yang, J., Luvsanjav, D., Yu, W., Selaru, F.M., Hutfless, S., Lazarev, M., Kwon, J.H., Brant, S.R., Marohn, M.R., Hutcheon, D.F., Duncan, M.D., Goel, A., & Meltzer, S.J. (2011). Novel candidate colorectal cancer biomarkers identified by methylation microarray-based scanning.Endocrine Relationships of Cancer,18(4), 465-78.

Notterman, D.A., Alon, U., Sierk, A.J., & Levine, A.J. (2001). Transcriptional gene expression profiles of colorectal adenoma, adenocarcinoma, and normal tissue examined by oligonucleotide arrays, Cancer Research, 61(7), 3124-30

Osborn, N.K., & Ahlquist, D.A. (2005). Stool screening for colorectal cancer: molecular approaches, Gastroenterology, 128(1), 192-206.

Payne, S.R. (2010). From discovery to the clinic: the novel DNA methylation biomarker (m)SEPT9 for the detection of colorectal cancer in blood. Epigenomics, 2(4), 575-85.

Polley, A.C.J., Mulholland, F., Pin, C., Williams, E.A., Bradburn, D.M., Mills, S.J., Mathers, J.C., & Johnson, I.T. (2006). Proteonomic analysis reveals field-wide changes in protein expression in the morphologically normal mucosa of patients with colorectal neoplasia. Cancer Research, 66(13), 6553-6561.

Ransohoff, D.F, (2005). Colon cancer screening in 2005: status and challenges. Gastroneneterology 128(6),1685-1696.

Sieg, A. (2011). Colon capsule endoscopy compared with conventional colonoscopy for the detection of colorectal neoplasms, Expert Review of Medical Devices, 8(2), 257–261.

Smith, A.P., Chiu, Y.,S.Y. & Lee, N.M. (2012). Towards Universal Screening for Colon Cancer: A Cheap, Reliable, Non-invasive Test Using Gene Expression Analysis of Rectal Swabs Gastroenterology ISRN, in press

Sparks, A.B., Morin, P.J., Vogelstein, B., & Kinzler, K.W. (1998). Mutational analysis of the APC/beta-catenin/Tcf pathway in colorectal cancer, Cancer Research, 58(6), 1130-1134.

Spechler, S.J. (2000). Barrett's esophagus: an overrated cancer risk factor. Gastroenterology, 119(2), 587-589.

Sugiyama, Y., Farrow, B., Murillo, C., Li, J., Watanabe, H., Sugiyama, K., & Evers, B.M. (2005). Analysis of differential gene expression patterns in colon cancer and cancer stroma using microdissected tissues. Gastroenterology, 128(2), 480-486

Tagore, K.S., Lawson, M.J., Yucaitis, J.A., Gage, R., Orr, T., Shuber, A.P., & Ross, M.E. (2003). Sensitivity and specificity of a stool DNA multitarget assay panel for the detection of advanced colorectal neoplasia, Clinical Colorectal Cancer, 3(1), 47-53.

Traverso, G., Shuber, A., Levin, B., Johnson, C., Olsson, L., Schoetz, D.J. Jr, Hamilton, S.R., Boynton, K., Kinzler, K.W. and Vogelstein, B. (2002). Detection of APC mutations in fecal DNA from patients with colorectal tumors, New England Journal of Medicine, 346(5), 311-20.

van Soest, E.M., Dieleman, J. P., Siersema, P.D., Sturkenboom, M.C., & Kuipers, E.G. (2005). Increasing incidence of Barrett's esophagus in the general population, Gut, 54(8), 1062-1066.

Wang, J.Y., Yeh, C.S., Chen, Y.F., Wu, C.H., Hsieh, J.S., Huang, T.J., Huang, S.Y., & Lin, S.R. (2006). Development and evaluation of a colorimetric membrane-array method for the detection of circulating tumor cells in the peripheral blood of Taiwanese patients with colorectal cancer, International Journal of Molecular Medicine, 17(5), 737–747.

Warren, J.D., Xiong, W., Bunker, A.M., Vaughn, C.P., Furtado, L.V., Roberts, W.L., Fang, J.C., Samowitz, W,S., &Heichman, K.A. (2011). Septin 9 methylated DNA is a sensitive and specific blood test for colorectal cancer, BMC Medicine, 14(9) 133.

Woo, H.D., &Kim, J. (2012). Global DNA hypomethylation in peripheral blood leukocytes as a biomarker for cancer risk: a meta-analysis, PLoS One, 7(4), e34615.

Yang, J., Luan, J., Yu, Y., Li, C., DePinho, R.A., Chin, L., & Richmond, A. (2001). Induction of melanoma in murine macrophage inflammatory protein 2 transgenic mice heterozygous for inhibitor of kinase/alternate reading frame, Cancer Research, 61(22), 8150-7.

Zhang, Z., & DuBois, R.N. (2001). Detection of differentially expressed genes in human colon carcinoma cells treated with a selective COX-2 inhibitor, Oncogene, 20(33), 4450-6.

Zhang, H.Y., Spechler, S.J., &Souza, R.F. (2009). Esophageal adenocarcinoma arising in Barrett esophagus. Cancer Letters, 275(2), 170-177.

Zou, H., Taylor, W.R., Harrington, J.J., Hussain, F.T., Cao, X., Loprinzi, C.L., Levine, T.R., Rex, D.K., Ahnen, D., Knigge. K.L., Lance, P., Jiang, X., Smith, D.I., &Ahlquist, D.A. (2009). High detection rates of colorectal neoplasia by stool DNA testing with a novel digital melt curve assay, Gastroenterology. 136(2):459-470.

# Timing of Initiation of Chemotherapy after Primary Colorectal Cancer Resection

Yoichiro Yoshida
*Department of Gastroenterological Surgery*
*Fukuoka University, Japan*

Seiichiro Hoshino
*Department of Gastroenterological Surgery*
*Fukuoka University, Japan*

Yuichi Yamashita
*Department of Gastroenterological Surgery*
*Fukuoka University, Japan*

# 1    Introduction

Colorectal cancer (CRC) is the third leading cause of cancer mortality in the Western world (Parkin *et al.*, 2005). While surgical resection remains the cornerstone of management for patients with stage I–III disease, a considerable proportion of patients will ultimately relapse and die from their disease. Large, randomized clinical trials of adjuvant chemotherapy (AC) after curative resection of CRC have consistently demonstrated improvement in survival, which dictates the current standard of care (National Institutes of Health.1990).Adjuvant chemotherapy is routinely recommended after curative surgical resection of stage II and III rectal cancer, stage III (node-positive) colon cancer, and stage II (node-negative) colon cancer in which high-risk features are present (Benson *et al.*, 2004; Figueredo *et al.*, 2004). However, the optimal time from surgery to the start of chemotherapy in CRC is not known.

The surgical resection of asymptomatic primary colorectal cancer with unresectable synchronous metastases is controversial. Among patients with severe intestinal symptoms, resection is mandatory before starting systemic chemotherapy (Joffe *et al.*, 1981; Longo *et al.*, 1988; Rosen *et al.*, 2000). Palliative resection of the primary tumor is also reported to improve the efficacy of systemic chemotherapy (Temple *et al.*, 2004) and prolong the duration of chemotherapy (Kaufman *et al.*, 2008). A recent review article suggested that noncurative resection of asymptomatic primary colorectal tumors may prolong survival in patients with metastatic colorectal cancer (Eisenberger *et al.*, 2008). However, another article concluded that chemotherapy should be started initially, with resection of the primary tumor reserved for the small proportion of patients who develop major complications from the primary tumor. This is because resection of an asymptomatic primary tumor provides only minimal palliative benefits (Scheer *et al.*, 2008). The National Comprehensive Cancer Network currently recommends that patients with metastatic colorectal cancer undergo surgical intervention if they have a bowel obstruction, an impending obstruction, or metastases that are potentially resectable.

The purpose of the surgical resection of primary tumors is the prevention of hemorrhage, perforation, and bowel obstruction. In many cases, patients cannot continue chemotherapy treatments because of complications such as bleeding, perforation, and bowel obstruction when chemotherapy is initiated without prior surgical resection of the primary tumor. Surgical removal of the primary tumor therefore seems necessary to continue chemotherapy with few complications. In the past, some investigators have recommended routine resection of the primary tumor to prevent the need for urgent surgical procedures because of local complications (Joffe *et al.*, 1981; Longo *et al.*, 1988). Ruo reported that 30 (29%) of the 103 patients who were initially managed without bowel resection required a subsequent surgery for the palliation of complications (Ruo *et al.*, 2003). Recently, some authors have suggested the elective resection of asymptomatic colorectal cancers in at least a subset of patients with less advanced stage IV disease (Rosen *et al.*, 2000; Ruo *et al.*, 2003). Other authors have suggested deferring the resection of minimally symptomatic colorectal tumors because most of these patients succumb to progressive systemic disease rather than complications related to the intact primary lesion (Ruo *et al.*, 2003; Benoist *et al.*, 2005; Yoshida *et al.*, 2011). However, surgical resection may delay the start of chemotherapy (Benoist *et al.*, 2005). Generally, an interval of 4 weeks after surgery is considered necessary before the initiation of chemotherapy treatments such as folinic acid, fluorouracil (5-FU), and oxaliplatin (FOLFOX); folinic acid, 5-FU, and irinotecan (FOLFIRI); and capecitabine and oxaliplatin (XELOX). Most clinical trials exclude patients who have undergone an operation within 4 weeks. However, there is no apparent evidence for this delay. A metastatic tumor can grow rapidly before the start of chemotherapy and possibly lead to patient death (Figure 1).

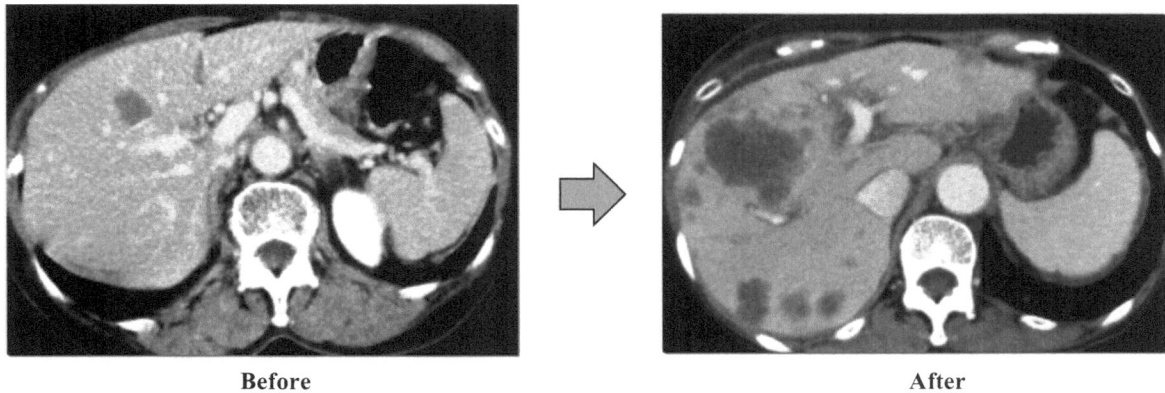

**Before**                                          **After**

**Figure1:** Liver metastases before and after resection of primary colon cancer. (Borrowed from Dr. Kohei Shitara)

Because the significance of this postoperative 4-week delay before the start of chemotherapy is unclear, we evaluated the feasibility and safety of an early chemotherapy start in patients who had undergone colorectal surgery for colorectal cancer and who had multiple, distant, synchronous metastases.

## 2    Demerit of Resection

It was recently reported that the growth rate of liver metastases was significantly higher in patients in whom the primary colorectal tumor had been resected than in patients in whom the primary tumor was still in situ (Peeters *et al.*, 2004; Simpson-Herren *et al.*, 1976). In addition, immunohistochemical analysis revealed an increased proliferation rate and increased vessel density in the metastases in the absence of the primary tumor. These data suggest that outgrowth of metastatic disease may be partially controlled by the primary tumor (Peeters *et al.*, 2006).In animal models, primary tumor–mediated inhibition of metastatic vascularization and outgrowth is an established concept in tumor biology. Research in this area was initiated by the observation that in the Lewis lung carcinoma mouse model, resection of the primary tumor led to increased vascularization and accelerated growth of distant metastases that had previously remained microscopic. O'Reilly *et al.* demonstrated in a murine model that the primary tumor produced the potent antiangiogenic compound angiostatin, which prevented vascularization and thereby the growth of metastases (O'Reilly *et al.*, 1994). More recently, it was demonstrated that irradiation of murine angiostatin-producing primary tumors was subsequently followed by rapid growth of the metastases, suggesting a similar phenomenon (Camphausen *et al.*, 2001; von Essen., 1991). Moreover, when angiostatin was replaced immediately after regression of the primary tumor, outgrowth of the metastases did not occur (Camphausen *et al.*, 2001).

Although only a limited number of patients were included, a significant increase in [18]F-FDG/uptake of colorectal liver metastases after resection of the primary tumor (Scheer *et al.*, 2008). In contrast, [18]F-FDG uptake in liver metastases remained stable in 2 subsequent [18]F-FDG positron emission tomography (PET) scans of patients without any surgery or other therapeutic intervention between the scans. These results suggest that in humans, as in animal models, the primary tumor can inhibit the growth of its metastases. This inhibitory effect on secondary tumor growth is reversed when the primary tumor is resected. For example, Li *et al.* demonstrated increased microvessel density, a higher cell proliferation index in tumor cells, and a decreased apoptotic index after resection of a primary tumor in a mouse model compared with a sham operation (Li *et al.*, 2001).

On the other hand, the increased metabolic activity observed after resection of the primary colorectal tumor may also be caused by the surgical trauma of the resection itself. Surgery alone could stimulate proinflammatory cytokines (interleukin-6 (IL-6) and IL-1β) resulting in enhanced expression of vascular endothelial growth factor and angiogenesis (Nagengast *et al.*, 2007). The data cannot differentiate between these 2 hypotheses. Another explanation for the outgrowth of the metastases could be that the increase in $^{18}$F-FDG uptake is merely time-dependent progression, and that synchronous liver metastases (group A) would grow faster than metachronous liver metastases (most patients in group B). This explanation, however, is unlikely because the initial standard uptake values (SUVs) in both groups were identical and the interval between the 2 serial $^{18}$F-FDG positron emission tomography (PET) scans was even longer in group B than in group A. Furthermore, increased retention of $^{18}$F-FDG may be the result of the increased size of the lesion; however, our results did not show a correlation between the alteration in tumor size and the change in SUV.

Although the precise mechanism of increased metabolic activity after resection of the primary colorectal tumor—as observed in our study—remains to be clarified, the slowing of this accelerated growth by angiogenesis inhibitors seems promising. The present approach of serial $^{18}$F-FDG PET scans before and after resection of the primary tumor would possibly allow direct measurement of the therapeutic effect of such antiangiogenic therapy. Such studies might provide insight into the use of adjuvant antiangiogenic agents to prevent accelerated outgrowth of distant metastases after resection of the primary colorectal tumor.

## 3   5-FU

Surgeons are reluctant to prescribe 5-FU in the immediate postoperative period. This is primarily because of the belief that 5-FU will increase the anastomotic leakage rate. This can result in the need for reoperation, the creation of a colostomy, and the need for a future takedown, or even death. It is estimated that 1 out of 3 postoperative deaths after colonic surgery are caused by leaking anastomosis (Debas *et al.*, 1972). The dangers of postoperative 5-FU are well documented. Several animal studies have reported weaker anastomosis and an increased risk of anastomotic rupture when systemic 5-FU is given as a bolus immediately after surgery (Goldman *et al.*, 1969; Morris., 1979). Immediate intraperitoneal 5-FU also increases the risk of anastomotic dehiscence (Weiber *et al.*, 1994). Continuous infusion of 5-FU allows higher daily dosages and appears to be safer than bolus 5-FU (Lokich *et al.*, 1989). Continuous infusion avoids the peak serum levels of 5-FU that are caused by bolus dosing, and it may therefore be effective for colorectal cancer without increasing the rate of anastomotic leakage. The oral fluoropyrimidine, UFT, and capecitabine have been developed to improve tolerability and patient convenience and have replaced the continuous infusion of 5-FU in many treatment regimens (Bennouna *et al.*, 2009). Oral fluoropyrimidine is a promising alternative to the constant infusion of 5-FU, and pharmacokinetic studies have found that consecutive oral administrations of UFT as tegafur (370 $mg \cdot m^{-2} \cdot d^{-1}$) provide a steady-state concentration of 5-FU that is comparable to that achieved by a 5-day constant infusion at 250 $mg \cdot m^{-2} \cdot d^{-1}$. In addition, injecting a bolus of 5-FU results in ultra-high concentrations followed by rapid disappearance (Ho *et al.*, 1998; Borner *et al.*, 2002). We therefore selected the XELOX regimen for this study.

# 4    Adjuvant Chemotherapy for CRC

The amount of time before the initiation of AC is an important parameter. Timely access to AC is often cited and tracked as a quality indicator (Systemic treatment wait times. 2011).Furthermore, beyond a certain time period after surgery, such as the often-quoted 12 weeks, it is uncertain whether the adjuvant benefit diminishes or is even lost entirely. To address this important gap in the literature, we undertook a formal systematic literature review and a meta-analysis to identify studies that assessed the relationship between time to AC and survival in CRC.

The effect of AC on survival is thought to be the eradication of micrometastatic deposits in a proportion of patients who would otherwise eventually experience cancer recurrence. There is a substantial theoretical rationale to the prompt initiation of AC after curative surgery. Studies in animal models suggest that surgery may increase the numbers of circulating tumor cells and potentiate the growth of metastatic deposits. This increase in metastatic growth is thought to correlate with a reduction in angiogenesis inhibitors such as angiostatin following removal of the primary tumor (McCulloch *et al.*, 1994; Filder *et al.*, 1994; Folkman *et al.*, 1990; Gunduz *et al.*, 1979). Surgery has also been shown to enhance production of oncogenic growth factors such as transforming growth factor α that can increase tumor growth (Ono *et al.*, 1994; Eggermont *et al.*, 1987). Furthermore, the classic mathematical model by Goldie and Coldmanpredicts that the probability of mutations that lead to drug resistance increases over time (Goldie *et al.*, 1979) and is dependent on mutation rate and tumor size. Whether the more recent discovery of pluripotent colon cancer stem cells may also play a role in relapse following AC awaits further investigation (Dalerba *et al.*, 2007; O'Brien *et al.*, 2007; Ricci-Vitiani *et al.*, 2007).

If we apply the findings to a patient who is ready to initiate AC 4 weeks after surgery but is delayed for logistical rather than medical reasons, that patient would have a 14% increased risk of mortality if treated at 8 weeks and a 30% increased risk of mortality at 12 weeks (James *et al.*,2011). The following hypothetical example makes use of Adjuvant! Onlineto illustrate the potential effect that the time-to-AC parameter may have on patient outcome (Adjuvant! Online. 2010): a 65-year-old man in good general health, with T3N2 moderately differentiated colon cancer is treated with fluorouracil-based chemotherapy and has an estimated 5-year survival probability of 60%. If we assume this estimate is made on the basis of a time to AC of 4 weeks (which is reasonable because Adjuvant! Online is based on clinical trials that have strict time-to-AC limits), then a delay to 8 weeks and to 12 weeks would reduce his 5-year survival prognoses to 54% and 48%, respectively. In perspective, the survival effect of a shorter time to AC would be comparable to the magnitude of benefit seen with the addition of oxaliplatin to fluoropyrimidine chemotherapy in the adjuvant setting (André *et al.*, 2004; Kuebler *et al.*, 2007).

# 5    Bevacizumab

Wound-healing complications with bevacizumab therapy were first recognized during the pivotal phase III trial of bevacizumab, which was conducted in 813 previously untreated patients with metastatic colorectal cancer (Hurwitz *et al.*, 2004). The control arm of the study comprised patients who received irinotecan, 5-FU, and leucovorin (LV), while the treatment arm added bevacizumab as targeted therapy. In patients who underwent surgery after beginning study treatment, 15% (6/39) of patients in the treatment armexperienced wound healing or bleeding complications, compared with 4% (1/25) in the control arm (Avastin prescribing information. 2010). To investigate how the interval between bevacizumab therapy and surgery affects the risk of wound-healing complications, Scappaticci *et al.* performed a meta-analysis that included patients from the pivotal phase III trial (Scappaticci *et al.*, 2005), as well as patients from a trial comparing 5-FU and LV with or without bevacizumab (Kabbinavar *et al.*, 2005). In patients who underwent surgery after beginning study treatment, 3.4% (1/29) experienced wound-healing complications in the arm receiving chemotherapy alone compared with 13% (10/75) of patients receiving bevacizumab and chemotherapy; however, this difference did not reach significance ($P < .28$). Of the 10 patients who experienced wound-healing complications after surgery with bevacizumab and chemotherapy, the time interval between bevacizumab and surgery was 0 to 29 days for 5 patients and 30 to 59 days for 5 patients. D'Angelica *et al.* also found no significant difference in postoperative complications in patients who were treated with bevacizumab an average of 6.9 weeks before surgery or 7.4 weeks after surgery when compared with a group of matched historical controls (D'Angelica *et al.*, 2007). Currently, the precise timing to initiate bevacizumab treatment before or after surgery to avoid postoperative wound-healing complications is not clear (Nordlinger *et al.*, 2009), but an interval of 5 to 8 weeks has been suggested (Gruenberger *et al.*, 2008; Ellis *et al.*, 2005; Reddy *et al.*, 2008).

## 6   Chemotherapy for mCRC

Resection of the primary tumor significantly increased the hospital stay and delayed the initiation of chemotherapy; however, there was no evidence to suggest that this delay was associated with reduced response rates leading to curative resection or reduced survival. Recently, it was reported that the growth rate of liver metastases in patients in whom the primary colorectal tumor had been resected was significantly higher than the growth rate of liver metastases in patients in whom the primary tumor was still in situ (Peeters *et al.,* 2004; Simpson-Herren *et al.*, 1976). In addition, immunohistochemical analysis revealed an increased proliferation rate and increased vessel density in the metastases in the absence of the primary tumor. These data suggest that outgrowth of metastatic disease may be partially controlled by the primary tumor (Peeters *et al.*, 2006). Patients may therefore die if they are not able to initiate chemotherapy because of the rapid postoperative progression of a metastatic tumor (Makino *et al.*, 2006; Tajima *et al.*, 2006). We reported a case involving an early initiation of chemotherapy in a patient who had undergone a right hemicolectomy for multiple synchronous liver metastases (Yoshida *et al.*, 2011). He survived for 22 months despite large liver metastases. We began the prospective study to confirm the feasibility of an early initiation of chemotherapy after surgery(Trial registration: UMIN000004361). To the best of our knowledge, this was the first pilot study to determine the feasibility of an early initiation to chemotherapy after resection of a primary colorectal cancer with distant metastases, and it was undertaken only in a small cohort of well-selected patients. Five patients were enrolled. They received XELOX therapy (130 mg/m2 of oxaliplatin on day 1 plus 1,000 mg/m2 of capecitabine twice daily on days 1 – 14) on the 7th postoperative day and XELOX+bevacizumab (7.5 mg/kg of bevacizumab on day 1) after the 2nd cycle of chemotherapy.The procedures included right hemicolectomy in 1 patient, sigmoidectomy in 2 patients, high anterior resection in 1 patient, and Hartmann procedure in 1 patient. All patients started chemotherapy on postoperative day 7. The median number of cycles of chemotherapy was 11 (8 – 22). No postoperative complications were observed. The tumor reduction rate was 44.3% (32.0 – 66.6%). Progression-free survival was 10.3 months. An early initiation of chemotherapy after surgery may be safe and may improve the prognosis of colorectal cancer patients with synchronous metastases. These findings suggest the potential for changes in the suggested time of initiation of chemotherapy after surgery in the future. We have already begun a new phase II trial to confirm the effects of the early initiation of chemotherapy after surgery.

Enhanced recovery after surgery (ERAS) protocols aim to reduce the surgical stress response and optimize recovery to reduce the length of hospital stays (Lassen *et al.*, 2009). All ERAS parameters have been shown to improve patient outcome individually. The development of ERAS enabled an early start to chemotherapy after surgery. An early initiation of chemotherapy after surgery may therefore prevent tumor growth. Resection of colorectal tumors with severe stenosis and bleeding is the first treatment step in preventing complications related to colorectal tumors. The European multicenter COlon cancer Laparoscopic or Open Resection (COLOR) trial assessed the short-term and long-term outcomes after laparoscopic surgery or open surgery for colon cancer (Veldkamp *et al.*, 2005; Buunen *et al.*, 2009). Allaix *et al.*reported a higher percentage of patients submitted to adjuvant chemotherapy within8 weeks in laparoscopic surgery group, due to a shorter hospital stay and a quicker return to preoperative performance status (Allaix *et al.*, 2012). The opportunity of an early onset of adjuvant chemotherapy could represent a further theoretical advantage of minimally invasive surgery in metastatic CRC patients compared with open surgery. An earlier administration will be made possible using this minimally invasive surgery for the treatment of advanced colon cancer. This early chemotherapy may extend the prognosis for patients who undergo laparoscopic surgery for colon cancer.

Recently, the use of the self-expandable metal stent (SEMS) as a nonsurgical alternative for relief of obstructing colorectal cancer has increased. The effects of chemotherapy after SEMS placement are controversial. One study was closed prematurely because of chemotherapy-induced colonic perforation in 54% (6/11) of patients (van Hooft *et al.,* 2008). Another report found, in contrast, that complications including perforation and stent migration were not associated with additional chemotherapy (Fernandez-Esparrach *et al.*, 2010). However, these results were limited by the small numbers of patients included. Yoon *et al.* reported that 126 patients who achieved immediate clinical success from palliative SEM-placement, cumulative long-term clinical failure occurred more frequently in patients who did not receive post-stentchemotherapy than in those who received chemotherapy (Yoon *et al.*, 2011). In other words, receiving additional chemotherapy after palliative stenting contributed to long-term clinical success. This may have been caused by the effects of tumorshrinkage from chemotherapy (Im *et al.*, 2008). This hypothesis was indirectly supported by the subanalysis. Although there was no difference in the long-term clinical failure rate according to cancer subtype, differentiated cancers (well-differentiated and moderately differentiated adenocarcinoma) had a lower long-term clinical failure rate than undifferentiated cancers (poorly differentiated adenocarcinoma, signet-ring cell carcinoma, etc), which are generally regarded as rapidly progressive and lesschemotherapy responsive tumors.

# 7    Discussion

The National Comprehensive Cancer Network currently recommends that patients with metastatic colorectal cancer undergo surgical intervention if they have a bowel obstruction, an impending obstruction, or metastases that are potentially resectable. Complications from the primary lesion are uncommon in these circumstances, and the removal of the lesion delays the initiation of systemic chemotherapy. The precise timing for starting treatment with chemotherapeutic agents prior to and/or after surgery in order to avoid postoperative complications is not clear, but an at least 4-week interval has been suggested. In most clinical trials, patients who had undergone an operation within 4 weeks were excluded. Resection of the primary tumor significantly increased the hospital stay and delayed the initiation of chemotherapy; however, there was no evidence to suggest that this delay was associated with reduced response rates leading to curative resection or reduced survival. However, there is a chance that patients may die if they are not able to start chemotherapy because of the rapid postoperative progression of a metastatic tumor.

We have carried out the prospective study to confirm the feasibility of an early start of chemotherapy after surgery, and a phase II trial should be performed to confirm the safety and effects of the early start of chemotherapy after surgery.

# 8   Conclusion

An early start of chemotherapy after surgery is feasible and safe. These findings suggest possible changes in the start time of chemotherapy after surgery in the future. We have already started a new phase II trial to confirm the effects of the early start of chemotherapy after surgery.

# References

Adjuvant! Online: Decision making tools for health care professionals. http://www.adjuvantonline.com. Accessed October 8, 2010

André, T., Boni, C., Mounedji-Boudiaf, L., et al. (2004). Multicenter International Study of Oxaliplatin/ 5-Fluorouracil/Leucovorin in the Adjuvant Treatment of Colon Cancer (MOSAIC) Investigators. Oxaliplatin, fluorouracil, and leucovorin as adjuvant treatment for colon cancer. N Engl J Med, 350,2343-2351

Allaix, ME., Degiuli, M., Giraudo, G., Marano, A., & Morino, M. (2012). Laparoscopic versus open colorectal resections in patients with symptomatic stage IV colorectal cancer. Surg Endosc, 26, 2609-2616.

Avastin (bevacizumab) prescribing information. Available at: http://www.gene.com/gene/products/information/pdf/avastinprescribing.pdf Accessed October 4, 2010.

Bennouna, J., Saunders, M., &Douillard, JY. (2009). The role of UFT in metastatic colorectal cancer. Oncology, 76,301-310.

Benoist, S., Pautrat, K., Mitry, E., Rougier, P., Penna, C., & Nordlinger, B. (2005). Treatment strategy for patients with colorectal cancer and synchronous irresectable liver metastases. Br J Surg, 92,1155-1160.

Benson, AB III., Schrag, D., Somerfield, MR., et al. (2004). American Society of Clinical Oncology recommendations on adjuvant chemotherapy for stage II colon cancer. J Clin Oncol, 22,3408-3419.

Borner, MM., Schoffski, P., de Wit, R., Caponigro, F., Comella, G., Sulkes, A., Greim, G., Peters, GJ., van der Born, K., Wanders, J., de Boer, RF., Martin, C., &Fumoleau, P. (2002). Patient preference and pharmacokinetics of oral modulated UFT versus intravenous fluorouracil and leucovorin: a randomised crossover trial in advanced colorectal cancer. Eur J Cancer, 38,349-358.

Camphausen, K., Moses, MA., Beecken, WD., Khan, MK., Folkman, J., O'Reilly, MS. (2001). Radiation therapy to a primary tumor accelerates metastatic growth in mice. Cancer Res, 61:2207–2211.

Colon Cancer Laparoscopic or Open Resection Study Group, Buunen, M., Veldkamp, R., Hop, WC., Kuhry, E., Jeekel, J., Haglind, E., Påhlman, L., Cuesta, MA., Msika, S., Morino, M., Lacy, A., &Bonjer, HJ. (2009). Survival after laparoscopic surgery versus open surgery for colon cancer: long-term outcome of a randomised clinical trial. Lancet Oncol, 10,44-52.

Dalerba, P., Dylla, SJ., Park, IK., et al. (2007).Phenotypic characterization of human colorectal cancer stem cells. Proc Natl

Acad Sci U S A, 104,10158-10163.

D'Angelica, M., Kornprat, P., Gonen, M., et al. (2007). Lack of evidence for increased operative morbidity after hepatectomy with perioperative use of bevacizumab: a matched case-control study. Ann Surg Oncol,14,759-765.

Debas, HT., & Thomson, FB. (1972). A critical review of colectomy with anastomosis.Surg Gynecol Obstet, 135,747-752.

Eggermont, AM., Steller, EP., &Sugarbaker, PH. (1987). Laparotomy enhances intraperitoneal tumor growth and abrogates the antitumor effects of interleukin-2 and lymphokine-activated killer cells. Surgery, 102,71-78

Eisenberger, A., Whelan, RL., & Neugut, AI. (2008). Survival and symptomatic benefit from palliative primary tumor resection in patients with metastatic colorectal cancer: A review. Int J Colorectal Dis, 23,559-568.

Ellis, LM., Curley, SA., &Grothey, A. (2005). Surgical resection after downsizing of colorectal liver metastasis in the era of bevacizumab. J Clin Oncol,23,4853-4855.

Fernández-Esparrach, G., Bordas, JM., Giráldez, MD., et al. (2010).Severe complications limit long-term clinical success of self-expanding metal stents in patients with obstructive colorectal cancer. Am J Gastroenterol, 105,1087–1093.

Fidler, IJ., &Ellis, LM. (1994). The implications of angiogenesis for the biology and therapy of cancer metastasis. Cell, 79,185-188.

Figueredo, A., Charette, ML., Maroun, J., Brouwers, MC., &Zuraw, L. (2004). Adjuvant therapy for stage II colon cancer: a systematic review from the Cancer Care Ontario Program in evidence-based care's gastrointestinal cancer disease site group. J Clin Oncol, 22,3395-3407.

Folkman J. (1990). What is the evidence that tumors are angiogenesis dependent? J Natl Cancer Inst, 82,4-6.

Goldie, JH., &Coldman AJ. (1979). A mathematic model for relating the drug sensitivity of tumors to their spontaneous mutation rate. Cancer Treat Rep, 63,1727-1733

Goldman, LI., Lowe, S., & al-Saleem, T. (1969). Effect of fluorouracil on intestinal anastomoses in the rat.Arch Surg, 98,303-304.

Gruenberger, B., Tamandl, D., Schueller, J., et al. (2008).Bevacizumab, capecitabine, and oxaliplatin as neoadjuvant therapy for patients with potentially curable metastatic colorectal cancer. J Clin Oncol,26,1830-1835.

Gunduz, N., Fisher, B., &Saffer, EA. (1979). Effect of surgical removal on the growth and kinetics of residual tumor. Cancer Res, 39,3861-3865

Ho, DH., Pazdur, R., Covington, W., Brown, N., Huo, YY., Lassere, Y., &Kuritani, J. (1998). Comparison of 5-fluorouracil pharmacokinetics in patients receiving continuous 5-fluorouracil infusion and oral uracil plus N1-(2'-tetrahydrofuryl)-5-fluorouracil. Clin Cancer Res, 4,2085-2088.

Hurwitz, H., Fehrenbacher, L., Novotny, W., et al.(2004). Bevacizumab plus irinotecan, fluorouracil, and leucovorin for metastatic colorectal cancer. N Engl J Med,350,2335-2342.

Im, JP., Kim, SG., Kang, HWet al.(2008). Clinical outcomes and patency of self-expanding metal stents in patients with malignant colorectal obstruction: a prospective single center study.Int J Colorectal Dis, 23, 789–794.

James, JB., Michael, JR., William, JM., Weidong, K., Will, DK.,&Christopher, MB.(2011). Association Between Time to Initiation of Adjuvant Chemotherapy and Survival in Colorectal CancerA Systematic Review and Meta-analysis. JAMA,305,2335-2342.

Joffe, J., &Gordon, PH.(1981). Palliative resection for colorectal carcinoma. Dis Colon Rectum, 24,355-360.

Kabbinavar, FF., Schulz, J., McCleod, M., et al. (2005). Addition of bevacizumab to bolus fluorouracil and leucovorin in firstline metastatic colorectal cancer: results of a randomized phase II trial. J Clin Oncol,23,3697-3705.

Kaufman, MS., Radhakrishnan, N., Roy, R., Gecelter, G., Tsang, J., Thomas, A., Nissel-Horowitz, S., & Mehrotra, B. (2008). Influence of palliative surgical resection on overall survival in patients with advanced colorectal cancer: A retrospective single institutional study. Colorectal Dis, 10,498-502.

Kuebler, JP., Wieand, HS., O'Connell, MJ., et al.(2007). Oxaliplatin combined with weekly bolus fluorouracil and leucovorin as surgical adjuvant chemotherapy for stage II and III colon cancer: results from NSABP C-07. J Clin Oncol,
25,2198-2204.

Lassen, K., Soop, M., Nygren, J., Cox, PB., Hendry, PO., Spies, C., von Meyenfeldt, MF., Fearon, KC., Revhaug, A.,
Norderval, S., Ljungqvist, O., Lobo, DN., & Dejong, CH. (2009). Enhanced Recovery After Surgery (ERAS) Group:
Consensus review of optimal perioperative care in colorectal surgery: Enhanced recovery after surgery (ERAS) group
recommendations. Arch Surg, 144,961-969.

Li, TS., Kaneda, Y., Ueda, K., Hamano, K., Zempo, N., &Esato, K. (2001). The influence of tumour resection on angiostatin levels and tumour growth: an experimental study in tumour-bearing mice. Eur J Cancer, 37,2283–2288.

Lokich, JJ., Ahlgren, JD., Gullo, JJ., Philips, JA., & Fryer, JG. (1989) A prospective randomized comparison of continuous
infusion fluorouracil with a conventional bolus schedule in metastatic colorectal carcinoma: a Mid-Atlantic Oncology
Program Study. J Clin Oncol, 7,425-432.

Longo, WE., Ballantyne, GH., Bilchik, AJ., & Modlin, IM.(1998). Advanced rectal cancer. What is the best palliation? Dis
Colon Rectum, 31,842-847.

Makino, T., Mishima, H., Ikenaga, M., Tsujinaka, T., Takeda, M., &Mano M. (2006).Clinicopathologic features of signet-
ring cell carcinoma of the colon and rectum. Jpn J Gastroenterol Surg, 39,16-22.

McCulloch, P., &Choy, A. (1994). Effect of menstrual phase on surgical treatment of breast cancer. Lancet, 344,402-403

Morris T. (1979). Retardation of healing of large-bowel anastomoses by 5-fluorouracil.Aust N Z J Surg, 49,743-745.

Nagengast, WB., de Vries, EG., Hospers, GA., et al. (2007) In vivo VEGF imaging with radiolabeled bevacizumab in a
human ovarian tumor xenograft. J Nucl Med, 48,1313–1319.

National Institutes of Health. Adjuvant Therapy for Patients With Colon and Rectum Cancer: NIH Consensus State-
ment.Vol 8. Bethesda, MD: National Institutes of Health; 1990:1-25

Parkin, DM., Bray, F., Ferlay, J., &Pisani, P. (2005).Global cancer statistics.CA Cancer J Clin, 55,74-108.

Nordlinger, B., Van Cutsem, E., Gruenberger, T., et al. (2009). Combination of surgery and chemotherapy and the role of
targeted agents in the treatment of patients with colorectal liver metastases: recommendations from an expert panel.
Ann Oncol,20,985-992.

O'Brien, CA., Pollett, A., Gallinger, S., &Dick, JE. (2007). A human colon cancer cell capable of initiating tumour growth
in immunodeficient mice. Nature, 445,106-110.

Ono, I., Gunji, H., Suda, K., Iwatsuki, K., &Kaneko, F. (1994). Evaluation of cytokines in donor site wound fluids. Scand J
Plast Reconstr Surg Hand Surg, 28,269-273.

O'Reilly, MS., Holmgren, L., Shing, Y., et al.(1994). Angiostatin: a novel angiogenesis inhibitor that mediates the suppression of metastases by a Lewis lung carcinoma. Cell, 79,315–328.

Peeters, CF., Westphal, JR., de Waal, RM., Ruiter, DJ., Wobbes, T., &Ruers, TJ. (2004). Vascular density in colorectal
liver metastases increases after removal of the primary tumor in human cancer patients. Int J Cancer, 112,554–559.

Peeters, CF., de Waal, RM., Wobbes, T., Westphal, JR., &Ruers, TJ. (2006). Outgrowth of human liver metastases after
resection of the primary colorectal tumor: a shift in the balance between apoptosis and proliferation. Int J Cancer,
119,1249–1253.

Reddy, SK., Morse, MA., Hurwitz, HI., et al. (2008).Addition of bevacizumab to irinotecan- and oxaliplatin-based preoperative chemotherapy regimens does not increase morbidity after resection of colorectal liver metastases. J Am
Coll Surg,206,96-106.

Ricci-Vitiani, L., Lombardi, DG., Pilozzi, E., et al. (2007).Identification and expansion of human colon-cancer-initiating cells. Nature, 445,111-115

Rosen, SA., Buell, JF., Yoshida, A., Kazsuba, S., Hurst, R., Michelassi, F., Millis, JM., &Posner, MC.(2000). Initial presentation with stage IV colorectal cancer: how aggressive should we be? Arch Surg, 135,530-534.

Ruo, L., Gougoutas, C., Paty, PB., Guillem, JG., Cohen, AM., &Wong, WD.(2003). Elective bowel resection for incurable stage IV colorectal cancer: Prognostic variables for asyptomatic patients. J Am Coll Surg, 196,722-728.

Scappaticci, FA., Fehrenbacher, L., Cartwright, T., et al. (2005). Surgical wound healing complications in metastatic colorectal cancer patients treated with bevacizumab. J Surg Oncol,91,173-180.

Scheer, MG., Sloots, CE., van der Wilt, GJ.,& Ruers, TJ. (2008). Management of patients with asymptomatic colorectal cancer and synchronous irresectable metastases. Ann Oncol, 19,1829-1835.

Scheer, MG., Stollman, TH., Vogel, WV., Boerman, OC., Oyen, WJ., &Ruers, TJ. (2008).Increased metabolic activity of indolent liver metastases after resection of a primary colorectal tumor.J Nucl Med, 49,887-91.

Simpson-Herren, L., Sanford, AH., &Holmquist, JP. (1976). Effects of surgery on the cell kinetics of residual tumor. Cancer Treat Rep, 60,1749–1760.

Systemic treatment wait times. Cancer Care Ontario, Action Cancer Ontario. http://www.cancercare.on.ca/cms/One.aspx?portalId=1377&pageId=8888. Accessed May 13, 2011.

Tajima, T., Mukai, M., Hinoki, T., Ootani, Y., Sato, S., Nakasaki, H., &Makuuchi, H. (2006).A case of poorly differentiated carcinoma of the ascending colon with rapid postoperative progression suggesting disseminated carcinomatosis of the bone marrow. Jpn J Gastroenterol Surg, 39,265-270.

Temple, LK., Hsieh, L., Wong, WD., Saltz, L.,& Schrag D. (2004). Use of surgery among elderly patients with stage IV colorectal cancer. J Clin Oncol, 22,3475-3484.

van Hooft, JE., Fockens, P., Marinelli, AW., Timmer, R., van Berkel, AM., Bossuyt, PM., & Bemelman, WA. (2008). Early closure of a multicenter randomized clinical trial of endoscopic stenting versus surgery for stage IV left-sided colorectal cancer.Endoscopy, 40,184-191.

Veldkamp, R., Kuhry, E., Hop, WC., Jeekel, J., Kazemier, G., Bonjer, HJ., Haglind, E., Påhlman, L., Cuesta, MA., Msika, S., Morino, M., & Lacy, AM. (2005). Laparoscopic surgery versus open surgery for colon cancer: short-term outcomes of a randomised trial.Lancet Oncol, 6,477-484.

von Essen, CF. (1991) Radiation enhancement of metastasis: a review. Clin Exp Metastasis, 9,77–104.

Weiber, S., Graf, W., Glimelius, B., Jiborn, H., Påhlman, L., & Zederfeldt, B. (1994). Experimental colonic healing in relation to timing of 5-fluorouracil therapy.Br J Surg, 81,1677-1680.

Yoshida, Y., Hoshino, S., Shiwaku, H., Beppu, R., Tanimura, S., Tanaka, S., Yamashita, Y. (2011).Early start of chemotherapy after resection of primary colon cancer with synchronous multiple liver metastases: a case report.Case Rep Oncol, 4,250-254.

Yoon, JY., Jung, YS., Hong, SP., Kim, TI., Kim WH., &Cheon, JH. (2011). Clinical outcomes and risk factors for technical and clinical failures of self-expandable metal stent insertion for malignant colorectal obstruction. Gastrointest Endosc74,858–868

# Intestinal Microbiota around Colorectal Cancer Genesis

Giovanni Brandi, Francesco De Rosa, Giuseppina Liguori
Valentina Agostini, Stefania Di Girolamo
*L. and A. Seràgnoli Department of Hematology and Oncological Sciences*
*Sant'Orsola-Malpighi Hospital, University of Bologna, Italy*

Valerie Gaboriau-Routhiau
*INSERM, U989*
*Universite´ Paris Descartes, Paris, France*

Pierre Raibaud
*Unité d'Écologie et Physiologie du Systéme Digestif, INRA, France*

Guido Biasco
*L. and A. Seràgnoli Department of Hematology and Oncological Sciences*
*Sant'Orsola-Malpighi Hospital, University of Bologna, Italy*

# 1   Introduction

Colorectal cancer (CRC) pathogenesis is well known from a molecular perspective, but how endoluminal colonic factors interact with mucosal genome remains to be determined. Moreover, when referring to them, often only diet components reaching the large intestine are considered, forgetting about a silent, important player: intestinal microflora, or microbiota.

In fact, the gut in newborns is considered sterile, but bacterial colonization occurs quickly and the adult human intestinal tract hosts a complex microbial system, the number of which overcomes by a log the entire number of host eukaryotic cells, playing a crucial role in the regulation of both enteric and systemic homeostasis. Even though the beneficial relationship between the host and the microbiota is largely demonstrated, and in certain conditions the intestinal microflora can increase the risk of carcinogenesis and promote the tumoral growth.

In fact, intestinal autochthonous bacteria are involved in the catabolism of several elements derived from diet or from endogenous secretions, they can modulate the expression of host genes participating in several pathological functions and can interfere with the immune system and the inflammation mechanisms. Furthermore, the gut microbiota is involved in redox stress damages, motility, angiogenesis, proliferation, differentiation, and fat storage regulation (Huycke & Gaskins, 2004).

The application of DNA-based molecular methods has helped to reduce many of the logistical problems associated with the identification of autochthonous microorganisms by cultural-based methods, but at the moment a significant part of the intestinal bacteria cannot be assigned to known genera or species (Bäckhed *et al.*, 2005).

In this review, we want to summarize the mechanisms thought to be involved in the bacterial carcinogenesis of CRC. In particular, we will focus on the difference in the role of intestinal microbiota (IM) in at-risk population with generic or familial/inherited risk factors (chromosomal instability pathway) and in subjects with chronic intestinal inflammatory disease (IBD-related pathway) (Figure 1).

In the first case, IM produces itself metabolites directly damaging DNA or affecting the expression of genes regulating cell cycle and proliferation; in the second, IM likely increases the level of oxidative stress of the mucosa, inducing a chronic inflammatory state, which over time can result in tissue hyperproliferation and dysplasia. An improved knowledge of the fundamental differences in pathogenetic mechanisms of the potential bacterial carcinogenesis could also influence prophylactic strategies for colon cancer.

# 2   Putative Role of Intestinal Microflora in the Development of Colorectal Cancer Related to Chromosomal Instability Pathway

## 2.1   Genetic Bases and Pathological Changes in Sporadic Colorectal Cancer

The pathologic mechanism underlying both sporadic and familial colorectal cancer is still in part referable to the model proposed by Fearon and Vogelstein in 1990. According to this model, progression from normal to dysplastic epithelium and finally to invasive carcinoma (the so-called adenoma-carcinoma sequence) is associated with the accumulation of multiple clonally selected genetic alterations (Beggs &Hodgson, 2008). Among these, allelic loss or loss of heterozygosity (LOH) in the APC tumour suppressor gene represents an early event in colorectal carcinogenesis, determining the precocious clonal expansion of the mutated cell and subsequent adenoma formation. Chromosome instability (characteristic

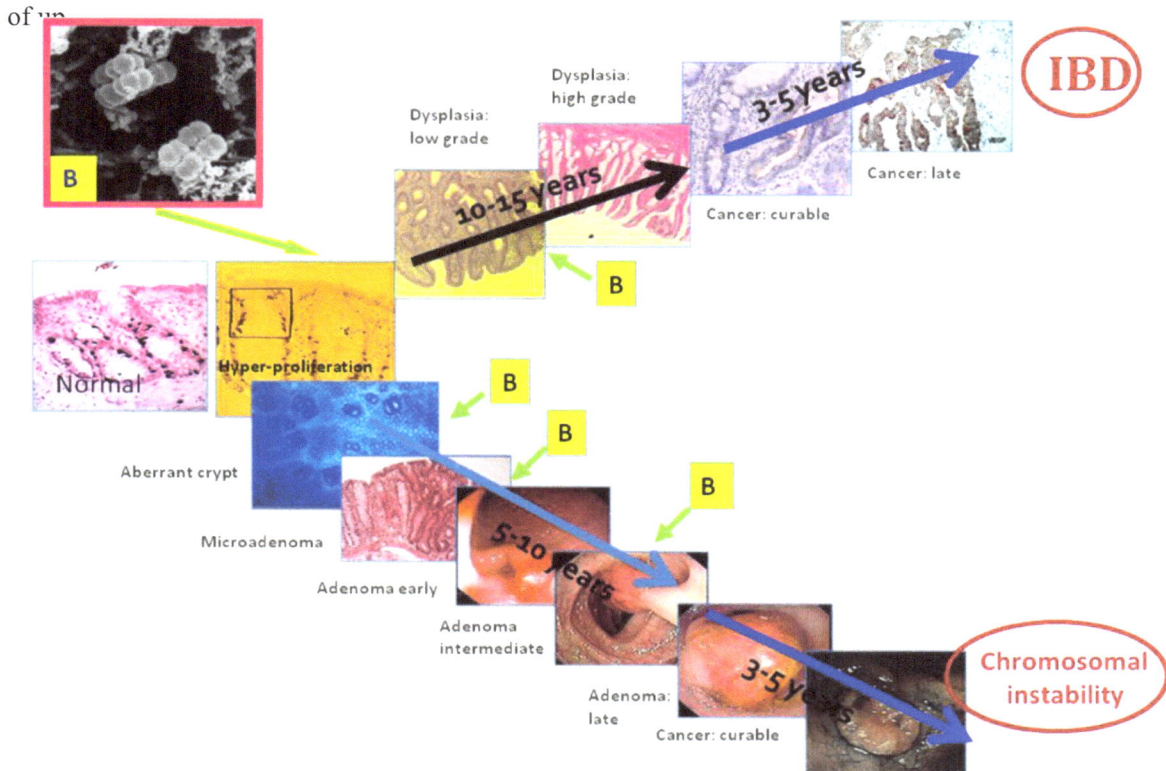

**Figure 1:** Sporadic and IBD-related colorectal cancer development. Here are described the phenotypic phases and the timing from normal mucosa to cancer through two different ways, linked to chromosomal instability (adenoma/carcinoma pathway) and to IBD, respectively. Genetic mutations are similar in these two pathways, although some genes are specific for CI cancer or act at different stage of disease (i.e. APC). 'B' indicates the crucial points where it has been demonstrated a participation of microbiota in the processes.

to 80% of sporadic cancer) is a cytogenetic feature of APC mutation, which, in turn, leads to ß-catenin accumulation in nucleus of epithelial cells. In the remaining cases, ß-catenin gene is directly mutated with its stabilization and final trigger of c-myc, c-jun and cycline genes. Activating mutations in the K-Ras (K-RASG12V and K-RASG13D), BRAF (BRAFV600E) and PIK3CA (PIK3CAH1074R) oncogenes, as well as functional inactivation of p53, SMAD2 and SMAD4 tumor suppressor genes, have been also reported to occur with high frequency during colorectal carcinogenesis, leading to uncontrolled cell proliferation (Beggs & Hodgson, 2008, De Roock *et al.*, 2010).

More recently, a comprehensive molecular characterization by whole genome-sequencing analysis has revealed additional recurrent mutations in colorectal cancer, involving ARID1A (that suppresses myc transcription) and FAM123B and SOX9 (both regulating WNT signaling) genes. Somatic mutations in polymerase e (POLE) gene, along with hypermethylation and silencing of MLH1 gene, have been also detected, leading to high microsatellite instability in this type of cancer (The Cancer Genome Atlas, 2012).

In any case, gene sequencing of different cancers has shown that most mutations found in cancer are rare, and different authors pointed out that the phenotype of the cancer cells could probably be produced by the typical aneuploid karyotype of the cancer cells itself, because an altered number of chromosomes unbalances at once the expression of thousands of genes and proteins (Duesberg*et al.*, 2011). In fact, this suggestion is confirmed by a whole genome-sequencing analysis showing a recurrent copy-number amplifications of ERBB2 and IGF2 genes, as well as recurrent chromosomal translocation, due to the fusion between NAV2 and the WNT pathway member TCF7L1 (The Cancer Genome Atlas Network. 2012).

Bacteria can play a role in this molecular dynamic process. Some sporadic data suggest the role of different bacteria not only in mutation rate but also in chromosome aberrations and in downregulation of DNA mismatch repair protein (Cuevas-Ramos *et al.*, 2010; Maddocks *et al.*, 2009).

Human adenocarcinoma would phenotypically evolve trough aberrant crypt foci (ACF) both preceded by unchecked cell proliferation. The fast enterocytes turnover suggests that stem cells on crypt fundus, and not the mature ones, are the target of oncogenic mutations. In particular, the CD133 cell, barely detectable in the normal colon but more frequent in cancer (2,5% of the population), is responsible for cancer initiation and propagation. Two models try to explain tumoral formation: the so-called bottom-up model states that the initially mutated cell is on the bottom of the crypt, thus proliferating in the luminal direction. On the contrary, by the top-down model the first mutation hits a cell on the apex between two crypts (i.e. on the luminal surface) which then proliferates towards crypt fundus. Interestingly, some putative "oncogenic bacteria" are found in the bottom of the crypts, near the stem cell regions (Maddocks *et al.*, 2009).

One of the first events in colonic carcinogenesis is crypt fission, i.e. the division of a hyperproliferating crypt in two "daughter" crypts. This is responsible of aberrant crypt foci formation. Aberrant crypt foci (ACF) density is variable in relation to the age of the patient and pathology: it is low in patients with benign pathologies of the large bowel; *vice versa*, it is high in patients with adenomatous polyposis and colorectal neoplasia. The presence of ACF seems to be a good marker of colon cancer risk, since there is a strict correlation between the number of ACF and the prevalence of adenomatous polypoid lesions and colon cancer.

## 2.2    Endoluminal Factors

Endoluminal factors have a great impact on various local and distant parameters, and probably they also influence individual CRC risk together with the genetic background. The most important endoluminal risk factors are the diet and IM; their interplay is summarized in Figure 2.

## 2.3    Diet

The geographic differences in CRC incidence, investigated in several migrant and dynamic studies performed since early Seventies, is largely due to environmental factors, especially diet (Flood *et al.*, 2000). With the word "diet", we mean nutrition in its different sides, such as food composition and variety, global energetic balance, body weight and other anthropometric characteristics. Various observational and randomised, controlled studies evaluated the relationship between these different aspects and CRC, but results has not been conclusive (Martínez *et al.*, 2008).

Colorectal cancer risk seems to increase with energy intake (Franceschi *et al.*, 1997). The EPIC study, a large epidemiologic survey on nutritional risk factors, showed that people with large waist circumference or waist/hip ratio have an increased CRC risk (Pischon *et al.*, 2006). Chronic hyperinsulinaemia is likely one of the most important risk factor, as many nutritional factor implicated in CRC genesis seem to elevate insulinaemia (Giovannucci, 2002). However, epidemiologic studies' results do not always support this hypothesis (Larsson *et al.,* 2007). Interestingly, the enzyme fatty acid synthase is physiologically regulated by energy balance, and its tumoral overexpression has been linked with survival in colorectal cancer patients in a body mass index-dependent manner (Ogino *et al.,* 2008). Recently, Park *et al.* suggest a strong linkage between obesity and liver or colon tumorigenesis, by enhancing IL-6, TNFα and STAT-3, although, these factors do not induce cancer on their own, but permit progression of already initiated lesions (Park *et al.,* 2010).

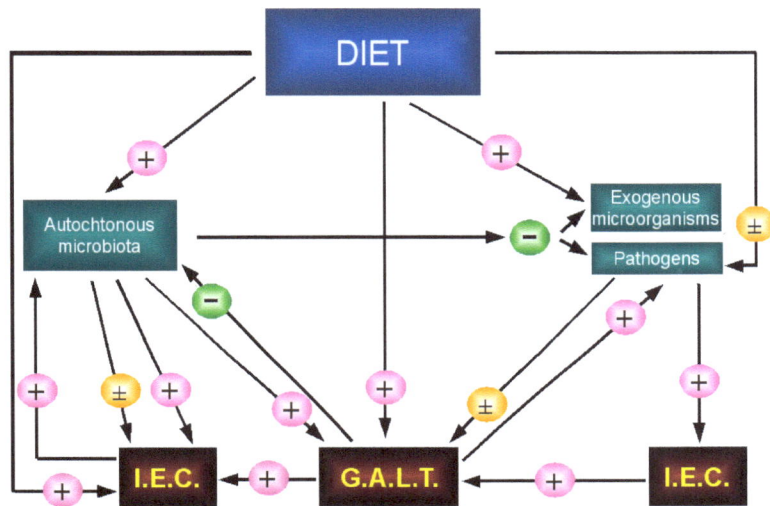

**Figure 2**: The complex interplay between diet, microbiota, pathogens and intestinal mucosa. Diet directly affects both the trophism of intestinal epithelium and its associated lymphoid tissue and the balance of autochtonous microbiota wich, in turn, strongly influences the I.E.C and G.A.L.T. Furthermore the diet is the way permitting the presence of alloctonous microflora and even pathogens inside the alimentary tract. Authoctonous microbiota plays an important protective role towards exogenous microorganisms and pathogens reducing their proliferation and their adhesion to the intestinal mucosa (the so-called barrier effect). Legend: I.E.C., intestinal epithelial cells; G.A.L.T., gut-associated lymphoid tissue; +positive interaction,- negative interaction).

Several studies focused on the role of meat, especially red and processed, as a risk factor in CRC. EPIC results are concordant, and show an increased CRC risk in subjects eating a lot of red and processed meat, confirmed in several metanalysis (Larsson & Wolk, 2006).

On the contrary, long-chain ω-3 fatty acids of fish seem to protect from CRC by reducing COX-2 formation and arachidonic acid-derived eicosanoids production (Hall *et al.,* 2008). Eicosanoids derived from long-chain ω-3 fatty acids possess an anti-inflammatory activity, and compete with pro-inflammatory arachidonic acid derived eicosanoids (Larsson *et al.,* 2004): FAT-1 transgenic mice, which convert ω-6 polyunsaturated fatty acids into ω-3, are less prone to develop colitis-associated CRC when treated with chemical carcinogens (Nowak *et al.,* 2007).

The most important alimentary protective factor seems to be represented by indigestible fibres, partly because they shorten the contact time between mucosa and potential nutritional carcinogens by favouring intestinal transit, and partly through the protective role of short chain fatty acids (SCFA), which regulate cellular proliferation and differentiation. The incidence of CRC is sixty-folds lower in native Africans than in Asian or Caucasian Americans. The former consume less protein and fat, and show a tenfold lower colonic crypt cell proliferation rate (O'Keefe *et al.*, 2007). Various observational studies, including EPIC, reported a reduced incidence of CRC in populations with a high fibre diet (Peters *et al.*, 2003); anyway, recent randomised trials on augmented fibre intake yielded conflicting results. In fact, both Wheat Bran Fibre Trial and Polyp prevention Trial did not find any significant difference in colorectal adenomas recurrence rate between the control and the study group with high fibre intake (Alberts *et al.*, 2000, Schatzkin *et al.*, 2000), while Toronto Polyp Prevention Trial showed a reduction of polyps in subjects with low fat, high fibre diet with respect to people keeping their usual diet (Asano & McLeod, 2002).

There are many hypotheses on the role of dietary calcium in the prevention of CRC. A recent systematic review by WCRF/AICR showed a significant inverse relation between total calcium intake and CRC risk, but modest in entity (World Cancer Research Fund/American Institute for Cancer Research, 2007), depending on the administered dose, on basal calcium reserves of the single subject and on the type of supplemental form (Martínez *et al.*, 2008).

## 3    Intestinal Microbiota

### 3.1    Description of Human Microbiota

In human colon are harboured up to $10^{13}$ bacteria (Savage, 1977), and this huge population may either reside within and colonize the gastrointestinal tract (i.e. autochthonous bacteria), or pass transiently through the gastrointestinal tract (i.e. allochthonous bacteria). Autochthonous bacteria can be classified into dominant or subdominant depending on their concentration. In the colon, anaerobic-aerobic ratio varies, being lower on mucosal surface and higher in the lumen (Eckburg *et al.*, 2005).

This heterogeneous population is traditionally studied with cultural methods, which allow ex vivo isolation of only a limited portion (40 – 60%) of our IM strains. Recently, molecular techniques permit a different approach to microbiota with identification of new species, which, however, cannot be further characterised. These molecular analyses are based on amplification of the 16S rRNA, a component of 30S small subunit of prokaryote ribosomes. The most utilized technique is polymerase chain reaction (PCR) employing an enzymatic reaction that allows in vitro amplification of a specific region of DNA providing extensive information about human microbial diversity and taxonomy (Kuczynski *et al.*, 2011).

In the last years, the increased interest about the relationship among bacteria has prompted to examine the microbiota by animal models and culture-independent genomic methods. Sequencing/metagenomics approaches (by 454 pyrosequencing and Illumina) provided greater information about the potential functional role of the microbes and their complex genome. More recently, to better understand the interactions between human microbiome and host, novel functional metagenomic approaches were developed. Transcriptomics and proteomics, including MS-based shotgun proteomics, identify a large spectrum of proteins produced by microbial genes, giving an important contribution to understand the interactions between microbiome and the human host (Kolmeder *et al.*, 2012).However, in certain contexts and, in particular, in the study of the role of individual bacterial species using gnotobiotic animal models, traditional methods are still necessary and not substitutable.

For long time, the organism is thought to be sterile before birth, although some recent findings suggest reconsidering the sterility of utero environment (Jiménez *et al.*, 2008).The newborn is quickly colonised by microbes coming from the environment and the mother, called pioneer bacteria. Such population is constituted by facultative anaerobes, which burn out all the oxygen in the colonic lumen and create the environmental conditions needed by strict anaerobes (Nicholson *et al.,* 2012). These ones will then become the vast majority, the other being only mere spectator and metabolically negligible (Fanaro *et al.*, 2003).

Only a restricted number of bacterial types colonise the gut. The dominant flora belongs to at least five bacterial phyla: *Firmicutes, Bacteroidetes, Actinobacteria, Proteobacteria* and *Fusobacteria*. There are six genera of strict anaerobes: *Bacteroides, Eubacteria, Bifidobacteria, Clostridia, Peptostreptococci* and *Ruminococci*, while most represented aerobic bacteria being of the genera *Escherichia, Enterococcus, Streptococcus* and *Klebsiella* (O'Hara & Shanahan, 2006). The number of bacterial species present in the human intestine is high, and 57 species are common to > 90% of subjects (Qin *et al.*, 2010).

A member of IM has to fulfil several features: a metabolic apparatus fit for available nutrients, the ability to escape host immune response and to replicate quickly enough to avoid expulsion through the anal canal. Mechanisms underlying bacterial homing have been extensively described for pathogens (migration and adhesion to mucus, other bacteria-expressed receptors), but are still obscure for autochthonous IM. In particular, epithelium-adherent bacteria are numerically irrelevant in human colon; the opposite is true in the case of rodents (Thompson-Chagoyán *et al.*, 2007).

Many studies have shown that significant inter-individually variability exists. A recent study of faecal 16S rRNA gene sequences collected from 14 unrelated adults over the course of a year showed large differences in microbial-community structure between individuals, while the community membership in each host was generally stable during this period. Conversely, the variability of IM composition is reduced in individuals living within the same family, but the relative influence of genetic and environmental factors, including diet, remains to be elucidated (Zoetendal *et al.*, 2001). Nonetheless, a recent study concluded that host genotype is probably a key factor (Khachatryan *et al.*, 2008).

Recently, by metagenomic approach, Arumugam *et al.* (Arumugam *et al.*, 2011) showed that intestinal microbiota, notwithstanding its interindividual variability, is not built in a random fashion, but is stratified along three main clusters (so called enterotypes) based on corresponding *Bacteroides, Prevotella* and *Ruminococcus* genera. Around these three main contributors, there are other bacteria, both dominant and subdominant. It is interesting to note that functional profiles are supported also by subdominant bacteria, assessing that defined functions are shared among different bacteria, indifferently by their numerousness. In this context, few numerous bacterial populations can regain, in the alimentary tract, a role so far neglected. Linked to it, is notable that these three enterotypes utilize different routes to extract energy from fermentable colonic substrates.

Most studies indicate that the intraindividual human flora of adult subjects is quite stable over prolonged periods of time with relative abundance of *Bifidobacteria* and *Clostridia* in adolescent (Zoetendal *et al.*, 1998). Interestingly, microbiota in old age is different to young age, and it is stable over limited time, although there is an imbalance of the main phyla with a decrease of *Firmicutes* and, in particular in the centenarians, of *Faecalibacterium prausnitzii*, which has anti-inflammatory properties.

Some temporal variability in relation to diet changes has been suggested; it happens during the first few weeks after birth, while in the adult life the diet-detected microflora fluctuations can be fully defined and may reflect changes in bacterial metabolic activity rather than changes in microbial composition. Population studies, conducted with metagenomic approaches, showed that changes in microbiota induced by diet are slow and that exists a stable metabolic core between individuals, despite changes in bacterial communities (Claesson *et al.*, 2012, Human microbiome project consortium, 2012).

As well as diet, there are some stresses that can influence the balance of microbiota; in particular, antibiotics modify microbiota, which is, after therapy, characterized by a different equilibrium respect to pre-treatment (Dethlefsen & Relman, 2011).

In each individual, intestinal microbiota is in a state of floating balance, thanks to an interconnecting network allowing minimal variations (Hughes & Sperandio, 2008). In such a state dominating bacterial strains are in steady growth phase, the exponential one being characteristic only of the post-implant period. Due to the intraindividual stability of IM in opposition to its extraordinary interindividual variability, every subject has a unique and distinct microbial pattern, like an adjunctive fingerprint. In fact, in every individual different genome are present and interact, one inherited from the parents and thousands of others from their microflora, but these latter ones are quite fortuitous, resulting from the uncontrolled entry of viable bacteria in his ecosystem.

## 3.2  Mucosa-Associated Bacteria

The majority of research has focused on microflora recovered from faecal samples or intestinal content, even in studying the aspects of host-microflora relation that imply mucosal proximity. In other sites, such as stomach, this is not a concern, since mucosa-associated bacteria and luminal flora are quite similar in number and typology as assessed by culture methods. Recent works have shown that this is not the case in the intestine.

In fact, in this enclave of the outside environment limited by a living wall, the microbial population reaches its own equilibrium thanks to interactions between biotic (intestinal secretions, bacteriocines etc.) and abiotic components (food, fibres, fermentation metabolites). Employing techniques of capture dissection laser and molecular methods, it has been realized that the distribution of the bacteria inside of the large intestine of rodents is not uniform and that some phyla are differently distributed in relation to the lumen or in the vicinity of the epithelium (Nava et al., 2011). The mucus layer and the innate immune system, at least in mice, actively contains microbiota mainly in the lumen, limiting penetration into the mucosa and avoiding excessive proinflammatory signaling (Artis, 2008). In particular, Paneth cells via MyD88/NF-kB pathway actively hamper bacterial penetration through antimicrobial peptide secretion (Vaishnava et al., 2008).

Zoetendal and colleagues analysed, through denaturing-gradient gel electrophoresis (DGGE), the 16S rRNA gene on faecal and bioptic samples from ten subjects, and reported that the number of bacteria in mucosal sample is quite uniform along the colon. Interestingly, the profiles at different location in the same individual are similar, indicating that such population is uniform also qualitatively. Finally, DGGE profiles from mucosal and faecal samples of the same individual were in most cases different, indicating that the two populations are not completely interchangeable (Zoetendal et al., 2002).

Another study by Green and colleagues (Green et al., 2006) focused on the characterisation of mucosa-adherent bacteria. Using the same method, they examined mucosal bioptic specimens from 33 healthy individuals and, by comparing DGGE profiles, they showed that samples from different sites of the same patient harboured very similar bacterial communities, confirming previous data, while all subjects had different profiles. According to a previous work that outlines the importance of genetic factors in this context (Zoetendal et al., 1998), this study suggests that host factors are important in modulating microflora composition. They also matched gene sequences of 16S rRNA DGGE bands with entries in the GeneBank data base, attributing most of them to uncultured species in the genera Bacteroides, Clostridium, Ruminococcus and Faecalibacterium.

Surprisingly, terminal ileum harbours a number of mucosa-associated bacteria higher than the colon (Ahmed *et al.*, 2007). This may be linked to the higher number of unidentified helical bacteria not found in the large bowel. Overall, bacterial number is quite similar in the whole colon length, but *Lactobacilli* are more prominent in the distal large intestine. *Bacteroides* and *Enterobacteriaceae* are uniformly distributed in ileal and colonic mucosa, while *Bifidobacteria* are more prominent in the colon. Moreover, the mucus plays a crucial role in regulating the relationships between bacteria and the colonic mucosa. Recently, it was found that the epithelium of the colon is protected by an inner mucus layer formed by Muc-2 mucin impervious for bacteria that, vice versa, can be found in the outer loose non-attached mucus layer (Johansson *et al.*, 2008). In case of Muc-2 mucin deficient mice, the bacteria are in close contact with epithelial cells and are even found in deep of crypt (i.e. near the stem cells of colon epithelium). The normal segregation of bacteria away from epithelium appears to play an important role in the genesis, or better, in the prevention of colon cancer, because it has been observed that mice lacking Muc-2 are prone to develop colon cancer (Velcich *et al.*, 2002).

Moreover, different strains of the same bacterial species can have different tendency to establish an association with the mucosa. It is not known if this characteristic found in pathogenic strains can also be present in autochthonous microflora. The use of FISH for the study of the microbiota in humans has shown that bacteria are localized (albeit, in a limited number of colonies) in the side of the intraluminal mucus layer with a composition similar to that of the faecal contents (Van der Waaij *et al.*, 2005). More refined molecular methods have then definitively established that bacterial populations related to the mucosa are different from those faecal (Eckburg *et al.*, 2005).

In normal human intestine, such mucosa-associated bacterial population is relatively small. Schultsz and colleagues (Schultsz *et al.*, 1999) performed bacterial rRNA in situ hybridization on bioptic specimens of inflammatory bowel disease (IBD) and non-IBD patients, mostly with irritable bowel syndrome. Interestingly, in normal individuals the number of bacteria in the mucus layer is very small: in the vast majority of sections, there were no bacteria at all. Swidsinski and colleagues, using FISH technique, have confirmed that the number of bacteria on the mucosa is low ($<10^7$ cfu) and that the mucus layer is often free from bacteria in over 80% of biopsies of normal subjects (Swidsinski *et al.*, 2007). We performed a similar study using scanning electron microscope and had analogous results (Brandi *et al.*, 1997). Moreover, our data showed that in mice there are many mucosa-associated bacteria. On the contrary, in human large bowel, bacteria are not in close contact with epithelium, and they are rarely found even in mucus layer. When present, they are clustered in small groups separated by wide areas with no bacteria at all. Studies performing quantitative evaluation with various techniques of mucosa-associated bacteria reported a concentration ($10^5 - 10^7$ colony forming units) lower than the faecal one, in subdominant position (Zoetendal *et al.*, 2002, Ahmed *et al.*, 2007). In conclusion, if the mucus of the human colon has a variable amount of bacteria, besides not fully corresponding to faecal microbiota, human colonic epithelium remains strictly germ-free under normal conditions.

## 3.3    Animal Models and Intestinal Microflora

### 3.3.1    Differences BetweenHuman and Rodent Microflora

Rodents are occasionally employed to study several characteristics of IM but some concerns exist in translating these data into humans. Differences can be identified both with classical and molecular approach; bacterial species likely belong to the same classes, while familiae and genera are host-specific. For example, in rodents, the number of endoluminal bacterial along the alimentary tract is substantially constant, ranging between $10^8$ to $10^9$ colony forming units (CFU)/ml. Conversely, in humans, the number of bacteria detectable in the small bowel is negligible (~$10^4$ – $10^5$ CFU/ml), increasing from the jejunum to the ileocecal valve and reaching the highest concentration in the cecum. Furthermore, the relationship between the bacterial flora and the intestinal epithelium could be substantially different between rodents and humans. In fact, in rodents there is an intimate relationship between the intestinal mucosa and a large amount of bacteria, often found to cluster over the mucus gel or in direct contact with epithelial cells, whereas in humans such correlation is lacking. These data and the difference in host-microbiota relationship between humans and mice constitute the major limitations of the murine model.

## 3.4     Molecular and Morpho-Functional Characteristics of Gastrointestinal Tract Induced by Microflora

The use of animal models without bacteria (germ-free) compared to those with normal microflora (holoxenic) has fostered the study of morpho-functional changes induced by the presence of microflora in the digestive tract and, therefore, of the main functions of this complex ecosystem. Some studies also focused on gnotobiotic rodents, i.e. animals with gut colonised by known, definite bacterial strains. Human flora-associated animals (HFA), belonging to this group, can be obtained by inoculating germfree animals (e.g. mice) with human faeces (Raibaud *et al.*, 1980). Human flora-associated mice and rats had and will undoubtedly have great importance in elucidating IM role in pathogenesis of intestinal diseases, but are also limited by various issues. Microflora obtained from faeces may not completely overlap with the intestinal one, and some bacterial strains may not colonise the murine gut; in particular, *Bifidobacteria* and *Lactobacilli* seem to be spontaneously eliminated (Raibaud *et al.*, 1980). On the other hand, a recent study has demonstrated that most constituents of IM are able to colonize rodents and are stable in time (Hirayama & Itoh, 2005).

Intestinal microflora inoculated in animal models should be standardized in order to obtain reproducible animal models, which are often associated to microflora coming from only one subject and thus are not directly comparable. Some studies are therefore focusing on definition of a reproducible average human flora to standardise bacterial strains employed in HFA models (Hirayama & Itoh, 2005). The difference of the relationship between bacteria and host mucosa in holoxenic mice, HFA ones and humans are showed in Figure3. However, animal models are our best chance to investigate the role of IM, in particular for practical and ethical limits of research on humans. Germ-free animals, when compared to holoxenic counterparts, present defects in the development of intestinal immune system, in the nutrient absorption and in the intestinal morphology and motility (Lee & Mazmanian, 2010). Germfree mice are characterised by a reduced thickness of the colonic wall, inadequate differentiation of the small intestine and inferior epithelial proliferation compared with controls. In particular, they show a defective development in GALT (gut-associated lymphoid tissues), fewer and smaller Peyer's patches and reduced expression of toll-like receptors (TLRs) and of CD4+ T cells in the lamina propria (Macpherson & Harris, 2004). In the absence of IM enterocyte cell cycle is prolonged and crypt cell proliferation rate is reduced (Alam *et al.*, 1994). The presence of bacteria in the intestinal lumen and mucosal surface can modify some cell kinetic parameters producing a condition of hyperproliferation compared to germfree life, but the type of IM is also important. This is evident in large bowel, where mucosal proliferation rate (evaluated by bromodeoxyuridine intraperitoneal injection 1 h before sacrifice) is significantly higher in holoxenic and HFA mice compared to germfree ones. Interestingly, human flora drives also higher mucosal proliferation rate than mice one (Brandi *et al.*, unpublished data).

The renewal of intestinal epithelium and even the building of aberrant crypts and adenomas follow a horizontal pattern, characterised by the production of new crypts through a phenomenon of fission (Li *et al.*, 1994). Differently from vertical renewal crypt pattern, the horizontal one seems independent from IM presence, as shown by comparisons between germfree and holoxenic rats (McCullogh *et al.*, 1998).

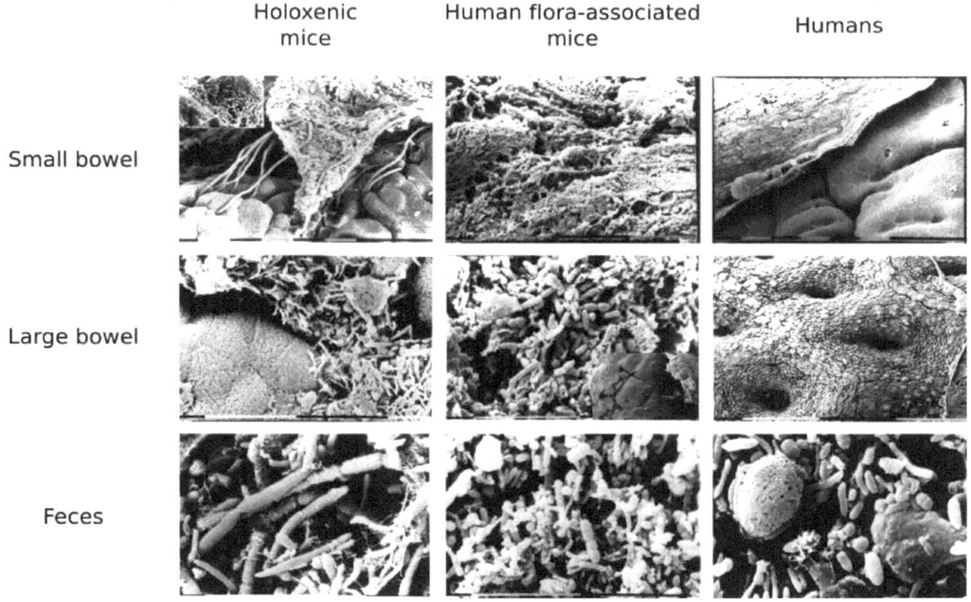

**Figure 3:** Scanning electron microscopy showing bacteria-mucosa relationship in humans and rodents along the gut. In mice, different types of bacteria can reach the epithelium cells both in small and in large bowel; while in humans bacteria are far from the epithelium and at the best they are found in the luminal part of the mucus. Even in HFA mice, bacteria do not reach epithelial surface, being embedded in mucus. In general, the amount of bacteria adhering to the mucosa is significantly lower as compared to their presence in faeces, thus suggesting that not all bacteria are able to adhere to the mucosa.

While pathogenic bacteria can induce or increase apoptosis of intestinal epithelium (Zychlinsky & Sansonetti, 1997), there is no specific knowledge about the capacity of autochthonous microbiota to directly affect epithelial apoptosis.

Hooper *et al.* investigated the role of IM in modulation of genes by laser capture microdissection and molecular array in *Bacteroides thetaiotaomicron*-monoassociated mice (Hooper *et al.*, 2001). The analysis of mRNA obtained from ileal mucosa after ten days of colonization showed an at least two fold variation in the expression of 118 probe sets. Among these genes, 95 resulted upregulated and 23 downregulated. This study demonstrated some fundamental consequences of commensal colonization, confirming results of observational studies. At different time (day 8 and day 60), most cell cycle genes induction was observed in both holoxenic and conventional mice compared to HFA mice inoculated at the same time. More than 100 genes were highly expressed including Sass6, E2f2, Hspa8, Aurka, Zwilch, Rad51 and Brca1, and also Cdc6, Exo1, Kntc1 and Cdc7 at day 60 (Gaboriau-Routhiau *et al.,* 2009).

Besides type, timing of arrival of microflora into the lumen seems also important. Conventionalized mice show high expression of 31 genes compared to holoxenic mice at day 60, indicating that cell cycle response is higher in these animals. The most affected gene signaling pathway at both time-points was the cell cycle pathway 'Role of APC in cell cycle regulation', which was highest in conventional animals at day eight, and in mouse flora-treated mice and axenic mice at day sixty. In this pathway, a polyubiquitin chain gets attached to a protein substrate by an ubiquitin-ligase, which targets it for degradation by the 26S proteasome. This is an important step in the cell cycle, as cell division progression is governed by degradation of different regulatory proteins in the ubiquitin-dependent pathway. Anaphase-promoting complex (APC) is an ubiquitin ligase that plays a key role in the cell cycle.

Around 50% of genes elicited in the ileal mucosa in response to bacterial colonization are linked to immune pathways. Transcriptomic analysis of terminal ileum mucosa from GF, holoxenic and HFA mice shows that cell cycles-specific genes are tenfold higher in HFA mice compared to holoxenic (Gaboriau-Routhiau *et al.*, 2009).

Bacterial presence and subsequent GALT TLRs activation are indeed fundamental for intestinal epithelium to achieve its normal trophism and gut-associated lymphoid tissue (GALT) to mature (Round & Mazmanian, 2009), but the type of IM is very important and only a restricted number of normal microbiota is able to stimulate the mucosal T-cell response. In particular human IM seems quite unable to stimulate the immune system in mice, and transcriptome analysis of immmune genes in HFA mice clustered with GF rather than holoxenic ones, supporting the impact of host-specific microbiota for immune stimulation (Gaboriau-Routhiau *et al.*, 2009). This observation was recently confirmed by Chung *et al.* that analysed immune maturation and gut microbiota composition of GF mice colonized at birth with rodents gut microbiota (MMb) and human gut microbiota (HMb), showing that HMb-colonized mice have a poorly developed small intestinal immune system, quite similar to that in GF mice, demonstrating that there is an essential interaction between specific microbe-host and the maturation of the intestinal immune system. Inducing infection of Salmonella enteric, these authors showed that HMb-colonized mice presented intestinal inflammation respect to MMb mouse, assessing that exists a host-specific microbiota that plays a critical role in modulation of immune system and GUT immune maturation (Chung *et al.*, 2012).

Members of microbiota as *Bacteroides fragilis* are important for the mucosal immune system stimulation of mammals (Mazmanian & Kasper, 2006). In particular, *Bacteroides fragilis* is able to prevent colitis in two different experimental models (Round & Mazmanian, 2010) and its capsular molecule Polysaccharide A (PSA) directs the differentiation of Interleukin-10 (IL-10)-secreting TReg cells (Mazmanian&Kasper, 2006). Furthermore, it has been demonstrated that oral treatment with purified PSA could reduce the expression of cytokine and the infiltration of lymphocyte, due to increased production of   IL-10 and Foxp3 expression (Round & Mazmanian, 2010).

Another bacterium, responsible to modulate the nature of the intestinal immune responses, is the *Segmented Filamentous bacteria* (SFB). This unculturable species detected in rodent intestine adheres to intestinal mucosa and stimulates a large spectrum of innate and adaptive immune responses, which notably mediate the abundance of lamina propria Th17 cells and the secretion of antimicrobial peptides (Gaboriau-Routhiau *et al.*, 2009, Ivanov *et al.*, 2009, Lee & Mazmanian, 2010). Furthermore, SFBs colonization plays a protective role against *Citrobacter rodentium*, an enteropathogenic bacterium that produces in rodent's intestinal inflammation similar to *E. Coli* (EPEC) in humans (Ivanov *et al.*, 2009).

Beyond the relationship with immune system, microbiota drives several other functions.

Some experiments also demonstrated that inoculation of a single dominant bacterial strain (e.g. *Bacteroides thetaiotaomicron*) in germfree mice causes complete epithelial differentiation and resumption of normal cellular proliferation (Umesaki *et al.*, 1995).

Monocolonization with this microorganism does not induce inflammation, contrary to *Salmonella enteritidis* that upregulates IL-8. The contemporary association of *B. thetaiotaomicron* and *S. enteritidis* is characterized by downregulation of IL-8, supporting the protective role of commensal microflora in infections. Expression of glutathione S-transferase and multidrug resistance protein 1a (MDR1a), involved in detoxification and elimination of various compounds, is also reduced. These data seem to support the hypothesis that colonised mucosa is less resistant to carcinogens and toxics in general, but it can't be excluded that lower level of expression of S-transferase and multidrug resistance protein 1a (MDR1a) may also be associated with a lower level of exposition to carcinogens of the epithelium, thus a lower need of expression of detoxifying proteins. Finally, colonization promotes angiogenesis by increasing angiogenin-3 expression (Hooper *et al.*, 2001).

### 3.5   Metabolic Functions of Intestinal Microflora

Intestinal microflora plays also an important role in the physiology of digestion and in metabolic functions. Wostmann and colleagues surprisingly showed that germ-free rats needed about 30% more caloric intake to keep their body weight with respect to their normal counterparts (Wostmann *et al.*, 1983), suggesting that intestinal microflora contributes to the digestion of nutritional elements introduced with diet rather than subtracting them.

Pioneeristic works showed that at least some bacterial species, especially of the genus *Bacteroides*, could degrade a lot of polysaccharides and glycans poorly digestible by humans (Salyers *et al.*, 1977, Salyers *et al.*, 1981) to mono- or disaccharides, well absorbable by enterocytes. Moreover, it has been shown in gnotobiotic mice that *B. thetaiotaomicron* can induce the host to synthetize glycans, which are then catabolized, by its enzymatic apparatus, this way obtaining metabolic substrates and energy (Sonnenburg *et al.*, 2005).

Moreover, IM, especially *Bacterioides*, seems to inhibit fasting-induced adipocyte factor (FIAF), a protein capable of inhibiting lipoprotein lipase, fat mass accumulation and inducing apoptosis (Bäckhed *et al.*, 2004). In addition, the reduced antiblastic chemotherapy toxicity in germfree mice is due to loss of FIAF inhibition, at least in part. Actually, FIAF favours apoptosis, and its inhibition thus limits tissue damage (Crawford & Gordon, 2005, Brandi *et al.*, 2006A).

*B. thetaiotaomicron* seems also to favour nutrient absorption by enhancing expression of digestive enzymes and transporters such as Na-glucose cotransporter (SGLT1), colypase and high affinity epithelial copper transporter (CRT1), thus suggesting that IM is important in utilisation of dietary macromolecules.

There are also evidences that, in humans, up to 20% of plasma lysine and threonine is synthetized in the gut by microflora and then absorbed (Metges *et al.*, 1999). In animal model it has been demonstrated that bacteria have a key role in nitrogen recycling in the gut, as urea generated in the host is hydrolysed into ammonia, which is available for amino acid synthesis (Forsythe & Parker, 1985).

Folate deficit has been suspected to be implicated in CRC genesis especially when combined with high alcohol intake, which lower folate levels and is metabolised to acetaldehyde, a well-known carcinogen. Intestinal microflora directly produces about 10% of intestinal folate and some ethanol by dietary glucides fermentation, so its role is uncertain: actually, a formal demonstration of a link between folate/ethanol metabolism and genetic changes of intestinal epithelium is still lacking (Giovannucci *et al.*, 1995). However, DNA methylation alteration is frequently reported in CRC (Selgrad *et al.*, 2008); folate deficit and consequent monocarbon unit transport impairment may influence this phenomenon.

Another important role of IM is much less beneficial for the host. In fact, bacterial metabolites produced in the human large intestine from endogenous secretion and excretion, as those produced by the liver, can be carcinogenic. The endoluminal concentration of such toxic metabolites depends upon the balance between dominant and subdominant bacterial strains and upon their presence in the intestine. The whole knowledge of metabolic pattern of microbiota and its interaction with host's physiology (even with central nervous system) is far to be reached, but research's field could be take off by "omics" approach.

## 3.6    Relationship between Diet and Human Microbiota

Although the influence of diet on IM composition is still debated, recent studies clearly support this cause-effect relationship. Several studies using animal models associated with human IM explored the changes in IM induced by dietary macrocomponents and dietary supplements as oligosaccharides and prebiotics. *Lactobacillus casei*-fermented milk is generally said to augment both the total bacteria and *Bifidobacteria* counts, and therefore alter the equilibrium among the dominant species. The same is true for dietary supplements as prebiotics (β-galactooligosaccharides and β-glucooligosaccharides), which do not affect total bacterial count (Djouzi *et al.*, 1997).

Focusing on cancer, significant changes in the composition of IM of HFA mice fed a high-bran or a high-meat diet have been reported (Hirayama *et al.*, 1994). Moreover, response of human IM to dietary components varies between populations, as demonstrated by investigating the effect of resistant starch on HFA rats inoculated with faeces of northern or southern European populations (Silvi *et al.,* 1999). Furthermore, different HFA microfloras in term of methanogens respond differently to seaweed (Andrieux *et al.*, 1998). HFA mice inoculated with faeces of meat-eaters or vegetarians show a strongly different impact on genotoxic effects of diet carcinogens (Kassie *et al.*, 2004), concordantly with previous observation (Hambly *et al.*, 1997), which shows an elevation of metabolic CRC biomarkers in HFA rodents fed with high-risk diet. The Gordon's group, using a metagenomic approach, shows that both luminal and mucosal adherent gut microbiota of HFA mice are quite different when animal are fed with low-fat or high-fat/sugar "Western" diet, with relative increase of bacteria belonging to *Firmicutes* phila in the latter one. Interestingly, the switching from a low-fat to "Western" diet shifted the structure of microbiota and changed its gene expression and metabolic pathways in few hours (Turnbaugh *et al.*, 2009A). A recent study, conducted through metagenomic approach in elderly people, suggests that changes in the microbiota associated with changes in diet seem less abrupt in humans, although the analysis on those individuals was not longitudinal, but, rather, for groups (Claesson *et al.*, 2012). The administration of "Western" diet restructures the distal gut bacterial community of rodents with a tremendous expansion of *Mollicutes*, not only at the expense of other members of the phylum *Firmicutes*, but also of *Bacteroidetes* that are reduced (Turnbaugh *et al.*, 2008). It seems also likely that the increase of these specific bacteria facilitates, besides the passage of calories from foods to host, also the metabolism of absorbed calories, with progressive development of obesity in the host. It has been established that the microbiota can play a role in obesity, as germ-free mice are resistant to obesity induced by "Western" diet, enhancing the level of circulating lipoprotein lipase (angiopoietin–like 4), finally increasing mitochondrial oxidation and the AMP kinase in liver and skeletal muscle (Backhed *et al.*, 2007). However, the interaction between microbiota, diet and obesity, exceed the simple relation to favour additional calories to its host by some specific bacteria, because the involvement of the intestinal immune system has been suggested. Vijay-Kumar *et al.*, show that knock-out mice for Toll- like receptors 5 (expressed by both intestinal epithelial cells and innate immune system with bacterial flagellin as ligand), are obese and with several aspects of metabolic syndrome (Vijay-Kumar *et al.*, 2010). The changes of normal interactions between GALT and bacteria alter the microbiota, which in turn promotes a mild inflammation by means of the feedback altered with the same GALT acting through MyD88. In this process, the key role of the gut microbiota of T5KO mice is demonstrated by its transfer in germ free mice that is necessary and sufficient to reproduce the metabolic phenotype. Furthermore, some bacterial products, as short chain fatty acids, peptidoglycan and lipopolysaccharides cross intestinal epithelium and active receptors of immune system (GPR43, NOD1, TLR4) (Maslowski *et al.*, 2009, Clarke *et al.*, 2010). Some animal models allow the dissection of the associated role of diet/obesity/inflammation and suggest that dietary factors are the real determinants of changes in the intestinal microbiota (Hildebrandt *et al.,* 2009). In fact, although some rats have an obesity-prone and others an obesity–resistant phenotype, the high fat diet induced identical microbiota changes in both groups, hence suggesting that other host factors might be involved in growth of intestinal permeability and induction of local inflammation (De La Serre *et al.*, 2010). The ob/ob mice (homozygous for the obesity's character) have an imbalance of the microbiota compared to the respective wild type, with increment of *Firmicutes* and decline of *Bacteroidetes*, hence the increased capacity to harvest energy from diet (Turnbaugh *et al.*, 2006). Interestingly, the obesity was even transmissible simply through transplant of faeces from obese to germ-free mice. According to mice models, Ley *et al.* observed a similar difference with a rise of microbiota ratio of *Firmicutes/Bacteroidetes* in human obese and consecutive re-equilibrium to the benefit of *Bacteroidetes* in case of fat restriction diet (Ley *et al.*, 2006).

However, this characteristic change of microbiota in relation to obesity has not been seen in all human studies, nevertheless, conducted with different methods. For example, the *Firmicutes* are equal in lean and obese twins; the *Bacteroidetes* can be the same in groups of obese or thin, or even increased in overweight (Turnbaugh *et al.*, 2009B; Schwiertz *et al.*, 2010). A metagenomic analysis of subjects of different countries/continents selects three clusters bacteria (so called enterotypes), which show no relationship between *Firmicutes/Bacteroidetes* ratio and BMI, however, some molecules conveyed by the intestinal microbiota correlate closely with this parameter, suggesting that functional aspects are more important than differences in the phila (Arumugam *et al.*, 2011). As a corollary of this, the metagenomic approach certifies definitively that populations with different diet and with different risk of colon cancer, have a dissimilar microbiota, as highlighted by studies conducted on children raised with rural african diet that, in comparison with those on western diet children, showing a decrease of *Firmicutes* and the enrichment of *Bacteroidetes*, *Prevotella* and even *Xilanibacter*, enabling genes allowing hydrolysis of cellulose and xilan (De Filippo *et al.*, 2010).

## 4   Specific Characteristics of IM in Adenoma or Cancer bearing Patients

The most active field of research about the possible role of microbiota in colon-rectum cancer genesis, searches gut bacteria putatively related with CRC by comparing their abundance among CRC/adenoma patients, high-risk population and healthy subjects. All studies are cross-sectional cohort study using coltural–based methods, or molecular-based ones, starting with DNA fingerprinting techniques until the high-throughput DNA sequencing with higher resolution level and expectance of fewer biases.

Some bacterial groups were supposed to positively or negatively influence CRC development based on their potentially dangerous enzymatic activities (7α-dehydroxylaseβ-glucuronidase, β-glucosidase, nitroreductase) or by their mere presence on the mucosa. Moore and Moore isolated and compared over 5 000 dominant bacterial strains from 18 polyp patients and 54 controls epidemiologically at different risk of CRC (North American Caucasian, Japanese-Hawaiians, native Africans and Japanese). IM of polyps patient, considered at high risk, and Japanese-Hawaiians are similar and significantly different from IM of low-risk native Americans and Japanese. Bacterial strains associated with high-risk subjects belong to the genera *Bacteroides*, *Eubacterium* and *Ruminococcus*, *Bifidobacterium* and

*Faecalibacterium prausnitzii* (Moore & Moore, 1995). O' Keefe *et al.* linked 7α-dehydroxylase bacteria to high CRC risk population, while *Lactobacillus plantarum* to low risk population (O'Keefe *et al.*, 2007).

The use of molecular methods (q-PCR for bacterial DNA and RNA), then confirmed by classical coltural methods, demonstrates that on the adenoma mucosa there is a lower number of bacteria compared to the normal colonic mucosa, while there is no difference between the concentration of bacterial DNA on the normal mucosa of patients with or without adenoma (Pagnini *et al.*, 2011). It is possible that the reduction of bacteria on the adenoma mucosa is linked to the activation of specific a-defensin antibacterial. Two consecutive case-control studies performed by the same group and using different molecular analysis (terminal restriction fragment length polymorphism, clonal sequencing and FISH, or more advanced sequencing technology and q-PCR) to investigate the bacterial communities of normal rectal mucosa in patients with polyps or controls, suggest differences in bacterial composition with a higher bacteria richness (i.e. the number of taxa in the sample) in cases, (87 more abundant taxa was found), without differences for evenness (i.e. taxa distribution within the sample) (Shen *et al.*, 2010, Sanapareddy *et al.*, 2012). Interestingly, the differences in richness are entirely due to low- abundance taxa and seem unrelated to diet. A bacterial profile of adenoma subjects is characterized by *Proteobacteria* increasing and *Bacteroidetes* decreasing without differences for *Firmicutes*, the most represented phylum. At genus level, polyps' subjects showed higher abundance of *Faecalibacterium*, *Shigella* and *Dorea spp* and reduction of *Bacteroides spp* and *Coprococcus* spp. The FISH analysis confirms that the outer mucus layer is the unique ecosystem of mucosa adherent-bacteria, even in normal mucosa of patients with adenoma. In a perspective of cause and effect, it can be assumed that changes in the bacterial population may have preceded the onset of adenoma formation.

Scanlan *et al.*, in two related studies using DNA fingerprinting techniques (DGGE, RIS, qPCR) and metabonomic tools, analysed interindividual and intraindividual variability of faecal microflora in healthy, colorectal cancer and polypectomyzed subjects (Scanlan *et al.,* 2008, Scanlan *et al.*, 2009). Only the polyp group shows significantly different interindividual DGGE profiles, in CRC patients significantly higher number of *Clostridiumcoccoides* and *Desulfovibriosp* (producer of hydrogen sulphide, a well know genotoxic agent) were found. No diversity has been detected concerning *Bacteroides* in the three groups. Using high-throughput DNA sequencing technology, faecal microbiota of CRC Caucasic (Sobhani *et al*., 2011) and Asiatic patients (Wang *et al.*, 2012) was compared to normal subjects, respectively, in a retrospective or prospective manner. Although the total number of bacteria was similar in CRC and controls (Sobhani *et al.*, 2011), both studies detect a differing faecal microbiota structure in cancer patients compared with controls. According to Sobhani, the *Bacteroides/Prevotella* are the only bacteria group higher in cancer patients, while other dominant or subdominant bacteria as *Bifidobacterium* genus, *Lactobacillus/Leuconostoc* group, *Clostridiumcoccoides/C leptum* group and *Faecalibacterium prausnitzii* did not show any differences. It is believed that the main changes of microbiota in CRC patients refer to depletion of butyrate-producing bacteria and to increase of opportunistic pathogens. Both *Clostridium coccoides/ C leptum* group and *Faecalibacterium prausnitzii* are strong producer of butyrate but their depletion are not constantly detected in different studies. Wang detects a reduction of *Clostridium coccoides* but not of *Faecalibacterium prausnitzii*. Vice versa, Balamurugan *et al.* (Balamurugan *et al.*, 2008) shows an important decrease of *Faecalibacterium prausnitzii* in patients with cancer. The *Bacteroides*, whose occurrence turned out to be unrelated to diet, are 1000 times more present in the faeces than in the mucosa but, above all, they correlate with constant increase in pro-inflammatory cytokine IL-17 in the mucosa (Sobhani *et al.*, 2011).

In Asiatic patients, Wang shows a separation of healthy and cancer patients based on lower abundance in the latter of OTUs (operational taxonomic units) belonging to butyrate producing bacteria (i.e *Roseburia* genus), to genera *Oscillibacter*, *Alistipes*, to *Clostriadiaes* order and concomitant higher abundance of *Escherichia/ Shigella*, *Klebsiella*, *Citrobacter*, *Streptococcus*, *Enterococcus*, *Peptostreptococcus*, *Fusobacterium* genera and *Bifidobacteriales* order. Differently from Sobhani, *Bacteroides spp* are less abundant in CRC subjects, although at species level, *Bacteroides* are either enriched (*B. fragilis*) or diminuted (*B. vulgatus*) in these patients.

Moreover, five studies analysed the mucosal microbiota of CRC patients. Using DNA fingerprinting and FISH methods, Ahmed *et al.,* showed that in normal mucosa of CRC patients, bacteria are found in the mucus layer without differences of overall bacterial number along the colon sites, but with an unexpected higher number in terminal ileum (Ahmed *et al.*, 2007). Marchesi J *et al.,* studying the microbiota of both tumoral and normal adjacent mucosa of caucasic patients by DNA fingerprinting and pyrosequencing of 16S rRNA genes indicated clear differences between two microbiotes. More *Bacteroidetes* and less *Firmicutes* phila are found on tumoral toward normal mucosa, in particular more butyrate producing bacteria (*Roseburia*, *Faecalibacterium*, and *Fusobacterium*) and less *Enterobacteriacee* (*Citrobacter*, *Shigella*; *Serratia*; *Salmonella*). These potential pathogens are quite absent on mucosa of normal subjects, and it is possible, that the CRC microenvironment is colonized by gut bacteria with antitumorigen and anticarcinogenic characteristic (Marchesi *et al.*, 2011). A similar pyrosequencing analysis was performed to determine the overall microbiote in Asiatic patients with CRC and health controls, investigating faecal and cancerous mucosa and matched non-cancerous normal tissue (Chen *et al.*, 2012). A strong difference on microbiota exists about lumen and cancerous tissue. In lumen, it was found more abundant phyla enhancing energy harvested from food, as *Firmicutes*, and less *Bacteroidetes* and *Proteobacteria*. The faecal and mucosa-adherent microbiotas differ in CRC compared to match ones of healthy subjects. In lumen, the bacterial phyla associated to metabolic exchange with host (*Prevotellaceae*, *Coriobacteriaceae*, and *Erysipelotrichaceae*) increases in cancer patients. Interestingly, these bacteria can represent the link between Western diet or obesity and CRC, due to their presence in obese humans or mice. In cancerous tissue, *Lactobacillaceae* increased while *Faecalibacterium* was reduced.

Finally, the normal mucosa of CRC patients in comparison with healthy subjects, show an increase number of *Fusobacterium*, *Peptostreptoccocus* and *Porphyromonas* and a corresponding decrease of *Bifidobacterium*, *Faecalibacterium* and *Blautia* genus.

Two independent reports, studying the same target (microbiota of cancer mucosa and matched adjacent normal tissues) and using the same methods (whole genome sequencing, qPCR, and respectively coltural or FISH) show a prevalence of *Fusobacterium* genus (and mainly *Fusobacterium nucleatum spp*) in cancer mucosa (Castellarin *et al.*, 2012; Kostic *et al.*, 2012). The first discovery phase of the two experiments on 11 and 9 patients affected by CRC through the 16S rDNA sequencing, showed that on the tumoral mucosa there is a depletion of *Firmicutes* and *Bacteroides* and, more interestingly, an increase (up to 10,000 times higher) of *Fusobacterium*. This figure was then validated in a larger sample (99 and 88 patients, respectively) by means of qPCR with specific probes for the *Fusobacterium*. The FISH analisys showed its plausible presence on the epithelium, and the *Fusobacterium nucleatum* isolated from the cancerous mucosa has even been found in lymph nodes and liver metastases, thus clearly suggesting its translocation.

Since the Kostic's patients were studied in parallel to the changes of the eukaryotic genome, it is interesting to note that in the presence of *Fusobacterium* coexist a high number of mutations and chromosomal rearrangements (Bass *et al.*, 2011). Finally, it must be emphasized that only a subset of patients affected by CRC shows an association with the presence of *Fusobacterium*, which, when present, can however, constitute 90% of the microbiota of the cancerous mucosa. This aspect resulted even more evident in the few cases in which the neoplastic mucosa was represented by the only adenoma (Castellarin *et al.*, 2012). Furthermore, the *Fusobacterium* has been found in the mucosa of IBD patients with invasive capacity of cellular lines (Strauss *et al.*, 2011, Dharmani *et al.*, 2011).

An interesting hypothesis about the relationship between microbiota and the development of cancer, suggests that one or more bacteria play a key role from the beginning to advance phases also modifying the microbiota setting (the alpha bugs hypothesis) (Sears, 2009). Other hypothesis, more on line to the recent data, forecasts that the development of CRC-microbiota linked is a dynamic process in which bacteria can change over time. In particular, the promoters are driven bacteria belonging to those able to directly interfere in host genome, thanks to a proinflammatory action directly on epithelium (i.e. *ETBF*, *E. coli*, *E. faecium* and perhaps *Fusobacterium spp.*). Over time, these promoters would no longer be present on mucosa because the development of neoplasia modifies the microenvironment, which becomes available to other bacteria (so-called passenger bacteria) (Tjalsma *et al.*, 2012).

| Authors/y. | N° of subjects | Bacteria in HS | | Bacteria in patients with Adenoma | | | Bacteria in CRC patients | | | Methods |
|---|---|---|---|---|---|---|---|---|---|---|
| | | Faeces | Mucosa | Faeces | Normal mucosa | Adenoma | Faeces | Normal mucosa | Cancer | |
| Moore and Moore 1995 | 88 | X | | X | | | | | | Coltural |
| O' Keefe 2007 | 52 | X | | | | | | | | Coltural |
| Shen 2010 | 44 | | X | X | | | | | | Sequencing/FISH |
| Pagnini 2011 | 51 | | X | X | | X | | | | FISH/qPCR |
| Sanapareddy 2012 | 71 | | X | X | | | | | | Pyrosequencing |
| Balamurugan 2008 | 37 | X | | | | | X | | | qPCR |
| Scanlan 2008 | 46 | X | | X | | | X | | | DGGE/RISA |
| Scanlan 2009 | 85 | X | | X | | | X | | | qPCR |
| Sobhani 2011 | 179 | X | | | | | X | X | | Pyrosequencing/qPCR |
| Wang 2012 | 102 | X | | | | | X | | | Pyrosequencing/qPCR |
| Ahmed 2007 | 26 | | | | | | X | | | DGGE/FISH |
| Marchesi 2011 | 6 | | | | | | X | | X | DGGE/Sequencing |
| Castellarin 2011 | 11 | | | | | | X | | X | WGSequencing/ qPCR/Coltural |
| Kostic 2012 | 18 | | | | | | X | | X | WGSequencing/FISH |
| Chen 2012 | 102 | X | X | | | | X | X | X | Pyrosequencing |

**Table 1**: Luminal and adherent mucosa microbiota in patients with adenoma or colorectal cancer and in health control subjects.

In summary, only the use of more performing high-throughpout DNA sequencing technology allows defining a microbiome associated to the presence of CRC, but the design of cross-sectional cohort study prevents discovering the causal relationship between microbiota and CRC. What is indispensable and we are still missing in order to define a cause-effect relationship, is to understand the changes in the intestinal microbiota in time and space, starting from the condition of normality and arriving to full blown CRC.

# 5   Animal Models, Intestinal Microflora and Sporadic Cancer Risk

Most studies on the relationship between IM and CRC have been conducted on rodent models, and are therefore biased by differences in the host-microbiota relationship between humans and animal. As a whole colorectal cancer tumor in rodent share many genetic and phenotypic features with human tumour (Corpet & Pierre, 2005). Studies often follow these schemes:

- Comparison among germfree, holoxenic and gnotobiotic rodents APC or carrier of other cancer-prone mutations;
- Comparison among germfree, holoxenic and gnotobiotic rodents treated with chemical carcinogens;
- Comparison among germfree, holoxenic and gnotobiotic rodents in capability of activating or inhibiting endogenous pro/co-carcinogens.

## 5.1   The Genetic Cancer-Prone Model (APC)

Since the serendipitous discover of APC mice in 1990 (Moser *et al.*, 1990), many animals genetically predisposed to gastrointestinal cancer have been studied to understand the pathogenetic bases of these tumours. In particular, the APC mouse has been the first and most studied model in investigating the putative role of IM in genetically prone subjects. Considering that mutations in Apc are not only responsibly for familial adenomatous polyposis syndrome (FAP) but frequently occur in the sporadic CRC, the Min mice provide an interesting in vivo model to study human colorectal cancer, although mice develop mainly adenomas in small bowel and human only in large bowel. In these APC Min/+mice usually Wnt/βcatenin, together with Cox2 and NOS hyper expression, plays a major role in tumorigenesis. However, in these mice tumors occur mainly in small bowel. Several mutant of genetically modified APC Min/+ exist with, like humans, different number of adenomas. In particular, the variant of APC MinIN/+mice with deletion of exon 14 shows a severe colon polyposis, thus better simulating the human FAP's condition.

As suggested by Dove's study, the microbial state in APC mice seems not to remarkably influence the development of multiple adenomas in small and large bowel, neither in number nor in quality, with just a higher trend to develop adenomas in jejunum in presence of microflora (Dove *et al.*, 1997). However, recently, Li *et al.* showed that a tumor load, either in small and large bowel of APC Min/+ mice, is strictly regulated by the presence of commensal microflora, which works, at least in part, by triggering the c-JUN/JNK and STAT3 signaling pathways (Li *et al.*, 2012). Thus, further studies supports the key role of My D88 dependent activation of NF-KB in myeloid cells for tumorigenesis in APC Min/+ mice (Rakoff-Nahoume *et al.*, 2007).

It is also true that some strains of bacteria seem to play a more critical role in CRC genesis of APC Min/+mice. For example, Newman and colleagues (Newman *et al.*, 2001) have demonstrated that APC mice infected with *C. Rodentium*, a murine pathogen strongly adherent to the epithelium trough a type III secretion system (a molecular syringe-like mechanism), develops a fourfold increased number of colic adenomas than uninfected APC mice. Furthermore, this study has shown that medium highness of dysplastic crypts is comparable with infected APC mice and infected wild type mice, demonstrating that even strong genetic background becomes negligible in case of *C. Rodentium* infection. The increased number of adenomas depends on the capability of this microorganism to induce hyperproliferation of epithelium (Barthold & Jonas, 1977), but its role in human gut is controversial. It is probable that the mechanism is similar to EHEC and EPEC pathogens, based on attaching and effacing lesions (AE). A comparison between germ-free and conventional mice infected with *C. Rodentium* shows that intestinal colonization does not require the type III secretion system in germ-free animals, and commensal bacteria are necessary to clear this pathogen from the mammalian intestine during infection, that occurs trough bacterial competition, by decreasing the number of anaerobes and increasing the number of *Proteobacteria* which compete with *C. Rodentium* for carbon sources (Kamada *et al.*, 2012).

Furthermore, if, a human colonic bacterium as enterotoxigenic *Bacteroides fragilis* (ETBF) (responsible of large amount of infective human diarrhoea but also asymptomatic, carried up to 35% of population) colonizes APC Min/+mic, triggers colitis and strongly induce colonic tumors. This is strictly due to its toxin: a protease able to bind colin epithelial cells and stimulate the E-cadherin cleavage, actually nontoxigenic *B. Fragilis* doesn't induce colonic tumor. Interestingly, ETBF induces adenoma or microadenoma early or very early after colonization, via both activation of Th17 in the lamina propria with IL-17 release and γδ-T cell with STAT3 pathway (Wu *et al.*, 2009). Indirectly, these data can explain the prevalence of adenoma in small bowel of APC Min/+mice, because the SFB housing this part of bowel induces a strong Th17/IL17 reaction (Gaboriau-Routhiau *et al.*, 2009).

Unfortunately, no sufficient data exist on intestinal microflora composition and relationship with mucosa of familial adenomatous polyposis patients. The unique, recent, exception suggests an unexpected characteristic: the presence of APC-like sequences in microbiota of FAP patients, thus suggesting a putative horizontal transfer of genetic information between eukaryotic and prokaryotic word (Holec *et al.*, 2012). In conclusion, although neither a very strong genetic pattern seems to be sufficient to develop adenomas in absence of commensal bacteria, this process is emphasized in presence of proinflammatory bacteria.

## 5.2    The Chemical Carcinogenesis Route

The most frequently used chemical cancerogenous in experimental models are cycasin and 1,2-dimethylhydrazine (DMH), both procarcinogens transformed in azoxymethane in the presence of, respectively, bacterial beta-glucosidase and bacterial or mucosal beta-glucuronidase.

As expected, cycasine is ineffective in inducing CRC in germfree rats, while DMH can induce colon neoplasia also in this population (Reddy *et al.*, 1975, Onoue *et al.*, 1977, Horie *et al.*, 1999A). Like humans, in several carcinogen- induced rodent tumors (in particular who's due to DMH/AOM) the Wnt/β-catenin pathway plays a back bone role, although the APC mutation is rare (Corpet & Pierre, 2005). Horie and Kanazawa evaluated the effect of intestinal microflora in the development of colonic neoplasia experimentally induced by DMH by comparing germ-free, holoxenic and gnotobiotic mice. In germfree rodents treated with DMH via subcutaneous route, the proliferation of crypts is higher than in holoxenic mice, but both the large/dysplastic adenoma and large/multiple ACF are significantly more represented in holoxenic than in germfree animals. The autochthonous microflora seems to have a suppressant effect on initiation of carcinogenesis induced by DMH. However, the size and the histopathological characteristics of adenomas developed in holoxenic animals suggest that bacterial flora may have an effect in promoting dysplastic transformation and tumoral growth (Horie *et al.*, 1999A).

Furthermore, every single bacterial species might be differently involved in the various phases of initiation and/or promotion of cancer. Even if in monoassociated gnotobiotic mice treated with DMH the number of adenoma is generally lower than in germfree (like in holoxenic ones), *Clostridium*-monoassociated adenomas are larger than in germfree or in gnotobiotics monoassociated with *B. longum* or *L. acidophilus*. In fact in pluriassociated gnotobiotic rats with a pool of *Clostridia* and *Bacterioides* species treated with DMH the total number of large ACF is significantly higher than in germfree rats, confirming that these genera have an important role in the progression of preneoplastic lesions. When *Bifidobacterium breve* is added to pluriassociated gnotobiotic rats, the number of large ACF and multiple ACF is lower (Onoue *et al.*, 1977, Horie H *et al.*, 1999B).

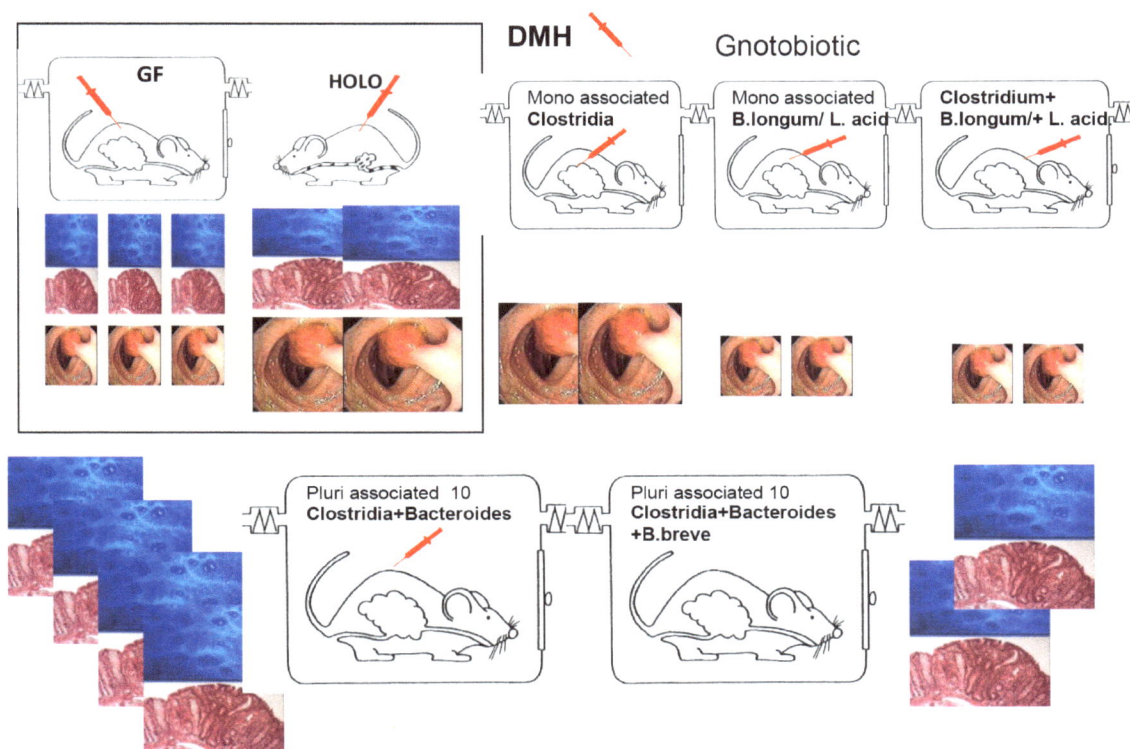

**Figure 4:** Role of bacteria in the activation of chemical pro-carcinogens. Some of these pro-carcinogens (cicasine), require an enzymatic bacterial action. Dymethil-hydrazine is activated by both procariotic and eucariotic Beta-glucuronidase, therefore DMH induces aberrant crypts and adenomas in germ-free animals. When bacteria are present, these pre-cancerous lesions are larger in conventional than in germ-free animals, because microbiota can have an ambivalent action: suppression of initiation processes and stimulation of promotion ones, and different bacterial species can have different roles in these processes of initation and promotion.

Eventually, some experiments linked genetic and chemical carcinogenetic routes. K-ras transgenic mice treated with DMH seem to have the same oncogenic potential both in germ free and in holoxenic mice, but number and size are slightly inferior in GF ones (Yamamoto *et al.*, 1996,Narushima *et al.*, 1998). Ohno and colleagues have demonstrated that number of CRC in DMH treated K-ras transgenic mice is inferior in mice supplemented with *Bifidobacterium longum* (Ohno *et al.*, 2001).

This data show that IM as a whole interacts with chemical carcinogens, while suggesting a different role for each bacterial strain, since some favour carcinogenesis and other do not or hamper it. However, these results are limited by differences between humans and rodents and by inadequate representation of multi-step adenoma-carcinoma sequence.

## 5.3    Intestinal Microflora and Endogenous Carcinogens

Intestinal bacteria has been involved in the tumoral process since it has hydrolytic and reductasic enzymatic activities (such as nitroreductase, azoreductase, beta-glucuronidase, beta-glucosidase, arylsulfatases and alcohol dehydrogenases) having the capacity to produce or activate cancerogenous metabolites from digestion products (McBain & Macfarlane, 1998). Some of these metabolites require an enzymatic action conduced by bacteria only and are not able to induce tumors in germ-free rodents.

A biunivocal relation seems to exist between bacterial enzymes and dietary carcinogenic metabolites: in fact, if it is demonstrated that metabolites are activated by IM, it is also true that diet can influence enzymatic activity. Hambly et al. evaluated the influence of high- and low-risk dietary regimens on enzymatic activity markers in HFA mice: high-risk diet increased 2.5 fold β-glucuronidase activity and halfed beta-glucosydasic activity (Hambly et al., 1997). Concomitantly ACF, preneoplastic precursors of CRC, also increase.

In the last years, many compounds modulated or metabolised by IM have been identified, investigated and seem to be involved in colorectal carcinogenesis: in the next sections, the main ones will be briefly outlined.

### 5.3.1    Heterocyclic Amines and other Products of Pyrolysis

The heterocyclic amines (HCA), which originate from fried or broiled proteinaceous foods, seem to be carcinogenic in mice, rats, and monkeys producing hepatic, intestinal, and mammary tumors (Schoeffner & Thorgeirsson, 2000). For example, one HCA, 2-amino-3-methyl-3H-imidazol [4,5-f]quinoline (IQ), produced through the pyrolysis of creatinine, can be converted into 2-amino-3-methyl-3H-imidazo[4,5-f]quinoline-7-one (HOIQ, a direct-acting mutagen) by bacterial β-glucuronidase (Carman et al., 1988). In fact, after absorption in the upper part of the gastrointestinal tract, IQ is mainly metabolized in the liver. Here UDP-glucuronosyl transferases lead to the formation of harmless glucuronidated derivatives. These metabolites are partly excreted via the bile into the digestive lumen, where they come into contact with the resident microflora (Kassie et al., 2001). In GF rats treated with a single dose of IQ the DNA damage in form of strand breaks (Comet Tail Test) is significantly lower than in conventional and human flora associated animals (Knasmüller et al., 2001). The Comet assay performed on colonocytes and hepatocytes showed that the presence of bacterical β-glucuronidase in the digestive lumen dramatically increased (3-fold) the genotoxicity of IQ in the colon (Humblot et al., 2007). When the DNA damage is measured by alkaline single-cell gel electrophoresis assay DNA, the test exhibits significantly fewer alkaline-labile breaks in GF rats than in rats colonized with conventional murine or human bacteria, and this happens not only in colon cells but also in hepatocytes (Kassie et al., 2001). The supplementation of the feed with Lactobacilli or Bifidobacteriumlongum seems to attenuate the induction of colon cancer by this same amine in a still unknown manner (Reddy & Rivenson, 1993, Knasmüller et al., 2001).

Other products of pyrolisis (such as benzopyrene), whose derivatives are inactive when joined to glucuronic acid, can be reactivated by the action of bacterial beta-glucuronidase, with successive damage to DNA (Renwick & Drasar, 1976). A very few bacterial strains bearing the ability to produce such metabolites in the intestinal lumen have been identified. This results from the fact that in vitro experiments using culture media frequently give different results than in vivo experiments using HFA rodents. For instance, our unpublished experience showed that human strains of *Clostridium* might express their β-glucuronidase activity in vitro, in vivo or both. This can be due to genetic organization of the β-glucoronidase gene, which differs according to the analized strain (*E. coli, L. gasseri, R. gnavus*) (Beaud *et al.*, 2005).

Benzopyrene originates from pyrolysis of organic material or food preparation at high temperature and is mutagenic and carcinogenic. This metabolite can be excreted as glucuronide (40%) and sulfate (9%) (Boroujerdi *et al.*, 1981) or can be oxidized in the liver to epoxides, which are conjugated to glutathione and excreted in the bile. In the gut biliary metabolites of benzopyrene are hydrolysed by IM (Renwick & Drasar, 1976). In fact fecal excretion of benzopyrene glucuronide is higher in germ-free rats than in conventional ones (Rafter *et al.*, 1987). Furthermore the DNA-benzopyrene adducts in colonic tissue seem to be produced only by bacterial β-glucuronidase hydrolysis of benzopyrene glucuronide (Kinoshita & Gelboin, 1978).

In summary, a western meat-rich diet may, apart the obesity risk, increase the risk of CRS, affecting the microbiota composition towards a profile with more effective metabolites of heterocyclic amines.

### 5.3.2    Secondary Biliary Acids and Diacylglycerol

Ileal bile salt transport is highly efficient (95%) but up to 800 mg of bile salts can escape the enterohepatic circulation daily and, in the colon, 7α-hydroxylating bacteria, such as *Clostridia*, convert primary biliary acids into secondary, e.g. deoxicolic (DCA) and lithocolic (LCA). Several observational studies suggest the role of faecal bile acids in CRC development (Tong *et al.*, 2008).

Secondary biliary acids can induce cell necrosis, hyperplasia, and alteration of the DNA synthesis and increase of genotoxic activity of several mutagens in vitro. Actually, most animal studies conclude that DCA is a promoter of the carcinogenesis process (Pereira *et al.,* 2004) and high concentration of secondary bile acids in faeces, blood and bile has been linked to the pathogenesis of CRC (McGarr *et al.,* 2005). Some researchers argue that bile acids may cause DNA damage and act as carcinogens in humans (Bernstein *et al.*, 2009) and it has been demonstrated that cell signaling pathways activated by DCA in mammalian epithelial cells include antiapoptotic cell signaling pathways involved in carcinogenesis, like protein kinase C (Zhu *et al.*, 2002), ERK 1/2 via the epidermal growth factor receptor (Rao et al., 2002); β-catenin (Pai *et al.*, 2004) and JNK 1/2 pathway (Gupta *et al.,* 2004). According to Pereira and colleagues, the fact that secondary bile acids cause apoptosis in colonic epithelial cells could exert selective pressure for emergence of epithelial cell mutants which are resistant to apoptosis (for example, via loss of p53) (Pereira *et al.*, 2004).

It is true also that a diet high in fat stimulates higher secretion rates of bile acids from the gallbladder, and the hypothesis that individuals who consume a high fat diet have higher levels of secondary bile acids in faeces has been confirmed in several studies (Hardison, 1978). An increased LCA/DCA ratio is also associated with a shift of the proliferative compartment towards the apex of colorectal crypts, an anomaly associated with cancer (Biasco *et al.*, 1991).

Presence of high deoxycolate's concentration enhances production of diacylglicerol (DAG), an activator of protein kinase C and, therefore, a promoter of carcinogenesis. DAG seems to be produced from phosphatidylcholine degradation through the action of bacterial enzymes. DAG formation in an acidic environment is negligible, therefore it has been hypothesized that Lactobacilli and Bifidobacteria exert a beneficial action on intestinal mucosa by reducing luminal pH (Vulevic *et al.*, 2004).

### 5.3.3   Sulphide

Sulphidogenic bacteria are commensals microrganism utilizing sulphate ($SO_4^{(-)}$) as energy source and oxidant agent with consequent production of sulphide ($S^{(-)}$) (Huycke & Gaskins, 2004); most of them belong to Proteobacteria phylum. Hydrogen sulphide concentration in the intestinal lumen is regulated on one hand by its bacteria production and on the other hand by the level of epithelial enzyme activity RHOD (thiolmethyltransferase and rhodanese), which degrades H2S.

Sulphide is a genotoxic agent, at 1 mM strongly increases crypt proliferation, and expands the proliferative zone to the upper crypt (Christl *et al.*, 1996). Furthermore, it stimulates cell cycle entry and can induce hypoxia-triggered proliferation in intestinal epithelial cells through an MAPK, Akt, ERK and p21-dependent mechanisms (Cai *et al.*, 2010). Furthermore, COX-2 is up-regulated in the epithelium after H2S challenge (Attene-Ramos *et al.*, 2010).

A recent study has showed that animals fed dextran sodium sulphate (DSS), a chemical toxic to the intestinal epithelium, develop low to high-grade dysplasia, as well as adenoma and carcinoma, while a control group fed dextran sodium sulphate and metronidazole displayed no dysplasia. This demonstrates that cancer development in animals fed a sulphate source is dependent on bacterial metabolism (Deplancke *et al.*, 2003).

Between sulphidogenic and metanogenic bacteria seems to be a substrate competition: the more is represented by the production of methane, the less is intestinal colonization of sulphidogenic bacteria (Strocchi *et al.*, 1994). The role IM plays in the production of sulphide and methane, considering possible interactions with diet and genetic background, remains to be defined.

### 5.3.4   Fecapentaenes

The fecapentaenes (FPs) are conjugated either lipids produced in the large bowel by *Bacteroides spp.* from polyunsaturated ether phospholipids (plasmalogens) whose natural origin and function are unknown. Their production is greatly enhanced by bile in an unknown manner. Fecapentaene-12 causes direct oxidative DNA damage via production of the reactive oxygen species O2-, $O_2^{(-)}$, and $OH^{(.)}$ (Szekely & Gates, 2006). FPs are strong mutagens (900 times more potent than N-methyl-N-nitrosurea), but there is no evidence for FPs as initiators and are considered promoters (Hinzman *et al.*, 1987). The potential of fecapentaene-12 (FP-12) to promote tumor development was tested in a rat colon carcinogenesis model using N-methyl-N-nitrosourea (MNU) as the initiating agent (Zarkovic *et al.*, 1993). The number of carcinoma-bearing rats as well as the average number of carcinomas per rat was significantly higher in the MNU + FP-12 group as compared to the MNU-alone values. Aberrant crypt foci (ACF) were found in all carcinogen-treated rats, including those that did not contain tumors, whereas none were observed in the FP-12 and control groups. The average number of ACF containing >10 aberrant crypts per focus was significantly higher in the MNU FP-12 group. These findings suggested that FP-12 could express promoting activity in chemical induced colon carcinogenesis.

Data reporting fecapentaenes excretion in man are apparently contradictory, since the excretion is higher in low risk subjects and lower in cancer patients: The FPs faecal excretion in groups at different risk of CRC is higher in vegetarian than in omnivores and lower in colon cancer patients than in controls (De Kok & Van Maanen, 2000). This apparent contradiction has been correlated to the lower exposition of intestinal mucosa to fecapentaenes in subjects with high excretion.

Due to these conflicting results, only few studies have been recently conducted on fecapentaenes role in colorectal carcinogensis, which currently seems negligible, but the existence of an interindividually variable mutagenic potential in the faeces seems reasonable.

### 5.3.5  Butyrate

The greatest part of intestinal microflora is strictly anaerobic, so the final products of its fermentative metabolism are short-chain fatty acids: in human colon, acetate, propionate and butyrate are the most represented (Høverstad *et al.*, 1984). In humans, short-chain fatty acids are absorbed and used as energy substrates, and butyrate represents the 60-70% of enterocytes' energy sources (Roediger, 1980). The main producers of butyrate are eubacteria, clostridia and roseburia (Nicholson *et al.*, 2012). Diet with high levels of non-digestible carbohydrates stimulates the growth of specific butyrate-producing bacteria, hence increased plasma levels of butyrate.

Butyrate regulates cellular proliferation and differentiation through various supposed mechanisms: basically it inhibits NF-kB and histone deacetylase (Gibson, 2000, Hamer *et al.*, 2008) and stimulates the detoxifying enzyme glutathione S-transferase (Ebert *et al.*, 2003). That is why it is supposed that butyrate is one of the principle mediators in the protective role of fibre (Bingham *et al.*, 2003). Some studies have supported the role of butyrate in colon carcinogenesis observing the down-regulation of butyrate transporters, like MCT1 and SMCT1, in neoplastic colonic tissue: this down-regulation could be responsible for reduced activity of butyrate in colonic mucosa and, consequently, for the increase in dysplastic alterations (Lambert *et al.*, 2003).

The suppression of NF-kB has an important anti-inflammatory effect and, consequently, has a role in the prevention of inflammation related cancer. In fact, NF-kB regulates the expression of cytokines, inflammatory enzymes, immune receptors and acute phase proteins and has a responsibility in colon cancerogenesis (Hamer *et al.*, 2008). The anti-inflammatory effect of butyrate could be due also to inhibition of interferon α production (Klampfer *et al.*, 2003) or to upregulatin of PPAR-γ (peroxisome proliferator-activated receptor γ) (Kinoshita *et al.*, 2002).

Histone deacetylase inhibition is responsible for the enhancement of the accessibility of transcription factor to DNA and for the modulation of fundamental apoptosis and cell cycle genes. Cancer cells seem to be more sensitive to this effect than normal cells, although there are no explanations for this different response (Dashwood *et al.*, 2006).

Other effects of butyrate are inhibition of tumor cell migration by decreasing DAF (decay accelerating factor) (Andoh *et al.*, 2002), inhibition of angiogenesis (Zgouras *et al.*, 2003) and inactivation of metalloproteinase. More in general butyrate seems to decrease proliferation on the upper side of the crypt, increasing contemporary proliferation on the basal compartment of the crypt. This peculiar activity, called the butyrate paradox, could support the protective role on dysplastic/neoplastic tissue and, at the same time, could introduce to the procancerogenic role of butyrate on in vitro nonneoplastic cells (Comalada *et al.*, 2006). The explanation of this double activity is still unknown.

It is important to note that fermentation of indigestible carbohydrates with consequent SCFA production takes place mostly in proximal colon, while protein fermentation occurs in its distal portion. This metabolic difference might be responsible for the prevalent distal localisation of most colic diseases. Human studies are needed to confirm the role of butyrate on cancer progression and/or prevention.

## 6  Bacteria and Inflammatory Bowel Disease – Associated Colorectal Cancer

Inflammatory bowel disease (IBD) is characterized by chronic, relapsing inflammation of the gastrointestinal tract. The two main types of IBD are Crohn's disease (CD) and ulcerative colitis (UC).

The first one can affect any portion of the gut, but usually the terminal ileum and the colon. Inflammation, often with granulomas, involves the whole thickness of the gut wall and can be destroying, leading to stenosis and fistulas. It is usually discontinuous, with areas affected separated by apparently normal mucosa. Ulcerative colitis, on the contrary, always affects the rectum, and inflammation can spread cranially in a continuous fashion up to the caecum. Only mucosa and submucosa are affected, and inflammation is characteristically non-granulomatous (Podolsky, 2002). Patients affecting to severe UC, refractory to medical therapy, often undergo to total colectomy with anal-ileal pouch anastomosis (IPAA). This surgical procedure is commonly followed by pouchitis, a nonspecific inflammation of the ileal pouch (Meagher *et al.*, 1998).

IBD is a strong risk factor for CRC development, with a prevalence of 2-3% at 10 years (Canavan *et al.,* 2006). In the following section, the role of bacteria in IBD pathogenesis and their implication in malignant transformation will be discussed. Actually many data, albeit often based on animal models, support these hypothesis.

## 6.1    Pathogenesis of IBD

The aetiology of the disease is largely unknown, although various factors have been implicated in its pathogenesis, including the influence of genetic, environmental and microbial factors (Xavier & Podolsky, 2007). Among others, there is increasing evidence showing an important role for bacteria, in particular defects in both immune response and microbial recognition genes are pivotal for IBD onset in genetically predisposed patients (Bouma & Strober, 2003). Four main mechanisms, not mutually exclusive, have been suggested in the pathogenesis of IBD in humans: microbial pathogens, alteration of commensal microflora, defect of host mucosal barrier function, defect of host immune regulation (Farrell & LaMont, 2002).

## 6.2    Microbial Pathogens

Over the years various microbial pathogens have been suggested as aetiologic factors in IBD: *Listeria monocitogenes*, *Helicobacter hepaticus*, *Chlamydia*, *Enterobacteriaceae*, *reoviruses* and *paramyxovirus* (Liu *et al.*, 1995). *Mycobacterium avium subspecies paratuberculosis*(MAP), which has been isolated in surgical specimens of Crohn's disease,was strongly suspected as an etiologic factor of IBD onset. Actually, MAP is an obligate intracellular pathogen that causes Johne's disease, a granulomatous inflammatory condition of the ruminants which affects the distal intestine, characterized by diarrhea and wasting and resembling human Crohn's disease (Chiodini, 1989).

The detection of this organism in those individuals with defective innate immunological defenses, such as CD patients by various techniques has been reported, including culture, PCR, FISH, or serology (Behr & Schurr, 2006); others have shown immune response against mycobacterial antigens (Ibbotson *et al.*, 1992). However, epidemiologic studies do not show increased prevalence of Crohn's disease in spouses of patients, physicians treating patients, or farmers and veterinarians working with infected animals (Farrell & LaMont, 2002). Moreover, anti-TNF therapy and corticosteroids, risk factors for disseminated mycobacterial infections (Wallis *et al.*, 2004), are effective in Crohn's disease, while clinical studies failed to demonstrate the efficacy of antimycobacterium triple antibiotic therapy in CD patients (Thomas *et al.*, 1998).

The most commonly IBD related bacterium is *E. Coli* belonging to the *Enterobacteriaceae*. In IBD patients, an increase of *E. Coli* was observed (Kotlowski *et al.*, 2007). The adherent invasive *E. coli* was associated with ileal mucosal lesions in CD patients, with increased number and capability to adhere to the intestinal epithelial cells, disrupting the intestinal barrier (Rolhion & Darfeuille-Michaud, 2007). This bacterium is more invasive in CD patients compared to UC patients (Sasaki *et al.*, 2007).

Further studies demonstrated that the pathotype adhesive and invasive *E. coli* stimulates the production of IL-8, an important proinflammatory cytokine produced by macrophages and other cell types (Martin *et al.*, 2004).

The different strains of *Fusobacterium nucleatum*, a gram-negative bacterial species of human mouth and gut, could have a pathogen role in IBD (Strauss *et al.*, 2011). Two pathogen strains of *F. nucleatum* are capable to adhere to the colonic mucosa and to up-regulate the expression of TNF-α mRNA (Ohkusa *et al.*, 2009). Furthermore, these pathogen strains have a role in regulating the expression of TNF-α, IL-10β mRNA and in the up-regulation MUC1 (4-fold) and MUC2 (12- to 15-fold) (Dharmani *et al.*, 2011). As a while, due to these conflicting data no single microbial agent has been proven so far to be the cause of IBD in humans.

## 6.3    Changes in Commensal Microflora

Notwithstanding the difficulties to assess the normal microflora per group of subjects due to the personal pattern of IM, many studies have reported changes in microflora in patients with IBD, especially Crohn's disease (Qin *et al.*, 2010). In particular, IBD patients are characterized by a reduction of dominant members of the gut microbiota.

Recent studie suggest a decreased in microbial diversity in the active phase of the disease, describing an increase relative number of *Enterobacteriaceae*, especially of the enteroinvasive strains, and a decrease of *Clostridium* and *Bacteroides* species, with no substantial differences between ulcerative colitis and Crohn's disease (Frank *et al.*, 2007, Baumgart *et al.*, 2007). While many studies agree with decreased *Clostridia* concentration (Gophna *et al.*, 2006, Manichanh *et al.*, 2006), for *Bacteroides* results are less clear, since some studies report an opposite pattern (Swidsinski *et al.*, 2005, Kleessen *et al.*, 2002).

Since *Bacteroides* and *Clostridia* produce butyrate and other short-chain fatty acids (Høverstad *et al.*, 1984), the major energetic substrates of colonocytes (Roediger, 1980), their reduction could explain the reduced short-chain fatty acids concentration in the feces of patients with IBD (Marchesi *et al.*, 2007). This, coupled with increased hydrogen sulphide production by other species – which inhibits short-chain fatty acid utilization – suggests the possibility of nutritional deficiency of colonocytes of IBD patients, which could lead to a loss of function. Actually, Roediger and colleagues hypothesized that ulcerative colitis can be the consequence of this mechanism (Roediger *et al.*, 1993).

The disequilibrium between bacteria with anti or proinflammatory properties (due to their own characteristics and/or relationship with intestinal epithelium) can be involved in IBD onset. A recent study confirmed these data and also showed that Faecalibacterium prausnitzii, a member of the *Clostridium* leptum phylogenic group, has interesting anti-inflammatory properties both in vitro and in vivo on murine models. Moreover, its reduction on ileal mucosa is associated with higher risk of postoperative recurrence of Crohn's disease (Sokol *et al.*, 2008). Therefore, the disequilibrium between bacteria showing anti or proinflammatory features (due to their own characteristics and/or their relationship with intestinal epithelium) can be involved in IBD onset.

Furthermore, *Escherichia coli* concentration is increased in both faeces and mucosa of IBD patients (Frank *et al.*, 2007, Baumgart *et al.*, 2007). It is also present in granulomas (Ryan *et al.*, 2004) and near ulcers and fistulae (Liu *et al.*, 1995). These invasive strains express virulence factors and can replicate within macrophages which, in turn, secrete large quantities of TNF (Glasser *et al.*, 2001), contributing to inflammation. Whether these changes are primary or secondary is still controversial.

The relationship amongst bacteria, mucus, mucose (epithelium and gut-associated lymphoid tissue [GALT]) seems to be very important: in IBD patients, significantly more bacteria harbors in the intestinal mucus layer. Actually in a light microscope study on bioptic specimens were not seen bacteria at all in most control sections, while in 42% of IBD patients more than 50 bacteria per mucosal surface area examined have been observed, and the type of bowel preparation before undergoing the endoscopic procedure does not significantly affect this result (Schultsz *et al.*, 1999).

## 6.4    Defect of Host Mucosal Barrier Function and Immune Regulation

Under physiologic conditions, the complex interaction between host and intestinal microflora is finely regulated. This ultimately leads to a tolerogenic response, while retaining the ability to mount an immune response against bacterial detrimental to the host (e.g. invasive pathogens). Any defect in this homeostatic system could result in an enhanced and inappropriate inflammatory response, which could itself damage the host.

An increase of bacterial translocation through the lamina propria triggers pattern recognition receptor (PRR), TRL stimulation and pro-inflammatory chemokine and cytokine secretion, which induce NF-kB pathway activation (Cario, 2010).

It has been demonstrated in vitro that proinflammatory cytokines induce a defect in epithelial barrier function via an apoptosis-independent mechanism (Bruewer *et al.*, 2003); in particular interferon-γ can induce internalization of tight junction proteins (occludin, JAM-A, claudin-1) (Bruewer *et al.*, 2005). This could allow non-invasive bacteria and gut antigens to cross epithelium and stimulate an immune response (Clark *et al.*, 2005).In fact, IBD is characterized by enhanced mucosal permeability, but it is not clear whether the defect is primary or secondary: actually TNF upregulates claudin 2 expression, which is involved in pore formation. Moreover, altered regulation of apoptosis and tight junction components, have been reported in active Crohn's disease (Zeissig *et al.*, 2007). Some studies suggest that the defect is primary: Hollander and colleagues reported enhanced intestinal permeability both in patients with Crohn's disease and their relatives, hypothesising an aetiologic role (Hollander *et al.*, 1986).

The pathogenetic mechanisms previously described can ultimately lead to tolerance rupture and chronic intestinal inflammation, as suggested by efficacy of fecal diversion in Crohn's disease relapse (Rutgeerts *et al.*, 1991), but some evidence supports also the hypothesis of a primary defect in the immune system. Crohn's disease patients have impaired microbial killing, which leads to overexposure of the microflora to the immune system and consequent activation of adaptive immunity (Korzenik, 2007).

This may be due to defective production of antimicrobial peptides such as α-defensin. Alpha-Defensins are peptides produced by Paneth cells in response to microbial products or proinflammatory cytokines. Their antibactericidial property is significantly efficacious against *Enterobacteriaceae* and *BacteroidesVulgatus*. Studies reported a significantly reduction of these peptides in association with ileal CD, in particular in patients with NOD-2 mutations (Nuding *et al.*, 2007).More generally, there is evidence for reduced mucosal antimicrobial activity in Crohn's disease. Genetic polymorphisms characterized by reduced synthesis of these proteins have been associated with Crohn's disease, such as reduced copy number of α-defensin 2 (Fellermann *et al.*, 2006) and NOD2/CARD15 variants (Hisamatsu *et al.*, 2003). Moreover, the tolerogenic molecule gp96 is underexpressed in Crohn's disease patients (Schreiter *et al.,* 2005).

A reduced level of secretory IgA (sIgA) in IBD could be the cause of an impaired microbial clearance. IgA plays a critical role in mucosal immunity. In the gut is produced by B cells and its primary functions are to entrap bacteria and dietary antigens in the mucus layer and to regulate microbial intestinal colonization (Peterson *et al.*, 2007).

In IBD the reduction of sIgA is balanced by an increased secretion of mucosal IgG, which induces the production of pro-inflammatory cytokine and multiple adaptive immune responses to the microbiota (Sartor, 2008).

The presence of dysbiosis in IBD could be due also to alteration in autophagy, which is used by macrophages to kill bacterial pathogens, including *Legionella*, *E. Coli*, *Streptococcus* and *Mycobacterium* species. Autophagy-related protein 16-1 is a protein encoded by ATG16L1 gene and plays a critical role in autophagy. Recently it has been shown a strictly relation between CD and mutation in ATG16L1, demonstrating an implication of bacterial defective autophagy in IBD (Kuballa *et al.*, 2008). Autophagy also plays an important role in innate and adaptive immunity and this defective mechanism could influence the immune adaptive response to bacteria, the antigen presentation by APC and the regulation of T cell death and proliferation (Dengjel *et al.*, 2005).

Studies have demonstrated the important role of two categories of innate immune receptors in intestinal inflammation and the development of colon cancer. These are Toll-like receptors (TLRs) and the nucleotide-binding domain, leucine-rich-repeat-containing proteins (NLR) (Akira *et al.*, 2006, Franchi *et al.*, 2006).

There is evidence for T-cell (Duchmann *et al.*, 1995) and serologic (Mow *et al.*, 2004) response against various bacterial antigens. In fact, lamina propria mononucleated cells from areas of IBD proliferate when co-cultured with autologous intestinal bacteria sonicates, while peripheral blood or noninflammed lamina propria mononucleated cells do not, further supporting the hypothesis of an interplay among IM, intestinal epithelium and GALT. An autoimmune response is less evident; however, commensal bacteria are recognized by anti-neutrophil cytoplasm antibodies (Seibold *et al.*, 1998); also some data support cross-reactivity between bacterial and human antigens (Polymeros *et al.*, 2006).

## 6.5    Animal Models in Inflammation – Associated Colorectal Cancer (CAC)

The study of animal models of inflammatory bowel disease provides evidence that commensal microflora is necessary to induce and maintain inflammation. Actually, in most murine models of the disease (genetically engineered rats with immunoregolatory defects predisposed to inflammation) inflammation does not develop in germ-free animals (Rath *et al.*, 1996) or is significantly milder than in corresponding controls with intestinal microflora (Bamias *et al.*, 2007).

During the last years, various mouse IBD-related carcinoma models have been created. Their evaluation suggests the strictly relationship between microbiota, inflammation and development of CAC, where commensal or pathogenic bacteria interact with intestinal immune system with pro-inflammatory mechanisms.

IL-10 deficient mice develop both inflammation and cancer. An interesting study was conducted by Uronis *et al.* (Uronis *et al.*, 2009) demonstrating that AOM-Wild Type mice did not develop colitis, while conventionalized AOM-IL-10-/-presented spontaneous colitis and CAC, where severity of colitis and cancer depends on bacterial-induced inflammation. These conditions are worsened by infection of *Helicobacter Hepaticus* (Kullberg *et al.*, 2001). Similar pathogenic role has *Helicobacter spp.*, which increases tumor development in IL-10-/- (Chichlowski *et al.*, 2008). Helicobacter infection is also necessary for carcinogenesis in SMAD3 -/- and Rag2 -/- mice, where SMAD3 is a regulator of TGF-β signaling and Rag2 (recombination encoding gene) play an important role in the generation of mature B and T lymphocytes (Maggio-Price *et al.*, 2006, Poutahidis *et al.*, 2007).

In T-cell receptor-β-chain and p53 double Knock-out mice, the development of inflammation and CAC depends on the microbiota. In fact, it has been shown that these mice do not present inflammation nor cancer in germ-free condition (Kado *et al.*, 2001). In a STAT3 inactivated mouse model, where STAT3 is a mediator of IL-10 signaling, the development inflammation and CAC is produced only in the presence of intestinal microflora (Deng *et al.*, 2010).

With an important study about these two categories of innate immune receptors, Allen *et al.* firstly demonstrated the protective role of NLRP3 and the inflammasome complex PYCARD/procaspase-1 in recurring gastrointestinal inflammation and tumorigenesis in experimentally induced colitis. The NLR inflammasome complex is composed by Apoptotic Speck protein containing a CARD (ASC/PYCARD), caspase-1 and NLRP3, which influence IL-1β and IL-18 processes, regulating inflammation and tumorigenesis via hematopoietic/myeloid system. The authors demonstrated lack of the inflammasome complex dramatically increases the development of colitis (both acute and recurring) and cancer (Allen *et al.*, 2010).

TRUC mice develop spontaneous colitis. Afterwards, it has been shown that the majority of TRUC mice developed a colonic dysplasia and rectal adenocarcinoma, due to an altered regulation of TNFα and depending on the commensal microbiota (Garrett *et al.*, 2009).

A strictly correlation between E. Coli and inflammation and cancer has been demonstrated by Arthur *et al.* based on the evidence that microbiota plays a critical role in the development of CAC in IL-10 deficient mice (Uronis *et al.*, 2009). In a recent study they analyzed germ-free IL-10 deficient mice, compared to wild-type mice (WT), showing that 100% of GF IL-10-/- mice develop spontaneous colitis and, after addition of AOM, 60-80% of them develop CAC, with respect to WT mice that did not presented colitis nor CRC. Sequencing analysis showed differences in fecal and mucosal microbiota between WT and IL-10 K.O. mice. In particular, an increase of more than 100 fold of *E. Coli* was detected. To better understand the role of this bacterium in the pathogenesis of colitis and cancer, the authors conducted an experiment on mono-associated GF IL-10 K.O. with *E. Coli pks* + (a genic island that encodes enzymes synthesizing genotoxic peptides). This system reproduces colitis and CAC in 80% of mice (when AOM is administered), clearly suggesting the key role of the *E. Coli* in the propagation of lesion previously iniziated by AOM. These results well fits with the experiments conducted on humans, were it has been shown that the prevalence of *E. Coli* (pks +) is 67% in CRC, 40% in IBD and only 20% in healthy subjects (Arthur *et al.*, 2012).

## 6.6   Colon Cancer via Inflammatory Pathways

In the XIX century, Rudolph Virchow had already hypothesized a link between chronic inflammation and cancer. Now, much evidence has grown up, and this causal relationship is becoming more and more accepted as studies give insight into the possible mechanisms (Coussens & Werb, 2002). Chronic inflammation is actually a source of injury for the organism through tissue infiltration by macrophages and their release of reactive oxygen and nitrogen species, cytokines and growth factors. This milieu can induce various consequences: it can influence cell growth, differentiation and apoptosis, damage DNA and promote angiogenesis. Actually, the incidence of colorectal cancer in IBD is increased both in ulcerative colitis and in Crohn's disease, which rank amongst the top risk factors together with familial adenomatous polyposis and hereditary nonpoliposis colorectal cancer. This appears to be inflammation-related.

However, there is a complex interplay between inflammation and cancer. Tumor cells can produce cytokines recruiting inflammatory cells (macrophages, lymphocytes and others) capable, in turn, to produce other cytokines and alter the tumor microenvironment. IL-6 and CSF-1, produced by neoplastic cells, can recruit myeloid precursors and induce a macrophage-like phenotype; moreover, dendritic cells recovered from tumors are often defective and unable to stimulate T cells (Allavena *et al.*, 2000). Tumor-associated macrophages can produce various cytokines and growth factors, stimulate angiogenesis, and thus have been implicated in disease progression (Schoppmann *et al.*, 2002). They also produce IL-10, which blunts the immune response, but interestingly may kill neoplastic cells after stimulation with IL-2, IL-12, or IFN-α (Brigati *et al.*, 2002).

A hypothesis explaining this complex relationship between inflammatory cells and cancer is that a causal relationship exists. In fact, many infectious agents have been recognized as carcinogenic (group 1 and 2A) by IARC, and 17.8% (1.9 million cases) of all the cancer in the year 2002 is attributable to chronic infections (Parkin, 2006). Persistent inflammation, characteristic of IBD, also causes overproduction of reactive oxygen and nitrogen species, which can damage DNA, and repeated tissue damage and repair. The observation that p53 point mutations have a similar incidence in cancers and in a chronic inflammatory condition such as rheumatoid arthritis further support this hypothesis. p53 mutation load and iNOS activity are increased in the colon of ulcerative colitis patients, supporting the link between inflammation and genetic damage (Hussain *et al.*, 2000). In Crohn's disease, p53 mutations are frequent and have been linked to dysplasia in a recent retrospective experience (Nathanson *et al.*, 2008). These changes are more frequent in area of active IBD.

A key factor in epithelial injury repair and inflammation is NF-kB, a transcription factor activated by a wide variety of proinflammatory stimuli. It forms dimers that are normally retained in the cytoplasm by inhibitors called IkB (Ghosh & Karin, 2002). Activating stimuli phosphorilate these proteins through Ikk complex and target them for ubiquitination and subsequent degradation by the proteasome. Unbound NF-kB can then translocate into the nucleus and affect the transcription of many genes (Karin *et al.*, 2000).

Activated NF-kB has been detected in many solid tumours (Amit & Ben-Neriah, 2003), where it can contribute to carcinogenesis and drug resistance by activating genes involved in cell survival and block of apoptosis (Karin *et al.*, 2002). As a key player in inflammatory response, activated NF-kB has been detected both in epithelial cells and in macrophages recovered from IBD patients (Rogler *et al.*, 1998), and also from colorectal cancer specimens (Lind *et al.*, 2001). Its activation seems to be precocious in colorectal carcinogenesis: actually APC inactivation, one of the first step in this process (Fearon & Vogelstein, 1990), can enhance IkB proteasomal degradation and thus result in NF-kB activation (Noubissi *et al.*, 2006). Notably, APC loss of function is a late event in IBD-associated cancer and its deletion occurs in less than 33% of these neoplasms: maybe the proliferative stimulus driven by this genetic lesion is not needed, due to NF-kB activation in the epithelium and the inflammatory microenvironment. Indirect evidence of involvement of this pathway also comes from the demonstration that non-steroidal anti-inflammatory drugs, effective in reducing colorectal cancer risk (Gupta & Dubois, 2001), inhibit both cyclooxygenases and IKKβ-dependent NF-kB signaling (Kopp & Ghosh, 1994, Yin *et al.*, 1998).

NF-kB might therefore link inflammation and carcinogenesis in IBD. This hypothesis has been tested in a mouse model characterized by IKKβ selective knockout in intestinal epithelial cells by Greten and colleagues. After a challenge of DSS plus azoxymethane they observed a decrease of 75% in tumor formation with respect to a control group. Tumors occurred in middle and distal colon, where DSS-induced inflammation is more severe. Actually, IKKβ deletion in enterocytes is associated with enhanced early p53-independent apoptosis, while its knockout in myeloid cells decreases tumor growth but does not affect apoptosis, suggesting a role for tumor-promoting paracrine factors (Greten *et al.*, 2004).

The control of NF-kB is mediated by inhibitors as TIR8 that belong to IL-1 receptor family. Deficiency or mutations in its gene encoding are associated to intestinal inflammation and cancer (Xiao *et al.*, 2007, Mantovani *et al.*, 2008).

These data are minutely described by Mantovani *et al.* The authors also explained the relationship between bone-marrow-derived components and carcinogenesis. In particular, leukocyte infiltration is characterized by the presence of tumor-associated macrophages (TAMs). It has been demonstrated that these receptor are involved in the promotion of tumor growth, angiogenesis and suppressing immunity (Mantovani *et al.*, 2002, Mantovani *et al.*, 2008).

These results, together with the previously discussed study by Rakoff-Nahoum and colleagues support the hypothesis of a dual function for NF-kB. Under steady-state condition it is activated through TLRs recognition of intestinal microflora, regulates epithelium turnover and protects the host from injury (Rakoff-Nahoum *et al.*, 2004), while in a chronic inflammatory milieu can promote tumorigenesis, as has been also suggested by Balkwill and Coussens (Balkwill & Coussens, 2004).

Furthermore, inflammation can drive to cancer not only in IBD but plays a role even in sporadic cancer. In the last years, the evidence of a correlation between diysbiosis/low grade inflammation and colon cancer, has been shown. In particular, a significant elevation of *Bacteroides/Prevotella* species in colon cancer has been detected (Sobhani *et al.*, 2011). These bacterial genera stimulate production of IL-17 and, more specifically, Bacteroides produce metalloprotease in CRC (Newman *et al.*, 2001), indicating a possible relationship of inflammation with cancer unrelated to IBD but related to chromosomal instability pathway.

Recently it has also been demonstrated the presence of *Fusobacteriumnucleatum* in CRC specimens and its association with lymph node metastasis (Kostic *et al.*, 2012, Castellarin *et al.*, 2012). The relationship between this bacterium and tumorigenesis is still unknown but is consistent its linkage with inflammatory bowel disease, stimulating host proinflammatory response.

This relation between the alterations of immune response, mucosal inflammation, increase of mucosal permeability and altered microbiota composition could clarify the chronic inflammation in IBD and its development to cancer (Fava *et al.*, 2011).

## 7   Conclusions

The microbiota and relative carriedgenes play a key role not only in physiology but also in many diseases of the human host. In the alimentary tract, microbiota plays a complex game with the diet and the host genome: on one hand it is modified by diet, on the other hand acquires a variable capacity to extract energy from food. So the oncogenic capacity or tumour-protective is related to the own composition of the microbiota.

Experimental evidences suggest a possible involvement of intestinal microbiota in some of the many steps eventually leading to colorectal carcinoma. In cancer related to chromosomal instability, IM is supposed to play a more important role in the promotion process rather than in the initiation one, while in IBD/CAC its role seems much more complex and pervasive, probably influencing both processes. However, a majority of these data comes mostly from animal models and cannot be directly translated into humans.

In humans, the data obtained bythe modern approaches (high-throughout DNA/RNA sequencing and molecular imaging) suggest a loss of the normal bacterial confinement away from colonic epithelium with progressive transformation of the mucosa and microbiota itself, in a dynamic process of carcinogenesis.

However, among several questions far from a definitive solution, the most intriguing remain those about the putative oncogenic or tumour-protective potential of different bacterial strains, as well as on the possible percentage of colorectal cancer, strongly linked to the microbiota action.

# References

Ahmed, S., Macfarlane, G. T., Fite, A., McBain, A. J., Gilbert, P., Macfarlane, S. (2007). Mucosa-associated bacterial diversity in relation to human terminal ileum and colonic biopsy samples. Appl Environ Microbiol, 73(22), 7435-7442.

Alam, M., Midtvedt, T., Uribe, A. (1994).Differential cell kinetics in the ileum and colon of germfree rats. Scand J Gastroenterol, 29, 445–451.

Alberts, D. S., Martínez, M. E., Roe, D. J., Guillén-Rodríguez, J. M., Marshall, J. R., van Leeuwen, J. B., Reid, M. E., Ritenbaugh, C., Vargas, P. A., Bhattacharyya, A. B., Earnest, D. L., Sampliner, R. E.(2000). Lack of effect of a high-fiber cereal supplement on the recurrence of colorectal adenomas.Phoenix Colon Cancer Prevention Physicians' Network. N Engl J Med, 342, 1156–1162.

Akira, S., Uematsu, S., Takeuchi, O. (2006). Pathogen recognition and innate immunity.Cell, 124, 783-801.

Allavena, P., Sica, A., Vecchi, A., Locati, M., Sozzani, S., Mantovani, A. (2000). The chemokine receptor switch paradigm and dendritic cell migration: its significance in tumor tissues. Immunol Rev, 177, 141–149.

Allen, I. C., TeKippe, E. M., Woodford, R. T., Uronis, J. M., Holle, E. K., Rogers, A. B., Hertfarth, H. H., Jobin, C., Ting, J. P. Y. (2010). The NLRP3 inflammasome functions as a negative regulator of tumorigenesis during colitis-associated cancer. J Exp Med, 207, 1045-1056.

Amit, S. & Ben-Neriah, Y. (2003).NF-kappaB activation in cancer: a challenge for ubiquitination- and proteasome-based therapeutic approach. Semin Cancer Biol, 13, 15–28.

Andoh, A., Shimada, M., Araki, Y., Fujiyama, Y., Bamba, T. (2002). Sodium butyrate enhances complement-mediated cell injury via down-regulation of decay-accelerating factor expression in colonic cancer cells. Cancer Immunol Immunother, 50, 663–672.

Andrieux, C., Hibert, A., Houari, A. M., Bensaada, M., Popot, F., Szylit, O. (1998). Ulva lactuca is poorly fermented but alters bacterial metabolism in rats inoculated with human faecal flora from methane and non-methane producers. J Sci Food Agric, 77, 25–30.

Arthur, J. C., Perez-Chanona, E., Mühlbauer, M., Tomkovich, S., Uronis, J. M., Fan, T. J., Campbell, B. J., Abujamel, T., Dogan, B., Rogers, A. B., Rhodes, J. M., Stintzi, A., Simpson, K. W., Hansen, J. J., Keku, T. O., Fodor, A. A., Jobin, C. (2012). Intestinal Inflammation Targets Cancer-Inducing Activity of the Microbiota. Science, Aug 16.

Artis, D. (2008). Epithelial-cell recognition of commensal bacteria and maintenance of immune homeostasis in the gut. Nat Rev Immunol, 8, 411–420.

Arumugam, M., Raes, J., Pelletier, E., Le Paslier, D., Yamada, T., Mende, D. R., Fernandes, G. R., Tap, J., Bruls, T., Batto, J. M., Bertalan, M., Borruel, N., Casellas, F., Fernandez, L., Gautier, L., Hansen, T., Hattori, M., Hayashi, T., Kleerebezem, M., Kurokawa, K., Leclerc, M., Levenez, F., Manichanh, C., Nielsen, H. B., Nielsen, T., Pons, N., Poulain, J., Qin, J., Sicheritz-Ponten, T., Tims, S., Torrents, D., Ugarte, E., Zoetendal, E. G., Wang, J., Guarner, F., Pedersen, O., De Vos, W. M., Brunak, S., Doré, J., MetaHIT Consortium, Antolín, M., Artiguenave, F., Blottiere, H. M., Almeida, M., Brechot, C., Cara, C., Chervaux, C., Cultrone, A., Delorme, C., Denariaz, G., Dervyn, R., Foerstner, K. U., Friss, C., van de Guchte, M., Guedon, E., Haimet, F., Huber, W., van Hylckama-Vlieg, J., Jamet, A., Juste, C., Kaci, G., Knol, J., Lakhdari, O., Layec, S., Le Roux, K., Maguin, E., Mérieux, A., Melo Minardi, R., M'rini, C., Muller, J., Oozeer, R., Parkhill, J., Renault, P., Rescigno, M., Sanchez, N., Sunagawa, S., Torrejon, A., Turner, K., Vandemeulebrouck, G., Varela, E., Winogradsky, Y., Zeller, G., Weissenbach, J., Ehrlich, S. D., Bork, P. (2011). Enterotypes of the human gut microbiome. Nature, 12, 473(7346),174-180. Erratum in: Nature, 30, 474(7353), 666.

Asano, T. & McLeod, R. S. (2002). Dietary fibre for the prevention of colorectal adenomas and carcinomas. Cochrane Database Syst Rev, (2), CD003430.

Attene-Ramos, M. S., Nava, G. M., Muellner, M. G., Wagner, E. D., Plewa, M. J., & Gaskins, H. R. (2010).DNA damage and toxicogenomic analyses of hydrogen sulfide in human intestinal epithelial FHs 74 Int cells. Environ Mol Mutagen, 51(4), 304-314.

Bäckhed, F., Ding, H., Wang, T., Hooper, L. V., Koh, G. Y., Nagy, A., Semenkovich, C. F., Gordon, J. I.(2004). The gut microbiota as an environmental factor that regulates fat storage. Proc Natl Acad Sci U S A, 101, 15718–15723.

Bäckhed, F., Ley, R. E., Sonnenburg, J. L., Peterson, D. A., Gordon, J. I. (2005).Host-bacterial mutualism in the human intestine. Science, 307, 1915–20.

Bäckhed, F., Manchester, J. K., Semenkovich, C. F., Gordon, J. I. (2007). Mechanisms underlying the resistance to diet-induced obesity in germ-free mice.Proc Natl Acad Sci U S A, 16, 104(3), 979-984.

Balamurugan, R., Rajendiran, E., George, S., Samuel, G. V., Ramakrishna, B. S. (2008).Real-time polymerase chain reaction quantification of specific butyrate-producing bacteria, Desulfovibrio and Enterococcus faecalis in the feces of patients with colorectal cancer. J Gastroenterol Hepatol, 23(8 Pt 1), 1298-1303.

Balkwill, F. & Coussens, L. M. (2004). Cancer: an inflammatory link. Nature, 431, 405–406.

Bamias, G., Okazawa, A., Rivera-Nieves, J., Arseneau, K. O., De La Rue, S. A., Pizarro, T. T., Cominelli, F. (2007). Commensal bacteria exacerbate intestinal inflammation but are not essential for the development of murine ileitis. J Immunol, 178, 1809–1818.

Barthold, S. W. & Jonas, A. M. (1977).Morphogenesis of early 1, 2-dimethylhydrazine-induced lesions and latent period reduction of colon carcinogenesis in mice by a variant of Citrobacter freundii. Cancer Res, 37, 4352–4360.

Bass, A. J., Lawrence, M. S., Brace, L. E., Ramos, A. H., Drier, Y., Cibulskis, K., Sougnez, C.,Voet, D., Saksena, G., Sivachenko, A., Jing, R., Parkin, M., Pugh, T., Verhaak, R. G., Stransky, N., Boutin, A. T., Barretina, J., Solit, D. B., Vakiani, E., Shao, W., Mishina, Y., Warmuth, M.,Jimenez, J., Chiang, D. Y., Signoretti, S., Kaelin, W. G., Spardy, N., Hahn, W. C., Hoshida, Y.,Ogino, S., Depinho, R. A., Chin, L., Garraway, L. A., Fuchs, C. S., Baselga, J., Tabernero, J., Gabriel, S., Lander, E. S., Getz, G., Meyerson, M. (2011). Genomic sequencing of colorectaladenocarcinomas identifies a recurrent VTI1A-TCF7L2 fusion. Nat Genet, 4, 43(10), 964-968.

Baumgart, M., Dogan, B., Rishniw, M., Weitzman, G., Bosworth, B., Yantiss, R., Orsi, R. H., Wiedmann, M., McDonough, P., Kim, S. G., Berg, D., Schukken, Y., Scherl, E., Simpson, K. W. (2007). Culture independent analysis of ileal mucosa reveals a selective increase in invasive *Escherichia coli* of novel phylogeny relative to depletion of Clostridiales in Crohn's disease involving the ileum. ISME J, 1, 403–418.

Beaud, D., Tailliez, P., Anba-Mondoloni, J. (2005).Genetic characterization of the beta-glucuronidase enzyme from a human intestinal bacterium, Ruminococcus *gnavus*. Microbiology, 151, 2323–2330.

Beggs, A. D. & Hodgson, S. V. (2008). The genomics of colorectal cancer: state of the art. Current Genomics, 9, 1-10.

Behr, M. A. & Schurr, E. (2006). Mycobacteria in Crohn's disease: a persistent hypothesis. Inflamm Bowel Dis, 12, 1000–1004.

Bernstein H, Bernstein C, Payne CM, Dvorak K. (2009). Bile acids as endogenous etiologic agents in gastrointestinal cancer. World J Gastroenterol, 15, 3329-3340.

Biagi, E., Nylund, L., Candela, M., Ostan, R., Bucci, L., Pini, E., Nikkïla, J., Monti, D., Satokari, R., Franceschi, C., Brigidi, P., De Vos, W. (2010). Through ageing, and beyond: gut microbiota and inflammatory status in seniors and centenarians. PLoS One, 17, 5(5), e10667. Erratum in: PLoS One, 5(6).

Biasco, G., Paganelli, G. M., Owen, R. W., Hill, M. J. (1991). Faecal bile acids and colorectal cell proliferation.The ECP Colon Cancer Working Group. Eur J Cancer Prev, 1 Suppl 2, 63–68.

Biasco, G., Nobili, E., Calabrese, C., Sassatelli, R., Camellini, L., Pantaleo, M. A., Bertoni, G., De Vivo, A., Ponz De Leon, M., Poggioli, G., Bedogni, G., Venesio, T., Varesco, L., Risio, M., Di Febo, G., Brandi, G.. (2006). Impact of surgery on the development of duodenal cancer in patients with familial adenomatous polyposis. Dis Colon Rectum, 49, 1860–1866.

Boroujerdi, M., Kung, H., Wilson, A. G., Anderson, M. W. (1981). Metabolism and DNA binding of benzo(a)pyrene in vivo in the rat. Cancer Res, 41, 951–957.

Bouma, G. & Strober, W. (2003).The immunological and genetic basis of inflammatory bowel disease.Nat Rev Immunol, 3, 521–533.

Brandi, G., Pisi, A. M., Biasco, G. (1997). Ultrastructure et Ecologie Microbienne du Tube Digestif Humain. EDRA edt, ISBN 88-86457-13-8.

Brandi, G., Mordenti, P., Calabrese, C., *et al.* (1999). Antral Cell Kinetics and Bacterial Overgrowth in the Human Hypochlorhydric Stomach.Prous Science.

Brandi, G., Dabard, J., Raibaud, P., Di Battista, M., Bridonneau, C., Pisi, A. M., Morselli Labate, A. M., Pantaleo, M. A., De Vivo, A., Biasco, G. (2006). Intestinal microflora and digestive toxicity of irinotecan in mice. Clin Cancer Res, 12, 1299–1307. (A).

Brigati, C., Noonan, D. M., Albini, A., Benelli, R. (2002). Tumors and inflammatory infiltrates: friends or foes? Clin Exp Metastasis, 19, 247–258.

Bruewer, M., Luegering, A., Kucharzik, T., Parkos, C. A., Madara, J. L., Hopkins, A. M., Nusrat, A. (2003). Proinflammatory cytokines disrupt epithelial barrier function by apoptosis-independent mechanisms. J Immunol, 171, 6164–6172.

Bruewer, M., Utech, M., Ivanov, A. I., Hopkins, A. M., Parkos, C. A., Nusrat, A. (2005). Interferon-gamma induces internalization of epithelial tight junction proteins via a macropinocytosis-like process. FASEB J, 19, 923–933.

Cai, W. J., Wang, M. J., Ju, L. H., Wang, C., Zhu, Y. C. (2010). Hydrogen sulfide induces human colon cancer cell proliferation: role of Akt, ERK and p21. Cell Biol Int, 14, 34(6), 565-572.

Canavan, C., Abrams, K. R., Mayberry, J. (2006). Meta-analysis: colorectal and small bowel cancer risk in patients with Crohn's disease. Aliment Pharmacol Ther, 23, 1097–1104.

Cario, E. (2010). Toll-like receptors in inflammatory bowel diseases: a decade later. Inflamm Bowel Dis, 16, 1583-1597.

Carman, R. J., Van Tassell, R. L., Kingston, D. G., Bashir, M., Wilkins, T. D. (1988).Conversion of IQ, a dietary pyrolysis carcinogen to a direct-acting mutagen by normal intestinal bacteria of humans. Mutat Res, 206, 335–342.

Castellarin, M., Warren, R. L., Freeman, J. D., Dreolini, L., Krzywinski, M., Strauss, J., Barnes, R., Watson, P., Allen-Vercoe, E., Moore, R. A., Holt, R. A. (2012). Fusobacterium nucleatuminfection is prevalent in human colorectal carcinoma. Genome Res, 22(2), 299-306.

Chen, W., Liu, F., Ling, Z., Tong, X., Xiang, C.(2012). Human intestinal lumen and mucosa-associated microbiota in patients with colorectal cancer. PLoS One, 7(6), e39743.

Chichlowski, M., Sharp, J. M., Vanderford, D. A., Myles, M. H., Hale, L. P. (2008).Helicobacter typhlonius and Helicobacter rodentium differentially affect the severity of colon inflammation and inflammation-associated neoplasia in IL10-deficient mice. Comp Med, 58(6), 534-541.

Chiodini, R. J. (1989). Crohn's disease and the mycobacterioses: a review and comparison of two disease entities. Clin Microbiol Rev, 2, 90–117.

Christl, S. U., Eisner, H. D., Dusel, G., Kasper, H., Scheppach, W. (1996). Antagonistic effects of sulfide and butyrate on proliferation of colonic mucosa: a potential role for these agents in the pathogenesis of ulcerative colitis. Dig Dis Sci, 41, 2477–2481.

Chung, H., Pamp, S. J., Hill, J. A., Surana, N. K., Edelman, S. M., Troy, E. B., Reading, N. C., Villablanca, E. J., Wang, S., Mora, J. R., Umesaki, Y., Mathis, D., Benoist, C., Relman, D. A., Kasper, D. L. (2012). Gut Immune Maturation Depends on Colonization with a Host-Specific Microbiota. Cell, 149, 1593–1608.

Claesson, M. J., Cusack, S., O'Sullivan, O., Greene-Diniz, R., de Weerd, H., Flannery, E., Marchesi, J. R., Falush, D., Dinan, T., Fitzgerald, G., Stanton, C., van Sinderen, D., O'Connor, M., Harnedy, N., O'Connor, K., Henry, C., O'Mahony, D., Fitzgerald, A. P., Shanahan, F., Twomey, C., Hill, C., Ross, R. P., O'Toole, P. W. (2011). Composition, variability, and temporal stability of the intestinal microbiota of the elderly. Proc Natl Acad Sci U S A, 15, 108 Suppl 1, 4586-4591.

Claesson, M. J., Jeffery, I. B., Conde, S., Power, S. E., O'Connor, E. M., Cusack, S., Harris, H. M., Coakley, M., Lakshminarayanan, B., O'Sullivan, O., Fitzgerald, G. F., Deane, J., O'Connor, M., Harnedy, N., O'Connor, K., O'Mahony, D., van Sinderen, D., Wallace, M., Brennan, L., Stanton, C., Marchesi, J. R., Fitzgerald, A. P., Shanahan, F., Hill, C., Ross, R. P., O'Toole, P. W. (2012). Gut microbiota composition correlates with diet and health in the elderly. Nature, 9, 488, 178-184.

Clark, E., Hoare, C., Tanianis-Hughes, J., Carlson, G. L., Warhurst, G. (2005). Interferon gamma induces translocation of commensal Escherichia coli across gut epithelial cells via a lipid raft-mediated process. Gastroenterology, 128, 1258–1267.

Clarke, T. B., Davis, K. M., Lysenko, E. S., Zhou, A. Y., Yu, Y., Weiser, J. N. (2010). Recognition of peptidoglycan from the microbiota by Nod1 enhances systemic innate immunity. Nat Med, 16(2), 228-231.

Comalada, M., Bailón, E., de Haro, O., Lara-Villoslada, F., Xaus, J., Zarzuelo, A., Gálvez, J. (2006). The effects of short-chain fatty acids on colon epithelial proliferation and survival depend on the cellular phenotype. J Cancer Res Clin Oncol, 132, 487–497.

Corpet, D. E. & Pierre, F. (2005). How good are rodent models of carcinogenesis in predicting efficacy in humans? A systematic review and meta-analysis of colon chemoprevention in rats, mice and men. Eur J Cancer, 41(13), 1911-1922.

Coussens, L. M. & Werb, Z. Inflammation and cancer. Nature, 420, 860–867.

Crawford, P. A. & Gordon, J. I. (2005).Microbial regulation of intestinal radiosensitivity. Proc Natl Acad Sci U S A, 102, 13254–13259.

Cuevas-Ramos, G., Petit, C. R., Marcq, I., Boury, M., Oswald, E., Nougayrède, J. P. (2010). *Escherichia coli* induces DNA damage in vivo and triggers genomic instability in mammalian cells. Proc Natl Acad Sci U S A, 107, 11537-11542.

Dashwood, R. H., Myzak, M. C., Ho, E. (2006). Dietary HDAC inhibitors: time to rethink weak ligands in cancer chemoprevention? Carcinogenesis, 27, 344–349.

De Filippo, C., Cavalieri, D., Di Paola, M., Ramazzotti, M., Poullet, J. B., Massart, S., Collini, S., Pieraccini, G., Lionetti, P. (2010). Impact of diet in shaping gut microbiota revealed by a comparative study in children from Europe and rural Africa. Proc Natl Acad Sci U S A, 17, 107(33), 14691-14696.

De Kok, T. M. & Van Maanen, J. M. (2000). Evaluation of fecal mutagenicity and colorectal cancer risk. Mutat Res, 463, 53–101.

De La Serre, C. B., Ellis, C. L., Lee, J., Hartman, A. L., Rutledge, J. C., Raybould, H. E. (2010). Propensity to high-fat diet-induced obesity in rats is associated with changes in the gut microbiota and gut inflammation. Am J Physiol Gastrointest Liver Physiol, 299, 440-448.

De Roock, W., Claes, B., Bernasconi, D., De Schutter, Jef., Biesmans, B., Fountzilas, G., Kalogeras, K. T., Kotoula, V., Papamichael, D., Puig, P. L., Llorca, F. P., Rougier, P., Vincenzi, B., Santini, D., Tonini, G., Cappuzzo, F., Frattini, M. , Molinari, F., Saletti, P. , De Dosso, S., Martini, M., Bardelli, A., Siena, S., Sartore-Bianchi, A., Tabernero, J., Macarulla, T., Di Fiore, F., Gangloff, A. O., Ciardiello, F., Pfeiffer, P., Qvortrup, C., Hansen, T. P., Van Cutsem, E., Piessevaux, H., Lambrechts, D., Delorenzi, M., &Tejpar, S. (2010). Effects of KRAS, BRAF, NRAS, and PIK3CA mutations on the efficacy of Cetuximab plus chemotherapy in chemotherapy-refractory metastatic colorectal cancer: a retrospective consortium analysis. Lancet Oncol, 11, 753-762.

Dharmani, P., Strauss, J., Ambrose, C., Allen-Vercoe, E., Chadee, K. (2011). Fusobacterium nucleatum infection of colonic cells stimulates MUC2 mucin and tumor necrosis factor alpha. Infect Immun, 79 (7), 2597-2607.

Deng, L., Zhou, J.F., Sellers, R.S., Li, J.F., Nguyen, A.V., Wang, Y., Orlofsky, A., Liu, Q., Hume, D.A., Pollard, J.W., Augenlicht, L., Lin, E.Y. (2010). A novel mouse model of inflammatory bowel disease links mammalian target of rapamycin-dependent hyperproliferation of colonic epithelium to inflammation-associated tumorigenesis.Am J Pathol, 176(2), 952-67.

Dengjel, J., Schoor, O., Fischer, R., Reich, M., Kraus, M., Müller, M., Kreymborg, K., Altenberend, F., Brandenburg, J., Albacher, H., Brock, R., Driessen, C., Rammensee, H. G., Stevanovic, S. (2005). Autophagy promotes MHC class II presentation of peptides from intracellular source proteins. Proc Natl Acad Sci USA, 102, 7922-7927.

Deplancke, B., Finster, K., Graham, W. V., Collier, C. T., Thurmond, J. E., Gaskins, H. R. (2003). Gastrointestinal and microbial responses to sulfate-supplemented drinking water in mice. Exp Biol Med (Maywood), 228, 424–433.

Dethlefsen, L. &Relman, D. A. (2011). Incomplete recovery and individualized responses of the human distal gut microbiota to repeated antibiotic perturbation. Proc Natl Acad Sci U S A, 108 Suppl 1, 455445-61.

Djouzi, Z. & Andrieux, C. (1997). Compared effects of three oligosaccharides on metabolism of intestinal microflora in rats inoculated with a human faecal flora. Br J Nutr, 78, 313–324.

Dove, W. F., Clipson, L., Gould, K. A., Luongo, C., Marshall, D. J., Moser, A. R., Newton, M. A., Jacoby, R.F. (1997).Intestinal neoplasia in the ApcMin mouse: independence from the microbial and natural killer (beige locus) status. Cancer Res, 1, 57(5), 812-814.

Duchmann, R., Kaiser, I., Hermann, E., Mayet, W., Ewe, K., zum Büschenfelde KHM. (1995). Tolerance exists towards resident intestinal flora but is broken in active inflammatory bowel disease (IBD). Clin Exp Immunol, 102, 448–455.

Duesberg, P., Mandrioli, D., McCormack, A., Nicholson, J. M. (2011). Is carcinogenesis a form of speciation? Cell Cycle, 10, 2100-2114.

Ebert, M. N., Klinder, A., Peters, W. H., Schäferhenrich, A., Sendt, W., Scheele, J., Pool-Zobel, B. L. (2003). Expression of glutathione S-transferases (GSTs) in human colon cells and inducibility of GSTM2 by butyrate. Carcinogenesis, 24, 1637–1644.

Eckburg, P. B., Bik, E. M., Bernstein, C. N., Purdom, E., Dethlefsen, L., Sargent, M., Gill, S. R., Nelson, K. E., Relman, D. A. (2005). Diversity of the human intestinal microbial flora. Science, 308, 1635–1638.

Fanaro, S., Chierici, R., Guerrini, P., Vigi, V. (2003). Intestinal microflora in early infancy: composition and development. Acta Paediatr Suppl, 91, 48–55.

Farrell, R. J. & LaMont, J. T. (2002). Microbial factors in inflammatory bowel disease. Gastroenterol Clin North Am, 31, 41–62.

Fava, F. & Danese, S. (2011). Intestinal microbiota in inflammatory bowel disease: friend or foe? World J Gastroenterol, 17, 557-566.

Fearon, E. R. & Vogelstein, B. (1990). A genetic model for colorectal tumorigenesis. Cell, 61, 759–767.

Fellermann, K., Stange, D. E., Schaeffeler, E., Schmalzl, H., Wehkamp, J., Bevins, C. L., Reinisch, W., Teml, A., Schwab, M., Lichter, P., Radlwimmer, B., Stange, E. F. (2006). A chromosome 8 gene-cluster polymorphism with low human beta-defensin 2 gene copy number predisposes to Crohn disease of the colon. Am J Hum Genet, 79, 439–448.

Flood, D. M., Weiss, N. S., Cook, L. S., Emerson, J. C., Schwartz, S. M., Potter, J. D. (2000). Colorectal cancer incidence in Asian migrants to the United States and their descendants. Cancer Causes Control, 11, 403–411.

Forsythe, S. J. & Parker, D. S. (1985).Nitrogen metabolism by the microbial flora of the rabbit caecum.J Appl Bacteriol, 58, 363–369.

Franceschi, S., Favero, A., Vecchia, C. L., Negri, E., Conti, E., Montella, M., Giacosa, A., Nanni, O., Decarli, A. (1997). Food groups and risk of colorectal cancer in Italy. Int J Cancer, 72, 56–61.

Franchi, L., McDonald, C., Kanneganti, T. D., Amer, A., Núñez, G. (2006). Nucleotide-binding oligomerization domain-like receptors: intracellular pattern recognition molecole for pathogen detection and host defense. J. Immunol, 177, 3507-3513.

Frank, D. N., Amand, A. L. S., Feldman, R. A., Boedeker, E. C., Harpaz, N., Pace, N. R. (2007). Molecular-phylogenetic characterization of microbial community imbalances in human inflammatory bowel diseases. Proc Natl Acad Sci U S A, 104, 13780–13785.

Gaboriau-Routhiau, V., Rakotobe, S., Lécuyer, E., Mulder, I., Lan, A., Bridonneau, C., Rochet, V., Pisi, A., De Paepe, M., Brandi, G., Eberl, G., Snel, J., Kelly, D., Cerf-Bensussan, N. (2009). The key role of segmented filamentous bacteria in the coordinated maturation of gut helper T cell responses. Immunity, 16, 31(4), 677-689.

Garrett, W. S., Punit, S., Gallini, C. A., Michaud, M., Zhang, D., Sigrist, K. S., Lord, G. M., Glickman, J. N., Glimcher, L. H. (2009). Colitis-associated colorectal cancer driven by T-bet deficiency in dendritic cells. Cancer Cell, 16, 208-219.

Ghosh, S. & Karin, M. (2002). Missing pieces in the NF-kappaB puzzle. Cell, 109 Suppl, S81–96.

Gibson, P. R. (2000). The intracellular target of butyrate's actions: HDAC or HDON'T? Gut, 46, 447–448.

Giovannucci, E., Rimm, E. B., Ascherio, A., Stampfer, M. J., Colditz, G. A., Willett, W. C. (1995). Alcohol, low-methionine–low-folate diets, and risk of colon cancer in men. J Natl Cancer Inst, 87, 265–273.

Giovannucci, E. (2002). Modifiable risk factors for colon cancer. Gastroenterol Clin North Am, 31, 925–943.

Glasser, A. L., Boudeau, J., Barnich, N., Perruchot, M. H., Colombel, J. F., Darfeuille-Michaud, A. (2001). Adherent invasive *Escherichia coli* strains from patients with Crohn's disease survive and replicate within macrophages without inducing host cell death. Infect Immun, 69, 5529–5537.

Gophna, U., Sommerfeld, K., Gophna, S., Doolittle, W. F., van Zanten, S. J. O. V. (2006). Differences between tissue-associated intestinal microfloras of patients with Crohn's disease and ulcerative colitis. J Clin Microbiol, 44, 4136–4141

Green, G. L., Brostoff, J., Hudspith, B., Michael, M., Mylonaki, M., Rayment, N., Staines, N., Sanderson, J., Rampton, D. S., Bruce, K. D. (2006). Molecular characterization of the bacteria adherent to human colorectal mucosa. J Appl Microbiol, 100, 460–469.

Greten, F. R., Eckmann, L. , Greten, T. F., Park, J. M., Li, Z. W., Egan, L. J., Kagnoff, M. F., Karin, M. (2004). IKKbeta links inflammation and tumorigenesis in a mouse model of colitis-associated cancer. Cell, 118, 285–296.

Gupta, R. A. & Dubois, R. N. (2001).Colorectal cancer prevention and treatment by inhibition of cyclooxygenase-2. Nat Rev Cancer, 1, 11–21.

Gupta, S., Natarajan, R., Payne, S. G., Studer, E. J., Spiegel, S., Dent, P., Hylemon, P. B. (2004). Deoxycholic acid activates the c-Jun N-terminal kinase pathway via FAS receptor activation in primary hepatocytes. Role of acidic sphingomyelinase-mediated ceramide generation in FAS receptor activation. J Biol Chem, 279, 5821–5828.

Hall, M. N., Chavarro, J. E., Lee, I. M., Willett, W. C., Ma, J. (2008).A 22-year prospective study of fish, n-3 fatty acid intake, and colorectal cancer risk in men. Cancer Epidemiol Biomarkers Prev, 17, 1136–1143.

Hambly, R. J., Rumney, C. J., Cunninghame, M., Fletcher, J. M., Rijken, P. J., Rowland, I. R. (1997). Influence of diets containing high and low risk factors for colon cancer on early stages of carcinogenesis in human flora-associated (HFA) rats. Carcinogenesis, 18, 1535–1539.

Hamer, H. M., Jonkers, D., Venema, K., Vanhoutvin, S., Troost, F. J., Brummer, R. J. (2008). Review article: the role of butyrate on colonic function. Aliment Pharmacol Ther, 27, 104–119.

Hardison, W. G. (1978). Hepatic taurine concentration and dietary taurine as regulators of bile acid conjugation with taurine. Gastroenterology, 75, 71–75.

Higgins, S. C., Lavelle, E. C., McCann, C., Keogh, B., McNeela, E., Byrne, P., O'Gorman, B., Jarnicki, A., McGuirk, P., Mills, K. H. (2003). Toll-like receptor 4-mediated innate IL-10 activates antigen-specific regulatory T cells and confers resistance to Bordetella pertussis by inhibiting inflammatory pathology. J Immunol, 171, 3119–3127.

Hildebrandt, M. A., Hoffmann, C., Sherrill-Mix, S. A., Keilbaugh, S. A., Hamady, M., Chen, Y. Y., Knight, R., Ahima, R. S., Bushman, F., Wu, G. D. (2009). High-fat diet determines the composition of the murine gut microbiome independently of obesity. Gastroenterology, 137(5), 1716-1724.

Hinzman, M. J., Novotny, C., Ullah, A., Shamsuddin, A. M. (1987). Fecal mutagen fecapentaene-12 damages mammalian colon epithelial DNA. Carcinogenesis, 8, 1475–1479.

Hirayama, K., Mishima, M., Kawamura, S., Itoh, K., Takahashi, E., Mitsuoka, T. (1994). Effects of dietary supplements on the composition of fecal flora of human-flora associated (HFA) mice. Bifidobacteria and Microflora, 13, 1–7.

Hirayama, K. & Itoh, K. (2005).Human flora-associated (HFA) animals as a model for studying the role of intestinal flora in human health and disease. Curr Issues Intest Microbiol, 6, 69–75.

Hisamatsu, T., Suzuki, M., Reinecker, H. C., Nadeau, W. J., McCormick, B. A., Podolsky, D. K. (2003). CARD15/NOD2 functions as an antibacterial factor in human intestinal epithelial cells. Gastroenterology, 124, 993–1000.

Holec, V., Ciernikova, S., Wachsmannova, L., Adamcikova, Z., Hainova, K., Mego, M., Stevurkova, V., Danihel, L., Liskova, A., Zajac, V. (2012). Analysis of bacteria from intestinal tract of FAP patients for the presence of APC-like sequences. Med Sci Monit, 18(8), 486-492.

Hollander, D., Vadheim, C. M., Brettholz, E., Petersen, G. M., Delahunty, T., Rotter, J. I. (1986). Increased intestinal permeability in patients with Crohn's disease and their relatives.A possible etiologic factor. Ann Intern Med, 105, 883–885.

Hooper, L. V., Wong, M. H., Thelin, A., Hansson, L., Falk, P. G., Gordon, J. I. (2001).Molecular analysis of commensal host-microbial relationships in the intestine. Science, 291, 881–884.

Horie, H., Kanazawa, K., Okada, M., Narushima, S., Itoh, K., Terada, A. (1999).Effects of intestinal bacteria on the development of colonic neoplasm: an experimental study. Eur J Cancer Prev, 8, 237–245. (A).

Horie, H., Kanazawa, K., Kobayashi, E., Okada, M., Fujimura, A., Yamagiwa, S., Abo, T. (1999).Effects of intestinal bacteria on the development of colonic neoplasm II.Changes in the immunological environment. Eur J Cancer Prev, 8, 533–537. (B).

Høverstad, T., Fausa, O., Bjørneklett, A., Bøhmer, T. (1984).Short-chain fatty acids in the normal human feces.Scand J Gastroenterol, 19, 375–381.

Hrelia, P., Fimognari, C., Maffei, F., Brandi, G., Biasco, G., Cantelli-Forti, G. (2002). Mutagenic and clastogenic activity of gastric juice in human gastric diseases. Mutat Res, 514, 125–132.

Hughes, D. T. & Sperandio, V. (2008). Inter-kingdom signalling: communication between bacteria and their hosts. Nat Rev Microbiol, 6, 111–120.

Human Microbiome Project Consortium.(2012). Structure, function and diversity of the healthy human microbiome. Nature, 486, 207-214.

Humblot, C., Murkovic, M., Rigottier-Gois, L., Bensaada, M., Bouclet, A., Andrieux, C., Anba, J., Rabot, S. (2007). Beta-glucuronidase in human intestinal microbiota is necessary for the colonic genotoxicity of the food-borne carcinogen 2-amino-3-methylimidazo[4,5-f]quinoline in rats. Carcinogenesis, 28, 2419–2425.

Hussain, S. P., Amstad, P., Raja, K., Ambs, S., Nagashima, M., Bennett, W. P., Shields, P. G., Ham, A. J., Swenberg, J. A., Marrogi, A. J., Harris, C. C. (2000). Increased p53 mutation load in noncancerous colon tissue from ulcerative colitis: a cancer-prone chronic inflammatory disease. Cancer Res, 60, 3333–3337.

Huycke, M. M. & Gaskins, H. R. (2004). Commensal bacteria, redox stress, and colorectal cancer: mechanisms and models. Exp Biol Med (Maywood), 229, 586–597.

Ibbotson, J. P., Lowes, J. R., Chahal, H., Gaston, J. S., Life, P., Kumararatne, D. S., Sharif, H., Alexander-Williams, J., Allan, R. N. (1992). Mucosal cell-mediated immunity to mycobacterial, enterobacterial and other microbial antigens in inflammatory bowel disease. Clin Exp Immunol, 87. 224–230.

Ivanov, I. I., Atarashi, K., Manel, N., Brodie, E. L., Shima, T., Karaoz, U., Wei, D., Goldfarb, K. C., Santee, C. A., Lynch, S. V., Tanoue, T., Imaoka, A., Itoh, K., Takeda, K., Umesaki, Y., Honda, K., Littman, D. R. (2009). Induction of intestinal Th17 cells by segmented filamentous bacteria. Cell, 139, 485–498.

Jiménez, E., Marín, M.L., Martín, R., Odriozola, J.M., Olivares, M., Xaus, J., Fernández, L., Rodríguez, J.M. (2008). Is meconium from healthy newborns actually sterile? Res Microbiol, 159, 187-193.

Johansson, M. E., Phillipson, M., Petersson, J., Velcich, A., Holm, L., Hansson, G. C. (2008).The inner of the two Muc2 mucin-dependent mucus layers in colon is devoid of bacteria. Proc Natl Acad Sci U S A, 105, 15064-15069.

Kado, S., Uchida, K., Funabashi, H., Iwata, S., Nagata, Y., Ando, M., Onoue, M., Matsuoka, Y., Ohwaki, M., Morotomi, M. (2001). Intestinal microflora are necessary for development of spontaneous adenocarcinoma of the large intestine in T-cell receptor beta chain and p53 double-knockout mice.Cancer Res, 15, 61(6), 2395-2398.

Kamada, N., Kim, Y. G., Sham, H. P., Vallance, B. A., Puente, J. L., Martens, E. C., Núñez, G. (2012). Regulated virulence controls the ability of a pathogen to compete with the gut microbiota. Science, 8, 336(6086), 1325-1329.

Karin, M. & Ben-Neriah, Y. (2000).Phosphorylation meets ubiquitination: the control of NF-[kappa]B activity. Annu Rev Immunol, 18, 621–663.

Karin, M., Cao, Y., Greten, F. R., Li, Z. W. (2002).NF-kappaB in cancer: from innocent bystander to major culprit. Nat Rev Cancer, 2, 301–310.

Kassie, F., Rabot, S., Kundi, M., Chabicovsky, M., Qin, H. M., Knasmüller, S. (2001). Intestinal microflora plays a crucial role in the genotoxicity of the cooked food mutagen 2-amino-3-methylimidazo [4,5-f]quinoline. Carcinogenesis, 22, 1721–1725.

Kassie, F., Lhoste, E. F., Bruneau, A., Zsivkovits, M., Ferk, F., Uhl, M., Zidek, T., Knasmüller, S. (2004). Effect of intestinal microfloras from vegetarians and meat eaters on the genotoxicity of 2-amino-3-methylimidazo[4,5-f]quinoline, a carcinogenic heterocyclic amine. J Chromatogr B Analyt Technol Biomed Life Sci, 802, 211–215.

Khachatryan, Z. A., Ktsoyan, Z. A., Manukyan, G. P., Kelly, D., Ghazaryan, K. A., Aminov, R. I. (2008). Predominant role of host genetics in controlling the composition of gut microbiota. PLoS ONE, 3:e3064.

Kinoshita, N. & Gelboin, H. V. (1978).beta-Glucuronidase catalyzed hydrolysis of benzo(a)pyrene-3-glucuronide and binding to DNA. Science, 199, 307–309.

Kinoshita, M., Suzuki, Y., Saito, Y. (2002).Butyrate reduces colonic paracellular permeability by enhancing PPARgamma activation. Biochem Biophys Res Commun, 293, 827–831.

Klampfer, L., Huang, J., Sasazuki, T., Shirasawa, S., Augenlicht, L. (2003).Inhibition of interferon gamma signaling by the short chain fatty acid butyrate.Mol Cancer Res, 1, 855–862.

Kleessen, B., Kroesen, A. J., Buhr, H. J., Blaut, M. (2002). Mucosal and invading bacteria in patients with inflammatory bowel disease compared with controls. Scand J Gastroenterol, 37, 1034–1041.

Knasmüller, S., Steinkellner, H., Hirschl, A. M., Rabot, S., Nobis, E. C., Kassie, F. (2001). Impact of bacteria in dairy products and of the intestinal microflora on the genotoxic and carcinogenic effects of heterocyclic aromatic amines. Mutat Res, 480-481, 129–138.

Kolmeder, C. A., de Been, M., Nikkilä, J., Ritamo, I., Mättö, J., Valmu, L., Salojärvi, J., Palva, A., Salonen, A., de Vos W. M. (2012). Comparative Metaproteomics and Diversity Analysis of Human Intestinal Microbiota Testifies for Its Temporal Stability and Expression of Core Functions. PLoS One, 7(1), e29913.

Kopp, E. & Ghosh, S. (1994). Inhibition of NF-kappa B by sodium salicylate and aspirin. Science, 265, 956–959.

Korzenik, J. R. (2007). Is Crohn's disease due to defective immunity? Gut, 56, 2–5.

Kostic, A. D., Gevers, D., Pedamallu, C. S., Michaud, M., Duke, F., Earl, A. M., Ojesina, A. I., Jung, J., Bass, A. J., Tabernero, J., Baselga, J., Liu, C., Shivdasani, R. A., Ogino, S., Birren, B. W., Huttenhower, C., Garrett, W. S., Meyerson, M. (2012). Genomic analysis identifies association of Fusobacterium with colorectal carcinoma. Genome Res, 22(2), 292-298.

Kotlowski, R., Bernstein, C. N., Sepehri, S., Krause, D. O. (2007). High prevalence of *Escherichia coli* belonging to the B2+D phylogenetic group in inflammatory bowel disease. Gut, 56, 669-675.

Kuballa, P., Huett, A., Rioux, J. D., Daly, M. J., Xavier, R. J. (2008). Impaired autophagy of an intracellular pathogen induced by a Crohn's disease associated ATG16L1 variant. PLoS One, 3, e3391.

Kuczynski, J., Lauber, C. L., Walters, W. A., Parfrey, L. W., Clemente, J. C., Gevers, D., & Knight, R. (2011). Experimental and analytical tools for studying the human microbiome. Nat Rev Genet, 16, 13(1), 47-58.

Kullberg, M.C., Rothfuchs, A.G., Jankovic, D., Kaspar, P., Wynn, T.A., Gorelick, P.L., Cheever, A.W., Sher, A. (2001). Helicobacter hepaticus-induced colitis in interleukin-10 deficient mice: cytokine requirements for the induction and maintenance of intestinal inflammation. Infect Immun, 69(7), 4232-4241.

Lambert, D. W., Wood, I. S., Ellis, A., Shirazi-Beechey, S. P. (2002). Molecular changes in the expression of human colonic nutrient transporters during the transition from normality to malignancy. Br J Cancer, 86, 1262–1269.

Larsson, S. C., Kumlin, M., Ingelman-Sundberg, M., Wolk, A. (2004). Dietary long-chain n-3 fatty acids for the prevention of cancer: a review of potential mechanisms. Am J Clin Nutr, 79, 935–945.

Larsson, S. C. & Wolk, A. (2006). Meat consumption and risk of colorectal cancer: a meta-analysis of prospective studies. Int J Cancer, 119, 2657–2664.

Larsson, S. C., Giovannucci, E., Wolk, A. (2007). Dietary carbohydrate, glycemic index, and glycemic load in relation to risk of colorectal cancer in women. Am J Epidemiol, 165, 256–261.

Lee, Y. K. & Mazmanian, S. K. (2010). Has the microbiota played a critical role in the evolution of theadaptive immune system? Science, 330, 1768–1773.

Leedham, S. J., Thliveris, A. T., Halberg, R. B., Newton, M. A., Wright, N. A. (2005). Gastrointestinal stem cells and cancer: bridging the molecular gap. Stem Cell Rev, 1, 233–241.

Leedham, S. J. & Wright, N. A. (2008). Expansion of a mutated clone: from stem cell to tumour. J Clin Pathol, 61, 164–171.

Ley, R. E., Turnbaugh, P. J., Klein, S., Gordon, J. I. (2006). Microbial ecology: human gut microbes associated with obesity. Nature, 21, 444(7122), 1022-1023.

Li, Y., Kundu, P., Seow, S. W., de Matos, C. T., Aronsson, L., Chin, K.C., Kärre, K., Pettersson, S., Greicius, G. (2012).Gut microbiota accelerate tumor growth via c-jun and STAT3 phosphorylation in APCMin/+ mice. Carcinogenesis, 33(6), 1231-1238.

Li, Y. Q., Roberts, S. A., Paulus, U., Loeffler, M., Potten, C. S. (1994).The crypt cycle in mouse small intestinal epithelium. J Cell Sci, 107 (Pt 12), 3271–3279.

Lind, D. S., Hochwald, S. N., Malaty, J., Rekkas, S., Hebig, P., Mishra, G., Moldawer, L. L., Copeland, E. M. 3rd, Mackay, S. (2001). Nuclear factor-kappa B is upregulated in colorectal cancer. Surgery, 130, 363–369.

Liu, Y., van Kruiningen, H. J., West, A. B., Cartun, R. W., Cortot, A., Colombel, J. F. (1995). Immunocytochemical evidence of *Listeria*, *Escherichia coli*, and *Streptococcus* antigens in Crohn's disease. Gastroenterology, 108,1396–1404.

Maddocks, O.D., Short, A.J., Donnenberg, M.S., Bader, S., Harrison, D.J. (2009). Attaching and effacing *Escherichia coli* downregulate DNA mismatch repair protein in vitro and are associated with colorectal adenocarcinomas in humans. PLoS One, 4, e5517.

Maggio-Price, L., Treuting, P., Zeng, W., Tsang, M., Bielefeldt-Ohmann, H., Iritani, B.M. (2006 ). Helicobacter infection is required for inflammation and colon cancer in SMAD3-deficient mice.Cancer Res, 15, 66(2), 828-838.

Manichanh, C., Rigottier-Gois, L., Bonnaud, E., Gloux, K., Pelletier, E., Frangeul, L., Nalin, R., Jarrin, C., Chardon, P., Marteau, P., Roca, J., Dore, J. (2006). Reduced diversity of faecal microbiota in Crohn's disease revealed by a metagenomic approach. Gut, 55, 205–211.

Mantovani, A., Sozzani, S., Locati, M., Allavena, P., Sica, A. (2002). Macrophage polarization: tumor-associated macrophages as a paradigm for polarized M2 mononuclear phagocytes.Trends Immunol, 23, 549-555.

Mantovani, A., Allavena, P., Sica, A., Balkwill, F. (2008). Cancer-related inflammation. Nature, 454, 436-444.

Marchesi, J. R., Holmes, E., Khan, F., Kochhar, S., Scanlan, P., Shanahan, F., Wilson, I. D., Wang, Y. (2007).Rapid and noninvasive metabonomic characterization of inflammatory bowel disease. J Proteome Res, 6, 546–551.

Marchesi, J. R., Dutilh, B. E., Hall, N., Peters, W. H., Roelofs, R., Boleij, A., Tjalsma, H. (2011). Towards the human colorectal cancer microbiome. PLoS One, 6(5), e20447.

Martin, H. M., Campbell, B. J., Hart, C. A., Mpofu, C., Nayar, M., Singh, R., Englyst, H., Williams, H. F., Rhodes, J. M. (2004).Enhanced *Escherichia coli* adherence and invasion in Crohn's disease and colon cancer. Gastroenterology, 127, 80-93.

Martínez, M. E., Marshall, J. R., Giovannucci, E. (2008). Diet and cancer prevention: the roles of observation and experimentation. Nat Rev Cancer, 8, 694-703.

Maslowski, K. M., Vieira, A. T., Ng, A., Kranich, J., Sierro, F., Yu, D., Schilter, H. C., Rolph, M. S., Mackay, F., Artis, D., Xavier, R. J., Teixeira, M. M., Mackay, C. R. (2009). Regulation of inflammatory responses by gut microbiota and chemoattractant receptor GPR43. Nature, 29, 461, 1282-1286.

Mazmanian, S. K. &Kasper, D. L. (2006). The love-hate relationship between bacterial polysaccharides and the host immune system. Nat Rev Immunol, 6, 849-858.

McBain, A. J. & Macfarlane, G. T. (1998).Ecological and physiological studies on large intestinal bacteria in relation to production of hydrolytic and reductive enzymes involved in formation of genotoxic metabolites. J Med Microbiol, 47, 407–416.

McCullogh, J. S., Ratcliffe, B., Mandir, N., Carr, K. E., Goodlad, R. A. (1998). Dietary fibre and intestinal microflora: effects on intestinal morphometry and crypt branching. Gut, 42(6), 799-806.

McGarr, S. E., Ridlon, J. M., Hylemon, P. B. (2005). Diet, anaerobic bacterial metabolism, and colon cancer: a review of the literature. J Clin Gastroenterol, 39, 98–109.

Macpherson, A. J. &Harris, N. L. (2004). Interactions between commensal intestinal bacteria and the immune system.Nat Rev Immunol, 4, 478-485.

Meagher, A. P., Farouk, R., Dozois, R. R., Kelly, K. A., Pemberton, J. H. (1998). J ileal pouch-anal anastomosis for chronic ulcerative colitis: complications and long-term outcome in 1310 patients. Br J Surg, 85,800–803.

Merritt, A. J., Gould, K. A., Dove, W. F. (1997). Polyclonal structure of intestinal adenomas in ApcMin/+ mice with concomitant loss of Apc+ from all tumor lineages. Proc Natl Acad Sci U S A, 94, 13927–13931.

Metges, C. C., El-Khoury, A. E., Henneman, L., Petzke, K. J., Grant, I., Bedri, S., Pereira, P. P., Ajami, A. M., Fuller, M. F., Young, V. R. (1999). Availability of intestinal microbial lysine for whole body lysine homeostasis in human subjects. Am J Physiol, 277, E597–607.

Mitsou, E.K., Kirtzalidou, E., Oikonomou, I., Liosis, G., Kyriacou, A. (2008). Fecal microflora of Greek healthy neonates.Anaerobe, 14, 94-101.

Moore, W. E. & Moore, L. H.(1995). Intestinal floras of populations that have a high risk of colon cancer. Appl Environ Microbiol, 61, 3202–3207.

Moser, A. R., Pitot, H. C., Dove, W. F. (1990). A dominant mutation that predisposes to multiple intestinal neoplasia in the mouse. Science, 247, 322–324.

Mow, W. S., Vasiliauskas, E. A., Lin, Y. C., Fleshner, P. R., Papadakis, K. A., Taylor, K. D., Landers, C. J., Abreu-Martin, M. T., Rotter, J. I., Yang, H., Targan, S. R. (2004). Association of antibody responses to microbial antigens and complications of small bowel Crohn's disease. Gastroenterology, 126, 414–424.

Narushima, S., Itoh, K., Mitsuoka, T., Nakayama, H., Itoh, T., Hioki, K., Nomura, T. (1998). Effect of mouse intestinal bacteria on incidence of colorectal tumors induced by 1,2-dimethylhydrazine injection in gnotobiotic transgenic mice harboring human prototype c-Ha-ras genes. Exp Anim, 47, 111–117.

Nathanson, J. W., Yadron, N. E., Farnan, J., Kinnear, S., Hart, J., Rubin, D. T. (2008).p53 mutations are associated with dysplasia and progression of dysplasia in patients with Crohn's disease. Dig Dis Sci, 53, 474–480.

Nava, G. M., Friedrichsen, H. J., Stappenbeck, T. S. (2011). Spatial organization of intestinal microbiota in the mouse ascending colon. ISME J, 5(4), 627-638.

Newman, J. V., Kosaka, T., Sheppard, B. J., Fox, J. G., Schauer, D. B. (2001). Bacterial infection promotes colon tumorigenesis in Apc(Min/+) mice. J Infect Dis, 184, 227–230.

Nicholson, J.K., Holmes, E., Kinross, J., Burcelin, R., Gibson, G., Jia, W., Pettersson, S. (2012).Host-gut microbiota metabolic interactions. Science, 8, 336,1262-1267.

Noubissi, F. K., Elcheva, I., Bhatia, N., Shakoori, A., Ougolkov, A., Liu, J., Minamoto, T., Ross, J., Fuchs, S. Y., Spiegelman, V. S. (2006). CRD-BP mediates stabilization of betaTrCP1 and c-myc mRNA in response to beta-catenin signalling. Nature, 441, 898–901.

Novelli, M. R., Williamson, J. A., Tomlinson, I. P., Elia, G., Hodgson, S. V., Talbot, I. C., Bodmer, W. F., Wright, N.A. (1996). Polyclonal origin of colonic adenomas in an XO/XY patient with FAP. Science, 272, 1187–1190.

Nowak, J., Weylandt, K. H., Habbel, P., Wang, J., Dignass, A., Glickman, J. N., Kang, J. X. (2007). Colitis-associated colon tumorigenesis is suppressed in transgenic mice rich in endogenous n-3 fatty acids. Carcinogenesis, 28, 1991–1995.

Nuding, S., Fellermann, K., Wehkamp, J., Stange, E. F. (2007).Reduced mucosal antimicrobial activity in Crohn's disease of the colon. Gut, 56, 1240–1247.

Ogino, S., Nosho, K., Meyerhardt, J. A., Kirkner, G. J., Chan, A. T., Kawasaki, T., Giovannucci, E. L., Loda, M., Fuchs, C. S. (2008). Cohort study of Fatty Acid synthase expression and patient survival in colon cancer. J Clin Oncol, 26, 5713–5720.

O'Hara, A. M. & Shanahan, F. (2006).The gut flora as a forgotten organ. EMBO Rep, 7, 688–693.

O'Keefe, S. J., Chung, D., Mahmoud, N., Sepulveda, A. R., Manafe, M., Arch, J., Adada, H., van der Merwe, T. (2007). Why do African Americans get more colon cancer than Native Africans? J Nutr, 137, 175S–182S.

Ohkusa, T., Yoshida, T., Sato, N., Watanabe, S., Tajiri, H., Okayasu, I. (2009). Commensal bacteria can enter colonic epithelial cells and induce proinflammatory cytokine secretion: a possible pathogenic mechanism of ulcerative colitis. J. Med. Microbiol, 58, 535–545.

Ohno, K., Narushima, S., Takeuchi, S., Itoh, K., Itoh, T., Hioki, K., Nomura, T. (2001). Effect of bacterial metabolism in the intestine on colorectal tumors induced by 1,2-dimethylhydrazine in transgenic mice harboring human prototype c-Ha-ras genes. J Exp Clin Cancer Res, 20, 51–56.

Onoue, M., Kado, S., Sakaitani, Y., Uchida, K., Morotomi, M. (1997).Specific species of intestinal bacteria influence the induction of aberrant crypt foci by 1,2-dimethylhydrazine in rats. Cancer Lett, 113, 179–186.

Pagnini, C., Corleto, V. D., Mangoni, M. L., Pilozzi, E., Torre, M. S., Marchese, R., Carnuccio, A., Giulio, E. D., Delle Fave, G. (2011). Alteration of local microflora and α-defensins hyper-production in colonic adenoma mucosa.J Clin Gastroenterol, 45(7), 602-610.

Pai, R., Tarnawski, A. S., Tran, T. (2004). Deoxycholic acid activates beta-catenin signaling pathway and increases colon cell cancer growth and invasiveness. Mol Biol Cell, 15, 2156–2163.

Park, E. J., Lee, J. H., Yu, G. Y., He, G., Ali, S. R., Holzer, R. G., Osterreicher, C. H., Takahashi, H., Karin, M.. (2010). Dietary and genetic obesity promote liver inflammation and tumorigenesis by enhancing IL-6 and TNF expression. Cell, 22, 140(2), 197-208.

Parkin, D. M. (2006).The global health burden of infection-associated cancers in the year 2002. Int J Cancer, 118, 3030–3044.

Pereira, M. A., Wang, W., Kramer, P. M., Tao, L. (2004). DNA hypomethylation induced by non-genotoxic carcinogens in mouse and rat colon. Cancer Lett, 212, 145–151.

Peters, U., Sinha, R., Chatterjee, N., Subar, A. F., Ziegler, R. G., Kulldorff, M., Bresalier, R., Weissfeld, J. L., Flood, A., Schatzkin, A., Hayes, R. B., Prostate, Lung, Colorectal, and Ovarian Cancer Screening Trial Project Team. (2003). Dietary fibre and colorectal adenoma in a colorectal cancer early detection programme. Lancet, 361, 1491–1495.

Peterson, D. A., McNulty, N. P., Guruge, J. L., Gordon, J. I. (2007). IgA response to symbiotic bacteria as a mediator of gut homeostasis. Cell Host Microbe, 2, 328-339.

Pischon, T., Lahmann, P. H., Boeing, H., Friedenreich, C., Norat, T., Tjønneland, A., Halkjaer, J., Overvad, K., Clavel-Chapelon, F., Boutron-Ruault, M. C., Guernec, G.,Bergmann, M. M., Linseisen, J., Becker, N., Trichopoulou, A., Trichopoulos, D., Sieri, S., Palli, D., Tumino, R., Vineis, P., Panico, S., Peeters, P. H., Bueno-de-Mesquita, H. B.,Boshuizen, H. C., Van Guelpen, B., Palmqvist, R., Berglund, G., Gonzalez, C. A., Dorronsoro, M., Barricarte, A., Navarro, C., Martinez, C., Quirós, J. R., Roddam, A., Allen, N., Bingham, S., Khaw, K. T., Ferrari, P., Kaaks, R., Slimani, N., Riboli, E. (2006). Body size and risk of colon and rectal cancer in the European Prospective Investigation Into Cancer and Nutrition (EPIC). J Natl Cancer Inst, 98, 920–931.

Podolsky, D. K. (2002).Inflammatory bowel disease. N Engl J Med, 347, 417–429.

Polymeros, D., Bogdanos, D. P., Day, R., Arioli, D., Vergani, D., Forbes, A. (2006). Does cross-reactivity between mycobacterium avium paratuberculosis and human intestinal antigens characterize Crohn's disease? Gastroenterology, 131, 85–96.

Potten, C. S. & Loeffler, M. (1990). Stem cells: attributes, cycles, spirals, pitfalls and uncertainties. Lessons for and from the crypt. Development, 110, 1001–1020.

Poutahidis, T., Haigis, K.M., Rao, V.P., Nambiar, P.R., Taylor, C.L., Ge, Z., Watanabe, K., Davidson, A., Horwitz, B.H., Fox, J.G., Erdman, S.E. (2007). Rapid reversal of interleukin-6-dependent epithelial invasion in a mouse model of microbially induced colon carcinoma. Carcinogenesis, 28(12), 2614-2623.

Preston, S. L., Wong, W. M., Chan, A. O., Poulsom, R., Jeffery, R., Goodlad, R. A., Mandir, N., Elia, G., Novelli, M., Bodmer, W. F., Tomlinson, I. P., Wright, N.A. (2003). Bottom-up histogenesis of colorectal adenomas: origin in the monocryptal adenoma and initial expansion by crypt fission. Cancer Res, 63, 3819–3825.

Qin, J., Li, R., Raes, J., Arumugam, M., Burgdorf, K. S., Manichanh, C., Nielsen, T., Pons, N., Levenez, F., Yamada, T., Mende, DR., Li, J., Xu, J., Li, S., Li, D., Cao, J., Wang, B., Liang, H., Zheng, H., Xie, Y., Tap, J., Lepage, P., Bertalan, M., Batto, J. M., Hansen, T., Le Paslier, D., Linneberg, A., Nielsen, H.B., Pelletier, E., Renault, P., Sicheritz-Ponten, T., Turner, K., Zhu, H., Yu, C., Li, S., Jian, M., Zhou, Y., Li, Y., Zhang, X., Li, S., Qin, N., Yang, H., Wang, J., Brunak, S., Doré, J., Guarner, F., Kristiansen, K., Pedersen, O., Parkhill, J., Weissenbach, J., MetaHIT Consortium, Bork, P., Ehrlich, S.D., & Wang, J. (2010). A human gut microbial gene catalogue established by metagenomic sequencing. Nature, 4, 464(7285), 59-65.

Rafter, J., Geltner, U., Bruce, R. (1987).Cellular toxicity of human faecal water–possible role in aetiology of colon cancer. Scand J Gastroenterol Suppl, 129, 245–250.

Raibaud, P., Ducluzeau, R., Dubos, F., Hudault, S., Bewa, H., Muller, M. C. (1980).Implantation of bacteria from the digestive tract of man and various animals into gnotobiotic mice.Am J Clin Nutr, 33, 2440–2447.

Rakoff-Nahoum, S., Paglino, J., Eslami-Varzaneh, F., Edberg, S., Medzhitov, R. (2004). Recognition of commensal microflora by toll-like receptors is required for intestinal homeostasis. Cell, 118, 229–241.

Rakoff-Nahoum, S.&Medzhitov, R. (2007). Regulation of spontaneous intestinal tumorigenesis through the adaptor protein MyD88. Science, 6, 317(5834), 124-127.

Rao, Y. P., Studer, E. J., Stravitz, R. T., Gupta, S., Qiao, L., Dent, P., Hylemon, P. B. (2002). Activation of the Raf-1/MEK/ERK cascade by bile acids occurs via the epidermal growth factor receptor in primary rat hepatocytes. Hepatology, 35, 307–314.

Rath, H. C., Herfarth, H. H., Ikeda, J. S., Grenther, W. B., Hamm, T. E. Jr., Balish, E., Taurog, J. D., Hammer, R. E., Wilson, K. H., Sartor, R. B. (1996). Normal luminal bacteria, especially Bacteroides species, mediate chronic colitis, gastritis, and arthritis in HLA-B27/human beta2 microglobulin transgenic rats. J Clin Invest, 98, 945–953.

Reddy, B. S., Narisawa, T., Maronpot, R., Weisburger, J. H., Wynder, E. L. (1975). Animal models for the study of dietary factors and cancer of the large bowel. Cancer Res, 35, 3421–3426.

Reddy, B. S. & Rivenson, A. (1993).Inhibitory effect of Bifidobacterium longum on colon, mammary, and liver carcinogenesis induced by 2-amino-3-methylimidazo[4,5-f]quinoline, a food mutagen. Cancer Res, 53, 3914–3918.

Renwick, A. G. & Drasar, B. S. (1976).Environmental carcinogens and large bowel cancer.Nature, 263, 234–235.

Ricci-Vitiani, L., Lombardi, D. G., Pilozzi, E., Biffoni, M., Todaro, M., Peschle, C., De Maria, R. (2007). Identification and expansion of human colon-cancer-initiating cells. Nature, 445, 111–115.

Roediger, W. E. (1980). Role of anaerobic bacteria in the metabolic welfare of the colonic mucosa in man.Gut, 21, 793–798.

Roediger, W. E., Duncan, A., Kapaniris, O., Millard, S. (1993). Reducing sulfur compounds of the colon impair colonocyte nutrition: implications for ulcerative colitis. Gastroenterology, 104, 802–809.

Rogler, G., Brand, K., Vogl, D., Page, S., Hofmeister, R., Andus, T., Knuechel, R., Baeuerle, P. A., Schölmerich, J., Gross, V. (1998). Nuclear factor kappaB is activated in macrophages and epithelial cells of inflamed intestinal mucosa. Gastroenterology, 115, 357–369.

Rolhion, N. & Darfeuille-Michaud, A. (2007). Adherent-invasive *Escherichia coli* in inflammatory bowel disease. Inflamm Bowel Dis, 13, 1277-1283.

Roncucci, L., Modica, S., Pedroni, M., Tamassia, M. G., Ghidoni, M., Losi, L., Fante, R., Di Gregorio, C., Manenti, A., Gafa, L., Ponz de Leon, M,.L. (1998). Aberrant crypt foci in patients with colorectal cancer. Br J Cancer, 77, 2343–2348.

Round, J. L. & Mazmanian, S. K. (2009). The gut microbiota shapes intestinal immune responses during health and disease. Nat Rev Immunol, 9, 313–323.

Round, J. L. & Mazmanian, S. K. (2010).Inducible Foxp3+ regulatory T-cell development by a commensal bacterium of the intestinal microbiota. Proc. Natl Acad. Sci. USA, 107, 12204–12209.

Rutgeerts, P., Goboes, K., Peeters, M., Hiele, M., Penninckx, F., Aerts, R., Kerremans, R., Vantrappen, G. (1991).Effect of faecal stream diversion on recurrence of Crohn's disease in the neoterminal ileum. Lancet, 338, 771–774.

Ryan, P., Kelly, R. G., Lee, G., Collins, J. K., O'Sullivan, G. C., O'Connell, J., Shanahan, F. (2004). Bacterial DNA within granulomas of patients with Crohn's disease–detection by laser capture microdissection and PCR. Am J Gastroenterol, 99, 1539–1543.

Salyers, A. A., Vercellotti, J. R., West, S. E., Wilkins, T. D. (1977). Fermentation of mucin and plant polysaccharides by strains of Bacteroides from the human colon. Appl Environ Microbiol, 33, 319–322.

Salyers, A. A., Gherardini, F., O'Brien, M. (1981).Utilization of xylan by two species of human colonic Bacteroides. Appl Environ Microbiol, 41, 1065–1068.

Sanapareddy, N., Legge, R. M., Jovov, B., McCoy, A., Burcal, L., Araujo-Perez, F., Randall, T. A., Galanko, J., Benson, A., Sandler, R. S., Rawls, J. F., Abdo, Z., Fodor, A. A., Keku, T. O. (2012). Increased rectal microbial richness is associated with the presence of colorectal adenomas in humans. ISME J, 6(10), 1858-1868.

Sartor, R. B. (2008). Microbial influences in inflammatory bowel dis- eases. Gastroenterology, 134, 577-594.

Sasaki, M., Sitaraman, S. V., Babbin, B. A., Gerner-Smidt, P., Ribot, E. M., Garrett, N., Alpern, J. A., Akyildiz, A., Theiss, A. L., Nusrat, A., Klapproth, J. M. (2007). Invasive *Escherichia coli* are a feature of Crohn's disease. Lab Invest, 87, 1042-1054.

Savage, D. C. (1977).Microbial ecology of the gastrointestinal tract. Annu Rev Microbiol, 31, 107–133.

Scanlan, P. D., Shanahan, F., Clune, Y., Collins, J. K., O'Sullivan, G. C., O'Riordan, M., Holmes, E., Wang, Y., Marchesi, J. R..(2008). Culture-independent analysis of the gut microbiota in colorectal cancer and polyposis.Environ Microbiol, 10, 789–798.

Scanlan, P. D., Shanahan, F., Marchesi, J. R. (2009). Culture-independent analysis of desulfovibrios in the human distal colon of healthy, colorectal cancer and polypectomized individuals. FEMS Microbiol Ecol, 69(2), 213-221.

Schatzkin, A., Lanza, E., Corle, D., Lance, P., Iber, F., Caan, B., Shike, M., Weissfeld, J., Burt, R., Cooper, M. R., Kikendall, J. W., Cahill, J. (2000). Lack of effect of a low-fat, high-fiber diet on the recurrence of colorectal adenomas. Polyp Prevention Trial Study Group. N Engl J Med, 342, 1149–1155.

Schoeffner, D. J. & Thorgeirsson, U. P. (2000). Susceptibility of nonhuman primates to carcinogens of human relevance.In Vivo, 14, 149–156.

Schoppmann, S. F., Birner, P., Stöckl, J., Kalt, R., Ullrich, R., Caucig, C., Kriehuber, E., Nagy, K., Alitalo, K., Kerjaschki, D. Tumor-associated macrophages express lymphatic endothelial growth factors and are related to peritumoral lymphangiogenesis. Am J Pathol, 161, 947–956.

Schreiter, K., Hausmann, M., Spoettl, T., Strauch, U. G., Bataille, F., Schoelmerich, J., Herfarth, H., Falk, W., Rogler, G. (2005). Glycoprotein (gp) 96 expression: induced during differentiation of intestinal macrophages but impaired in Crohn's disease. Gut, 54, 935–943.

Schultsz, C., Berg, F. M. V. D., Kate, F. W. T., Tytgat, G. N., Dankert, J. (1999). The intestinal mucus layer from patients with inflammatory bowel disease harbors high numbers of bacteria compared with controls. Gastroenterology, 117, 1089–1097.

Schwiertz, A., Taras, D., Schäfer, K., Beijer, S., Bos, N. A., Donus, C., Hardt, P. D. (2010). Microbiota and SCFA in lean and overweight healthy subjects. Obesity (Silver Spring), 18(1), 190-195.

Sears, C. L. (2009). Enterotoxigenic Bacteroides fragilis: a rogue among symbiotes.Clin microbiol Rev, 22: 349-369.

Seibold, F., Brandwein, S., Simpson, S., Terhorst, C., Elson, C. O. (1998). pANCA represents a cross-reactivity to enteric bacterial antigens. J Clin Immunol, 18, 153–160.

Selgrad, M., Malfertheiner, P., Fini, L., Goel, A., Boland, C. R., Ricciardiello, L. (2008). The role of viral and bacterial pathogens in gastrointestinal cancer.J Cell Physiol, 216, 378–388.

Shen, X. J., Rawls, J. F., Randall, T., Burcal, L., Mpande, C. N., Jenkins, N., Jovov, B., Abdo, Z., Sandler, R. S., Keku, T. O. (2010). Molecular characterization of mucosal adherent bacteria and associations with colorectal adenomas.Gut Microbes, 1(3), 138-147.

Shih, I. M., Wang, T. L., Traverso, G., Romans, K., Hamilton, S. R., Ben-Sasson, S., Kinzler, K. W., Vogelstein, B. (2001). Top-down morphogenesis of colorectal tumors. Proc Natl Acad Sci U S A, 98, 2640–2645.

Silvi, S., Rumney, C. J., Cresci, A., Rowland, I. R. (1999). Resistant starch modifies gut microflora and microbial metabolism in human flora-associated rats inoculated with faeces from Italian and UK donors. J Appl Microbiol, 86, 521–530.

Sobhani, I., Tap, J., Roudot-Thoraval, F., Roperch, J. P., Letulle, S., Langella, P., Corthier, G., Tran Van Nhieu, J., Furet, J. P. (2011). Microbial dysbiosis in colorectal cancer (CRC) patients. PLoS One, 27, 6(1), e16393.

Sokol, H., Pigneur, B., Watterlot, L., Lakhdari, O., Bermúdez-Humarán, L. G., Gratadoux, J. J., Blugeon, S., Bridonneau, C., Furet, J. P., Corthier, G., Grangette, C., Vasquez, N., Pochart, P., Trugnan, G., Thomas, G., Blottière, H. M., Doré, J., Marteau, P., Seksik, P., Langella, P. (2008). Faecalibacterium prausnitzii is an anti-inflammatory commensal bacterium identified by gut microbiota analysis of Crohn disease patients. Proc Natl Acad Sci U S A, 105, 16731–16736.

Sonnenburg, J. L., Xu, J., Leip, D. D., Chen, C. H., Westover, B. P., Weatherford, J., Buhler, J. D., Gordon, J. I.(2005). Glycan foraging in vivo by an intestine-adapted bacterial symbiont. Science, 307, 1955–1959.

Strauss, J., Kaplan, G. G., Beck, P. L., Rioux, K., Panaccione, R., Devinney, R., Lynch, T., Allen-Vercoe, E. (2011). Invasive potential of gut mucosa-derived Fusobacterium nucleatum positively correlates with IBD status of the host. Inflamm Bowel Dis, 17, 1971-1978.

Strocchi, A., Furne, J., Ellis, C., Levitt, M. D. (1994). Methanogens outcompete sulphate reducing bacteria for H2 in the human colon. Gut, 35, 1098–1101.

Swidsinski, A., Weber, J., Loening-Baucke, V., Hale, L. P., Lochs, H. (2005).Spatial organization and composition of the mucosal flora in patients with inflammatory bowel disease. J Clin Microbiol, 43, 3380–3389.

Swidsinski, A., Loening-Baucke, V., Theissig, F., Engelhardt, H., Bengmark, S., Koch, S., Lochs, H., Dörffel, Y. (2007). Comparative study of the intestinal mucus barrier in normal and inflamed colon. Gut, 56, 343-350.

Szekely, J. & Gates, K. S. (2006).Noncovalent DNA binding and the mechanism of oxidative DNA damage by fecapentaene-12. Chem Res Toxicol, 19, 117–121.

Takayama, T., Katsuki, S., Takahashi, Y., Ohi, M., Nojiri, S., Sakamaki, S., Kato, J., Kogawa, K., Miyake, H., Niitsu, Y. (1998). Aberrant crypt foci of the colon as precursors of adenoma and cancer. N Engl J Med, 339, 1277–1284.

The Cancer Genome Atlas Network.Comprehensive molecular characterization of human colon and rectal cancer. (2012). Nature, 487, 330-337.

Thompson-Chagoyán, O. C., Maldonado, J., Gil, A. (2007).Colonization and impact of disease and other factors on intestinal microbiota. Dig Dis Sci, 52, 2069–2077.

Thomas, G. A., Swift, G. L., Green, J. T., Newcombe, R. G., Braniff-Mathews, C., Rhodes, J., Wilkinson, S., Strohmeyer, G., Kreuzpainter, G. (1998). Controlled trial of antituberculous chemotherapy in Crohn's disease: a five year follow up study. Gut, 42, 497–500.

Tjalsma, H., Boleij, A., Marchesi, J. R., Dutilh, B. E. (2012). A bacterial driver-passenger model for colorectal cancer: beyond the usual suspects. Nat Rev Microbiol, 10, 575-582.

Tong, J.L., Ran, Z.H., Shen, J., Fan, G.Q., Xiao, S.D. (2008). Association between fecal bile acids and colorectal cancer: a meta-analysis of observational studies. Yonsei Med J, 31, 49(5), 792-803.

Turnbaugh, P. J., Ley, R. E., Mahowald, M. A., Magrini, V., Mardis, E. R., Gordon, J. I. (2006). An obesity-associated gut microbiome with increased capacity for energy harvest. Nature, 21, 444, 1027-1031.

Turnbaugh, P.J., Bäckhed, F., Fulton, L., Gordon, J.I. (2008). Diet-induced obesity is linked to marked but reversible alterations in the mouse distal gut microbiome. Cell Host Microbe, 17, 3, 213-223.

Turnbaugh, P.J., Ridaura, V.K., Faith, J.J., Rey, F.E., Knight, R., Gordon, J.I. (2009). The effect of diet on the human gut microbiome: a metagenomic analysis in humanized gnotobiotic mice. Sci Transl Med, 11, 1, 6ra14. (A).

Turnbaugh, P. J., Hamady, M., Yatsunenko, T., Cantarel, B. L., Duncan, A., Ley, R. E., Sogin, M. L, Jones, W. J., Roe, B. A., Affourtit, J. P., Egholm, M., Henrissat, B., Heath, A.C., Knight, R., Gordon, J.I. (2009). A core gut microbiome in obese and lean twins. Nature, 22, 457, 480-484. (B).

Umesaki, Y., Okada, Y., Matsumoto, S., Imaoka, A., Setoyama, H. (1995). Segmented filamentous bacteria are indigenous intestinal bacteria that activate intraepithelial lymphocytes and induce MHC class II molecules and fucosyl asialo GM1 glycolipids on the small intestinal epithelial cells in the ex-germ-free mouse. Microbiol Immunol, 39, 555–562.

Uronis, J.M., Mühlbauer, M., Herfarth, H.H., Rubinas, T.C., Jones, G.S., Jobin, C. (2009).Modulation of the intestinal microbiota alters colitis-associated colorectal cancer susceptibility. PLoS One, 24,4(6), e6026.

Vaishnava, S., Behrendt, C. L., Ismail, A. S., Eckmann, L., Hooper, L. V. (2008). Paneth cells directly sense gut commensals and maintain homeostasis at the intestinal host-microbial interface. Proc Natl Acad Sci U S A, 105, 20858–20863.

Van der Waaij, L. A., Harmsen, H. J., Madjipour, M., Kroese, F. G., Zwiers, M., van Dullemen, H. M., de Boer, N. K., Welling, G. W., Jansen, P. L. (2005). Bacterial population analysis of human colon and terminal ileum biopsies with 16S rRNA-based fluorescent probes: commensal bacteria live in suspension and have no direct contact with epithelial cells. Inflamm Bowel Dis, 11, 865-871.

Velcich, A., Yang, W., Heyer, J., Fragale, A., Nicholas, C., Viani, S., Kucherlapati, R., Lipkin, M., Yang, K., Augenlicht, L. (2002). Colorectal cancer in mice genetically deficient in the mucin Muc2. Science, 295, 1726-1729.

Vijay-Kumar, M., Aitken, J. D., Carvalho, F. A., Cullender, T. C., Mwangi, S., Srinivasan, S., Sitaraman, S. V., Knight, R., Ley, R. E., Gewirtz, A. T. (2010). Metabolic syndrome and altered gut microbiota in mice lacking Toll-like receptor 5. Science, 9, 328, 228-231.

Vulevic, J., McCartney, A. L., Gee, J. M., Johnson, I. T., Gibson, G. R. (2004). Microbial species involved in production of 1,2-sn-diacylglycerol and effects of phosphatidylcholine on human fecal microbiota. Appl Environ Microbiol, 70, 5659–5666.

Wallis, R. S., Broder, M. S., Wong, J. Y., Hanson, M. E., Beenhouwer, D. O. (2004). Granulomatous infectious diseases associated with tumor necrosis factor antagonists. Clin Infect Dis, 38,1261–1265.

Wang, T., Cai, G., Qiu, Y., Fei, N., Zhang, M., Pang, X., Jia, W., Cai, S., Zhao, L. (2012). Structural segregation of gut microbiota between colorectal cancer patients and healthy volunteers.ISME J, 6(2), 320-329.

World Cancer Research Fund/American Institute for Cancer Research. (2007). Food, Nutrition, Physical Activity, and the Prevention of Cancer: a Global Perspective. AICR, Washington DC.

Wostmann, B. S., Larkin, C., Moriarty, A., Bruckner-Kardoss, E. (1983).Dietary intake, energy metabolism, and excretory losses of adult male germfree Wistar rats. Lab Anim Sci, 33, 46–50.

Wu, S., Rhee, K. J., Albesiano, E., Rabizadeh, S., Wu, X., Yen, H. R., Huso, D. L., Brancati, F. L., Wick, E., McAllister, F., Housseau, F., Pardoll, D. M., Sears, C. L. (2009). A human colonic commensal promotes colon tumorigenesis via activation of T helper type 17 T cell responses. Nat Med, 15(9), 1016-1022.

Xavier, R. J. &Podolsky, D. K. (2007). Unravelling the pathogenesis of inflammatory bowel disease. Nature. 26, 448(7152), 427-434.

Xiao, H., Gulen, M. F., Qin, J., Yao, J., Bulek, K., Kish, D., Altuntas, C. Z., Wald, D., Ma, C., Zhou, H., Tuohy, V. K., Fairchild, R. L., de la Motte, C., Cua, D., Vallance, B. A., Li, X. (2007). The Toll-interleukin-1 receptor member SIGIRR regulates colonic epithelial homeostasis, inflammation, and tumorigenesis. Immunity, 26, 461-475.

Yamamoto, S., Mitsumori, K., Kodama, Y., Matsunuma, N., Manabe, S., Okamiya, H., Suzuki, H., Fukuda, T., Sakamaki, Y., Sunaga, M., Nomura, G., Hioki, K., Wakana, S., Nomura, T., Hayashi, Y. (1996). Rapid induction of more malignant tumors by various genotoxic carcinogens in transgenic mice harboring a human prototype c-Ha-ras gene than in control non-transgenic mice.Carcinogenesis, 17, 2455–2461.

Yin, M. J., Yamamoto, Y., Gaynor, R. B. (1998). The anti-inflammatory agents aspirin and salicylate inhibit the activity of I(kappa)B kinase-beta. Nature, 396, 77–80.

Zarkovic, M., Qin, X., Nakatsuru, Y., Oda, H., Nakamura, T., Shamsuddin, A. M., Ishikawa, T. (1993). Tumor promotion by fecapentaene-12 in a rat colon carcinogenesis model. Carcinogenesis, 14, 1261–1264.

Zeissig, S., Bürgel, N., Günzel, D., Richter, J., Mankertz, J., Wahnschaffe, U., Kroesen, A. J., Zeitz, M., Fromm, M., Schulzke, J. D. (2007). Changes in expression and distribution of claudin 2, 5 and 8 lead to discontinuous tight junctions and barrier dysfunction in active Crohn's disease. Gut, 56, 61–72.

Zgouras, D., Wächtershäuser, A., Frings, D., Stein, J. (2003). Butyrate impairs intestinal tumor cell-induced angiogenesis by inhibiting HIF-1alpha nuclear translocation. Biochem Biophys Res Commun, 300, 832–838.

Zoetendal, E. G., Akkermans, A. D., Vos, W. M. D. (1998). Temperature gradient gel electrophoresis analysis of 16S rRNA from human fecal samples reveals stable and host-specific communities of active bacteria. Appl Environ Microbiol, 64, 3854–3859.

Zoetendal, E. G., Ben-Amor, K., Akkermans, A. D., Abee, T., de Vos, W. M. (2001). DNA isolation protocols affect the detection limit of PCR approaches of bacteria in samples from the human gastrointestinal tract. Syst Appl Microbiol, 24, 405–410.

Zoetendal, E. G., von Wright, A., Vilpponen-Salmela, T., Ben-Amor, K., Akkermans, A. D. L., de Vos, W. M. (2002). Mucosa-associated bacteria in the human gastrointestinal tract are uniformly distributed along the colon and differ from the community recovered from feces. Appl Environ Microbiol, 68, 3401–3407.

Zhu, Y., Hua, P., Rafiq, S., Waffner, E. J., Duffey, M. E., Lance, P. (2002). Ca2+- and PKC-dependent stimulation of PGE2 synthesis by deoxycholic acid in human colonic fibroblasts. Am J Physiol Gastrointest Liver Physiol, 283, G503–510.

Zychlinsky, A. & Sansonetti, P. (1997). Perspectives series: host/pathogen interactions. Apoptosis in bacterial pathogenesis. J Clin Invest, 100, 493–495.

# Identification of a Novel Protein-Protein Interaction from an Integrative *in silico* Screening and Analysis

Ho-Jin Lee
*Department of Structural Biology*
*St. Jude Children's Research Hospital, USA*

Jie J. Zheng
*Department of Structural Biology*
*St. Jude Children's Research Hospital, USA*

## 1   Introduction

The completion of genome sequencing projects in humans and other species has resulted in the discovery of many putative and uncharacterized proteins. Structural identification and functional characterization of these proteins are greatly necessary to understanding various biological processes. Since most proteins show their biological functions through interaction with partner proteins (Pawson & Nash, 2003), characterization of protein-protein interactions (PPIs) in the global network is important to understanding protein function and biological processes (Ernst *et al.*, 2010; Gfeller *et al.*, 2011; Tonikian *et al.*, 2008). Several methods, such as co-immuno precipitation, yeast two-hybrid analysis, pull-down assays, protein microarrays, peptide libraries, and mass spectrometry-based proteomics, have been used to identify protein interaction networks (Aebersold & Mann, 2003; Kaushansky *et al.*, 2010; Lee & Zheng, 2010; Phizicky & Fields, 1995). Computational tools that predict the PPI partners *in silico* have been also developed (Hawkins *et al.*, 2012; McDowall *et al.*, 2009; Szklarczyk *et al.*, 2011; Yip *et al.*, 2011; Zhang *et al.*, 2012). Because much information on PPIs has been deposited in publicly available databases, this implies that optimal use of all the databases compiling the interactions will reduce the time necessary to explore the number of candidate proteins and enhance the efficiency of the investigations of new functions of a protein of interest.

In this chapter, we describe an approach used for identification of a novel PPI. We show that an uncharacterized protein, two-transmembrane protein 88 (TMEM88), is a binding partner of Dishevelled (Dvl/Dsh) by using a combination of techniques, including bioinformatics, biophysical, and biochemical methods (Lee *et al.*, 2010). We believe that the study presented here is a successful example of how existing knowledge can be applied to uncover a biologically relevant binding partner of a given protein, which will reveal new functions of proteins in novel signaling pathways.

## 2   Identification of Dvl PDZ-binding Protein: An Example Study

Wnt signaling plays important roles in cell development, growth, and tumorigenesis (Angers & Moon, 2009). At least three Wnt signaling pathways have been established, including canonical Wnt/β-catenin, non-canonical Wnt/planar cell polarity (PCP), and Wnt/Ca$^{2+}$ signaling pathways (Gao & Chen, 2010). The cytoplasmic protein Dvl (DVL1, DVL2, and DVL3 in mammals) is a key player in Wnt signaling pathways (Gao & Chen, 2010; Wallingford & Habas, 2005). In canonical Wnt signaling, the Wnt ligand binds to its co-receptors, Frizzled (Fz) and single-span transmembrane LDL receptor–related protein 5/6 (LRP5/6), resulting in the formation of Dvl-Fz complex and Axin is relocalized from the β-catenin destruction complex (Axin, GSK-3β, and APC tumor suppressor; they promote the destabilization of β-catenin) to the membrane (Zeng *et al.*, 2008). The activated Dvl proteins relay the Wnt signals to downstream components (Gao & Chen, 2010; Wallingford & Habas, 2005; Wharton, 2003). Accumulated β-catenin protein translocates into the nucleus and induces gene transcription by binding to TCF/LEF transcription factor (Figure 1a).

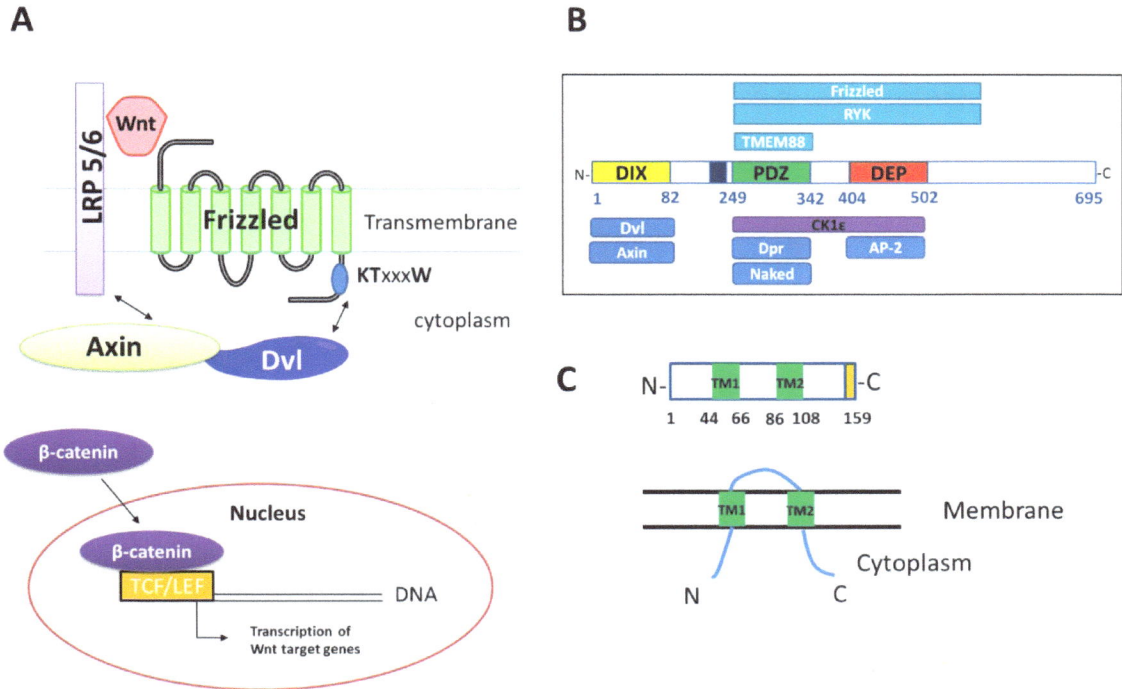

**Figure 1:** (A) Overview of the Wnt/β-catenin signaling pathway. The binding of Wnt ligand to the Fz-LRP5/6 receptor complex activates the Dvl, which then binds to the cytoplasmic C-terminus Fz. The activated Dvl also recruits Axin from the β-catenin destruction complex. Accumulated β-catenin protein translocates into the nucleus and induces gene transcription by binding to TCF/LEF transcription factor. (B) Schematic description of Dvl-1 and its binding partners. Mouse Dvl-1 is composed of three highly conserved domains: DIX, PDZ, and DEP domains. A number of proteins are known to be Dvl PDZ-binding proteins. (C) Schematic description of TMEM88, a two-transmembrane protein identified as a Dvl-binding protein by using a combinatorial approach including bioinformatics, biophysics, and biochemistry.

Dvl proteins consist of 3 highly conserved domains, the DIX (**DI**shevelled-a**X**in), PDZ (**P**ost synaptic density-95, **D**isc Large and **Z**onular Occludens-1), and DEP (**D**ishevelled-**E**GL10-**P**leckstrin) domains (Pan *et al.*, 2004; Park *et al.*, 2005; Schwarz-Romond *et al.*, 2007a; Schwarz-Romond *et al.*, 2007b; Simons *et al.*, 2009; Wong *et al.*, 2003; Wong *et al.*, 2000) (Fig. 1b). The Dvl PDZ domain is the PPI module, which is folded into a compact globular structure comprising six β-strands flanked by two α-helices (Lee & Zheng, 2010). The Dvl PDZ domain recognizes the extreme C-terminal and internal sequence of target proteins (N. X. Wang *et al.*, 2008). For example, the Dvl PDZ domain interacts with 7-transmembrane Wnt receptor Fz proteins through the internal sequence (Tauriello *et al.*, 2012; Wong *et al.*, 2003) and also the single-transmembrane receptor Tyr kinase Ryk through the extreme C-terminus (Angers & Moon, 2009; Sakurai *et al.*, 2009; Yoshikawa *et al.*, 2003). Thus, identification and characterization of Dvl PDZ-binding proteins are key steps toward understanding their biological functions in normal and cancer cells (Lee *et al.*, 2010).

## 2.1    Identification of Tripeptides Recognized by the PDZ Domain of Dishevelled

To identify novel PPIs, the binding interface of a given protein of interest should be fully investigated by several methods, such as nuclear magnetic resonance (NMR) and computational tools (Lee *et al.*, 2009a). NMR is useful for the study of weak PPIs in solution. A chemical shift perturbation NMR experiment that has been used to precisely map binding sites of target proteins is well suited to detecting weak but specific biologically relevant interactions (Pellecchia *et al.*, 2002). For computational tools, molecular dynamics (MD) is useful to understand the binding modes of the complex; the molecular mechanics Poisson-Boltzmann surface area (MM-PBSA) method may be applied to evaluate the relative binding free energies of the complex (Lee *et al.*, 2009a; W. Wang *et al.*, 2001).

We used tripeptides to investigate the binding properties of the Dvl1 PDZ domain. Tripeptides are drawing especially great attention in drug discovery because they are easy to modify and small (M.W. < 500 Da), which is consistent with typical small-molecule bioavailable oral drugs (Kannengiesser *et al.*, 2008; Lee *et al.*, 2007; Rifai *et al.*, 2008). In addition, the conformational properties of tripeptides have been explored to allow an understanding of the protein folding and intrinsic properties of amino acid residues in protein structures (Eker *et al.*, 2002; Eker *et al.*, 2004a, 2004b; Eker *et al.*, 2003; Schweitzer-Stenner *et al.*, 2003). Recent studies revealed that even short peptides could adopt a specific conformation in gas phase or in water solution, implying that they might serve as a model as well as a molecular scaffold for future drug design (Eker *et al.*, 2002; Eker *et al.*, 2004a, 2004b; Eker *et al.*, 2003; Hagarman *et al.*, 2006; Schweitzer-Stenner *et al.*, 2003; Schweitzer-Stenner *et al.*, 2006).

### 2.1.1    Tripeptide V-V-V Recognizes the Dvl1 PDZ Domain

To discover and optimize a Dvl PDZ-binding peptide, we chose the tripeptide VVV as a model because it has been reported to predominantly sample a β-strand structure in water solution and it resembles the PDZ-binding motif, such as S/T-X-Φ and Φ-X- Φ (X: any amino acid; Φ: hydrophobic residue) (Eker *et al.*, 2002; Lee & Zheng, 2010). To probe the interaction between the tripeptide VVV and the Dvl1 PDZ domain, we used NMR spectroscopy. The interaction of a protein and a short peptide can be easily detected by the chemical shift perturbations ($\Delta\delta_{binding}$) or peak broadening upon adding the unlabeled peptide to the $^{15}$N-labeled targeted protein. The large chemical shift perturbations resulting from the binding of the tripeptide VVV to the Dvl1 PDZ domain were observed for residues Ile264 and Ser265 in the βB-strand and the residues Arg322 and Val325 on the αB-helix structure of the Dvl1 PDZ domain. These peaks showed the continuous changes in chemical shifts in the $^{1}$H-$^{15}$N-HSQC spectra as the concentration of the tripeptide VVV was increased, indicating that its interaction is in the fast exchange range on the NMR time scale. As expected, the tripeptide VVV binds to the αB/βB-binding groove of the Dvl1 PDZ domain.

### 2.1.2    Evaluation of the Binding Free Energy of the Complex of Dvl1 PDZ and Model Tripeptide VXV

The observation of the direct interaction between the tripeptide VVV and the Dvl PDZ domain prompted us to investigate whether other similar tripeptides could bind to the Dvl PDZ domain. Because the tripeptide VVV resembles the typical PDZ-binding motif, investigating the role of a particular amino acid residue in binding was expected to provide valuable information to optimize a peptide bound to the Dvl1 PDZ domain. Because the P(-1) residue in the PDZ-binding peptide (position 0 referring to the extreme

C-terminal residue) has been found to play a role in enhancing binding in several cases(Appleton *et al.*, 2006; Runyon *et al.*, 2007; Skelton *et al.*, 2003), we virtually evaluated the binding affinities of Dvl PDZ with model tripeptides VXV (X: any amino acid residue except Pro) using the ICM empirical binding energy function (ICM Pro ver. 3.2). In this study, we used x-ray crystallographic data of the structure of the Xenopus Dishevelled PDZ (Xdsh PDZ)/Dapper peptide (SGSLKLMTTV) complex (PDB code: 1L6O:A) (Cheyette *et al.*, 2002). We used the coordinates of the last three amino acid residues (TTV) for the Dapper peptide in the complex structure to generate the model tripeptides. We assumed that all tripeptides bound to the PDZ domain adopt the β-strand that resembles the bound conformation of the Dapper peptide (Cheyette *et al.*, 2002). The side chain of each modeled tripeptide in the complex was optimized to escape a possible collapse of the side chain between Xdsh PDZ and the VXV tripeptide before calculating the binding free energy of the complex. The relative binding free energy ($\Delta\Delta G_{binding}$) of the Xdsh PDZ and model tripeptide VXV with respect to the tripeptide VVV ($\Delta G_{binding}$ is -21.8±3.3 kcal/mol) showed that the tripeptide VWV had the highest binding energy to the PDZ domain of Xdsh. Although the ICM empirical binding energy function has been validated for several cases (Schapira *et al.*, 1999), we wondered whether this would be the case for our model system. To confirm the theoretical result, we used an NMR-binding assay.

### 2.1.3    Tripeptide VWV Indeed Binds to the Dvl PDZ Domain

We chemically synthesized the tripeptide VWV and explored its interaction with the Dvl1 PDZ domain using NMR spectroscopy. Surprisingly, the residues I264, R322, and V325 began to disappear upon stepwise addition of the tripeptide VWV and reappeared at the saturated concentration. This indicates that the complex formation is in the intermediate exchange range on the NMR time scale. The two largest chemical shift perturbations were found in residues I264 ($\Delta\delta_{binding}$ = 0.565 ppm) on the βB-strand and R322 ($\Delta\delta_{binding}$ = 0.497 ppm) on the αB-helix of Dvl1 PDZ at the saturated concentration. They are much larger than the chemical shift perturbations in the same residues caused by the binding of the VVV peptide, indicating that the VWV peptide binds to the PDZ domain tighter than the VVV peptide.

We next determined the binding affinity (KD) of  tripeptides using fluorescence spectroscopy.In this study, wemade a fluorescence-labeled PDZ domain, 2-((5(6)-tetramethylrhodamine) carboxylamino)ethylethanethiosulfonate (TMR)-PDZ domain of Dvl1 (Shan *et al.*, 2005). The fluorescence intensity of the TMR-PDZ domain at 597 nm was monitored while the tripeptide VVV or VWV was added. The $K_D$ value was calculated from a reciprocal plot of fluorescence intensity quenching against the concentration of the peptide. The result showed that the binding affinity of the tripeptide VWV was 2 μM and that of the tripeptide VVV was 71 μM for the TMR-PDZ domain, which supports the ICM theoretical result that modification of the P(-1) position in the tripeptide can increase the binding affinity for the Dvl1 PDZ domain. Notice that the $K_D$ values of the tripeptides are much lesser than that of the organic molecule NSC668036, which was the first identified antagonist for targeting Dvl1 PDZ protein interactions (Shan *et al.*, 2005). Using the same binding assay, the $K_D$ value of NSC668036 and TMR-PDZ was found to be 237±31 μM (Shan *et al.*, 2005).

### 2.1.4    Structures of the Complex between the Dvl PDZ Domain and the VWV Peptide

To understand the greater affinity of the tripeptide VWV than of the tripeptide VVV for binding to the Dvl1 PDZ domain, we determined the three-dimensional structure of the Dvl1 PDZ/VWV complex. In the complex structure calculation, a total of 26 experimental restraints from intermolecular nuclear Overhauser effects (NOEs) between tripeptide VWV and the Dvl1 PDZ domain were used, including 22 intermolecular NOEs between the peptide and the protein and 4 intramolecular NOEs from the tripeptide VWV bound to the PDZ domain. Not surprisingly, the tripeptide VWV was fitted into the hydrophobic pocket of the Dvl1 PDZ domain and formed an additional β-strand with respect to the βB-structure. The lowest energy conformation of the PDZ/VWV complex shows that the side chains of P(0) and P(-2) contacted the hydrophobic residues within the binding site of the Dvl1 PDZ domain. The side chain of the P(-1) residue in the tripeptide was oriented to the βB- and βC-strand regions of the Dvl1 PDZ domain. The amino acid residues of the Dvl1 PDZ domain in proximity (<4.0 Å) to tripeptide V(-2)-W(-1)-V(0) were as follows: the residues Leu262, Gly263, Ile264, Val325, Arg322, Leu321, and Val318 were close to the residue V(0); the residues Ile266 and Val318 were close to the residue Val(-2); and Ser265 and Met284 were close to the W(-1) residue. The solution structure of the PDZ/VWV complex was in a good agreement with the complex structure used for the ICM calculations.

The structure of the PDZ/VWV complex implies that the difference in the binding affinity for the tripeptides VVV and VWV may result from the hydrophobic interaction between the side chain of the Ser265 or Met284 residues and the Trp side chain in the P(-1) position of the tripeptide VWV. However, it is difficult to quantitatively explain the linkage between the binding affinity of the tripeptide and the Dvl1 PDZ domain with the structural information.

### 2.1.5    Molecular Dynamics Simulation and MM-PBSA Calculation

To further understand the difference in the binding energies for the two complexes, we performed an MD simulation using AMBER software (Amber 8, Scripps Research Institute, La Jolla, CA). The starting structures of the complexes used were the lowest energy conformation. MD simulations were performed in explicit water for 2 ns. To analyze the stability of the MD simulations, we plotted the root-mean-square deviation (RMSD) values relative to the initial structures of the PDZ backbone atoms during the 2 ns MD simulation against time. The complexes of the Dvl1 PDZ domain with the VVV or VWV tripeptide reached convergence quickly and remained stable thereafter. We then calculated the binding free energy of the interaction between the Dvl1 PDZ domain and the tripeptides for the last 1 ns with the MM-PBSA method (W. Wang *et al.*, 2001). The individual energy terms that contribute to binding free energy are listed in Table 3. The predicted binding free energy (ΔG) of the Dvl1 PDZ/VVV complex was -5.52±0.80 kcal/mol and that of the Dvl1 PDZ/VWV complex was -7.15±1.20 kcal/mol, indicating that the binding of the tripeptide VWV to the Dvl1 PDZ domain is stronger than that of the tripeptide VVV. The relative binding free energies obtained from MM-PBSA calculations were in good agreement with experimental results (ΔG = -5.56 kcal/mol for TMR-PDZ/VVV and ΔG = -7.64 kcal/mol for TMR-PDZ/VWV). Besides ranking the binding free energies correctly, MM-PBSA allowed us to break down the total binding free energy into individual components, such as $E_{elec}$+PB and $E_{vdw}$, which enabled us to understand the binding interactions in detail. The $E_{elec}$+PB is the total electrostatic contribution, including solute-solute and solute-solvent interactions, and $E_{vdw}$ is the van der Waals contribution to the binding. The $E_{vdw}$ favors interaction of the Dvl1 PDZ domain with tripeptide VWV by 8.89 kcal/mol, whereas the electrostatic contribution resists the binding between the Dvl1 PDZ and VWV by 2.89 kcal/mol. The differences between the binding free energy of the two complexes therefore are largely controlled by the van der Waals contribution. This correlates well with the observation that the indole ring of the Trp(-1) residue in the tripeptide was close to the side chain of the S265 and M284 residues. The entropy contribution (TΔS) disfavors the binding of the PDZ/VWV due to orientational and positional restraints imposed by the larger side chain of the Trp residue; however, the overall binding free energy ($\Delta G_{overall}$) still promotes the binding of the PDZ/VWV complex over that of the PDZ/VVV complex.

## 2.2   Database Searches and Analysis

By conducting computational studies in combination with an NMR mapping assay, we identified and characterized the additional peptide sequences that bind to the Dvl PDZ domain (Lee *et al.*, 2009a). Given that the tripeptide VWV (Val-Trp-Val) is sufficient to recognize the Dvl PDZ domain, we reasoned that some proteins might have a VWV motif at their C-termini and regulate the Wnt signaling pathways by inhibiting the Fz-Dvl interaction.  Thus, we queried for proteins containing the VWV motif at the C-terminus in genome-wide database from ScanProsite (http://ca.expasy.org/tools/scanprosite) *(de Castro et al., 2006)*. We identified 294 proteins from invertebrates and vertebrates (protein fragments were excluded) in December 2009. To reduce the time and effort to verify PPIs, we focused on 5 proteins found in human (Accession No: P02743, Q5H8X8, Q6PEY1, Q6PEY1, and Q9NTI7).

Because putative Dvl-binding proteins must be co-expressed to interact in a physiological context, we examined the expression patterns and subcellular localizations of the 5 proteins from Ensembl (http://www.ensembl.org). In addition, since the human DVL proteins are located in the cytoplasm, ubiquitously expressed in fetal and adult tissues, and not secreted (Gray *et al.*, 2009; Semenov & Snyder, 1997), we can reduce the number of candidates. Among the 5 candidates, TMEM88, a 2-transmembrane protein, might be a binding partner of the Dvl PDZ domain because it should be localized in the cell membrane (Fig. 2c). Additional database searches such as GeneCards (http://www.genecards.org/) (Rebhan *et al.*, 1997; Stelzer *et al.*, 2011) and Gene Expression Atlas  (http://www.ebi.ac.uk/gxa) revealed that human TMEM88 is expressed in placenta, spleen, muscle, heart, bone, eye, kidney, and other tissues.

| Database | Website | Comments | Refs. |
|---|---|---|---|
| IMEx | http://www.imexconsortium.org | A non-redundant set of PPI data from a broad taxonomic range of organisms, which were curated from direct submissions or peer-reviewed journals. | Orchard *et al.*, 2012 |
| HIPPIE | http://cbdm.mdc-berlin.de/tools/hippie | Integrating PPI networks with experiment based quality scores. | Schaefer *et al.*, 2012 |
| STRING | http://string-db.org | Functional protein association networks. | Szklarczyk *et al.*, 2011 |
| PIPs | http://www.compbio.dundee.ac.uk/www-pips | Human PPI prediction database. | McDowall *et al.*, 2009 |
| DOMINO | http://mint.bio.uniroma2.it/domino/ | An open-access database comprising 3,900 annotated experiments describing PPIs. | Ceol *et al.*, 2007 |
| PDZBase | http://icb.med.cornell.edu/services/pdz/start | A manually curated PPI database developed specifically for PDZ PPIs. . | Beuming *et al.*, 2005 |
| I2D | http://ophid.utoronto.ca/ophidv2.201/index.jsp | Database of known and predicted mammalian and eukaryotic PPIs. | Brown & Jurisica, 2005 |

**Table 1:**  PPI Databases

Meanwhile, we also searched for PPI databases, such as I2D (Brown & Jurisica, 2005) and PDZBase that is a manually curated PPI database developed specifically for interactions involving PDZ domains (Beuming *et al.*, 2005), and for literature to ascertain possible binding partners of Dvl and found that no PPIs were reported (Table 1). This suggested that the interaction of TMEM88 and Dvl might be novel. During the course of this work, (Stiffler *et al.*, 2007) predicted 18,149 PDZ-peptide interactions from PDZ microarrays. Among them, 710 proteins were proposed to be binding partners for the Dvl PDZ domain, and TMEM88 was predicted to be a Dvl-3 PDZ binding protein. However, no other proteins predicted in this study were found. After this work, (Liu *et al.*, 2012) also predicted that TMEM88 was a Dvl-binding protein by using a web-based tool, "Sequence-based Protein Partner Search (http://mdl.shsmu.edu.cn/SPPS/)". Taken together, text-mining of the literature and prediction of PPI partners from web-based tools would be useful to make a further decision and guide researchers to design experiments.

## 2.3   Reanalysis of Microarray Data

Microarrays can monitor the expression of thousands of genes simultaneously to study the effects of drugs, developmental stages, or diseases (Kapushesky *et al.*, 2012; Parkinson *et al.*, 2011). As databases of gene expression profiles have increased dramatically in number and scope (Kapushesky *et al.*, 2012), we believe that a comprehensive analysis of microarray databases further facilitated the assessment of the function of a targeted gene. In this study, we downloaded raw data from a public database, GEO (http://www.ncbi.nlm.nih.gov/geo/), to find any correlation between *TMEM88* and Wnt signaling–related genes. We analyzed three embryonic mouse tissues, cardiac (GEO number: GSE1479), colon (GEO number: GSE5261), and small intestines (GEO number: GSE6383), because they had high TMEM88 expression and replicates. The analysis was performed on current Affymetrix GeneChip mouse genome 430 2.0 arrays. To stabilize variance, the MAS 5.0 signal was natural log-start transformed by the following formula: lin(MAS 5.0 signal +20). The transformed expression of each probe set on the array was correlated linearly with the transformed signal of *TMEM88* by using Pearson's coefficient ($\varrho$) using a script written for STATA software (version 10.1, College Station, TX) for each of the experiments. In brief, a correlation sums of the gene expression differences between any two genes across multiple arrays and then divides that sum by the total number of array experiments examined to give the Pearson's $\varrho$. $\varrho$ values, which measure the degree of association between variables, range from -1 to 1 (Lee *et al.*, 2010). The Pearson correlations of *TMEM88* with the upstream components of Wnt signaling were examined, showing strong Pearson correlations of *TMEM88* expression with that of several Wnt signaling–related genes in the embryonic small intestines: *Fzd1* ($\varrho$= 1.00), *Fzd2* ($\varrho$ = 1.00), *Fzd7* ($\varrho$ = 0.86), *Fzd9* ($\varrho$ = 0.90), *Frzb* ($\varrho$ = 0.89), *Dvl1* ($\varrho$ = 0.82), *Dvl2* ($\varrho$ = 0.89), and *Dvl3* ($\varrho$ = 0.92). We also observed modest Pearson correlations between the expression of *TMEM88* and that of the following Wnt signaling–related genes in other tissues: in embryonic mouse cardiac tissue, *ROR1* ($\varrho$ = 0.61); and in the colon, *Fzd1* ($\varrho$ = − 0.67), *Fzd2* ($\varrho$ = −0.49), and *Frzb* ($\varrho$ = −0.63). These findings suggest that *TMEM88* modulate Wnt signaling–related gene expression in a context-dependent manner.

## 2.4   Verification of PPI *in vitro*

On the basis of database screening and analysis and text-mining from the literature, we rationalized that TMEM88 might be a Dvl-binding partner and function in Wnt signaling. To verify and characterize the interaction of two proteins, TMEM88 and Dvl, we chemically synthesized a peptide derived from the C terminus of TMEM88 (TMEM88C, GSRSVPTPGKVWV, residues 147-159). We added TMEM88C peptide gradually into the uniformly $^{15}$N-labeled PDZ domain of Dvl-1 and recorded the $^{1}$H,$^{15}$N-heteronuclear single quantum coherence spectra. Some peaks disappeared and reappeared during the titration, suggesting that the binding is in the intermediate state on the NMR time scale (Pellecchia *et al.*, 2002). The result revealed that TMEM88C binds to the conventional peptide-binding groove in the Dvl-1 PDZ domain as expected. We compared the chemical-shift perturbations ($\Delta\delta_{binding}$) of the $^{15}$N Dvl PDZ domain caused by the binding of VWV tripeptide or that of the TMEM88C peptide, showing that the difference of $\Delta\delta_{binding}$ ($\Delta\Delta\delta_{binding}$) of the Dvl-1 PDZ domain for the 2 bound peptides was less than 0.03. The result showed that the last 3 residues at the extreme C terminus of TMEM88 would be crucial to determine the binding. We also performed the fluorescence experiment to get the binding affinity of Dvl PDZ to the TMEM88C and VWV peptides. We used an excitation wavelength of 280 nm and an emission wavelength of 360 nm to record the Trp fluorescent polarization of the Val-Trp-Val tripeptide and TMEM88C. The Trp fluorescence polarization data were measured during the titration of the Dvl1 PDZ domain and analyzed by Prism software (GraphPad, Inc.). The results showed that two peptides have a similar binding affinity. Together, biophysical methods such as NMR and fluorescence supported the interaction of TMEM88 and Dvl protein *in vitro*. We thus designed cell-based assays and *Xenopus* assays to characterize the PPI and the TMEM88 function.

## 2.5    Gain-of-function of TMEM88 on Wnt Signaling by Cell-based Assays

Since a direct interaction of the Dvl PDZ domain and the internal sequence of Fz protein is essential to activate Wnt signaling (Umbhauer *et al.*, 2000; Wong *et al.*, 2003), we reasoned that if TMEM88 binds to the Dvl PDZ domain in cells, then overexpressing TMEM88 might disrupt the Dvl-Fz interaction at the plasma membrane region, which, in turn, would suppress Wnt/β-catenin signaling. To test this hypothesis, we conducted a luciferase-based cell assay (Wong *et al.*, 2000). In HEK293 cells transfected with Wnt-1 plasmid, canonical Wnt signaling was activated, and luciferase activity was increased (Wong *et al.*, 2000). When TMEM88 was co-expressed with Wnt-1 in the HEK293 cells, Wnt-1–induced activation of Lef-1 was attenuated. The increased amount of TMEM88 expression plasmid resulted in substantial attenuation of Wnt-1–induced Lef-1 activity, suggesting that TMEM88 protein blocks Wnt signaling. To confirm this finding, we did the same experiment with TMEM88-ΔC4, which lacks 4 amino acid residues at the extreme C terminus. The loss of the PDZ-binding motif of TMEM88 caused little inhibitory effect on Wnt-1–induced signaling in a dose-dependent manner, indicating that the binding of TMEM88 to the Dvl-1 PDZ domain is essential to block Wnt signaling.

## 2.6    Loss-of-function of TMEM88 on Wnt Signaling by using RNA Interference Technique

To verify the role of TMEM88 in Wnt signaling, we designed a negative control experiment by using a TMEM88 RNA interference (RNAi) technique that can knock down expression of a specific gene (Fire *et al.*, 1998). On the basis of the expression profile of TMEM88, a few cell lines, such as IEC-6 (small intestine cell line), MRC-9 (lung cell line), or HEK293 (normal kidney cell line), might be candidates for further study. In this work, we chose the HEK293 cell line because this cell lines carry no known mutations in Wnt signaling components, because TMEM88 can inhibit Wnt-1–induced signaling in dose-dependent manner in this cell line, and because this cell-based assay is well-established in our collaborative laboratory. We treated TMEM88 RNAi to prevent endogenous expression of TMEM88 protein in HEK293 cells to investigate the effect of TMEM88 knockdown on Wnt activity. We preformed the luciferase report assay and found that luciferase reporter activity was more than 2-fold greater than that in the control. The result supported that endogenous TMEM88 indeed inhibits the canonical Wnt signaling in HEK293 cells.

## 2.7     Subcellular Localization of TMEM88 in *Xenopus*

Although TMEM88 was predicted to be a membrane protein, there was no direct evidence. We thus examined the subcellular distribution of TMEM88 in a *Xenopus* embryo system. We generated a fusion of the myc-epitope to the N-terminal region of TMEM88, myc-tagged TMEM88, and injected the mRNA of myc-tagged TMEM88 into the animal pole region of *Xenopus* embryos at the 4-cell stage. Animal cap explants were dissected at the late blastula stage and fixed. Then, immunofluorescent stainings were performed, and localization of myc-TMEM88 protein in *Xenopus* was examined by fluorescence confocal microscopy. As predicted, myc-TMEM88 proteins were essentially localized to the cell membrane, confirming that TMEM88 is a membrane protein.

## 2.8     Interaction of TMEM88 and Dvl Protein in *Xenopus*

Although TMEM88 is localized at the cell membrane, the question was raised whether the location of the N- and C-termini of human TMEM88 is in cytoplasm, although cell-based assays suggested that the C-terminal of TMEM88 is in the cytoplasmic region. We examined the effect of TMEM88 on the subcellular distribution of Dsh-GFP in *Xenopus* to confirm the interaction of TMEM88 with Dvl/Dsh.   Dsh-GFP was found in a punctuate, cytoplasm distribution in animal cap cells (Rothbacher *et al.*, 2000). Co-injection of TMEM88 leads to the recruitment of Dsh-GFP to the cell membrane, implying that the last C-terminal region of TMEM88 is located in the cytoplasmic region. To verify this finding, we generated TMEM88-ΔC that lacks the PDZ binding motif at the C-terminus and injected it along with Dsh-GFP mRNA. As expected, TMEM88-ΔC failed to recruit Dsh-GFP to the cell membrane, supporting that TMEM88 binds to Dvl protein through its last C-terminus residues in the cytoplasmic region.

## 2.9     Gain-of-function of TMEM88 in Wnt Signaling by using *Xenopus* Assays

Since the TMEM88 binds to Dvl, we further studied the role of TMEM88 in Wnt signaling in the *Xenopus* system. To confirm that TMEM88 blocks Wnt-1 induced signaling at the level of Dvl, we overexpressed Xdsh or β-catenin proteins without or with TMEM88 (Grandy *et al.*, 2009; Umbhauer *et al.*, 2000; Wong *et al.*, 2000). *Xenopus* Wnt target gene Siamois' promoter-driven luciferase reporter construct was injected alone or with synthetic Xdsh mRNA, Xdsh mRNA together with myc-tagged TMEM88 mRNA, β-catenin mRNA, or β-catenin mRNA plus myc-tagged TMEM88 mRNA in the animal pole region at the 2-cell stage (Grandy *et al.*, 2009; Lee *et al.*, 2009b).   Injected embryos were cultured, animal cap explants were dissected at the late-blastula stage, and luciferase assays were performed. Consistent with the results of the cell-based assays and binding data, TMEM88 inhibited Siamois promoter–driven luciferase activity induced by Xdsh but not by β-catenin, indicating that TMEM88 inhibits canonical Wnt signaling at the level of Xdsh.

To verify the role of TMEM88 in canonical Wnt signaling, we used the *Xenopus* secondary axis assay (Wong *et al.*, 2003). Xdsh mRNA injected into the ventro-vegetal region of a *Xenopus* ectodermal explant at the 4-cell stage induced a complete secondary axis in about 30% of *Xenopus* embryos and a partial secondary axis in about 40%. Co-injection of embryos with equal amounts of mRNAs of Xdsh and myc-tagged TMEM88 abolished the formation of a complete secondary axis, and only about 30% of embryos formed a partial secondary axis. The data also suggest that TMEM88 can negatively regulate canonical Wnt signaling.

## 2.10    Implication of TMEM88 functions in Disease

*TMEM88* may play an important role in diseases, including cancers. The human *TMEM88* gene is mapped to chromosome 17p13.1, from position 7,699,108 to 7,700,142 (Ensembl database). Several studies have shown that the loss of heterozygosity at 17p13.1 appears to be associated with an adverse disease course (Chang *et al.*, 2004; Cousin *et al.*, 2000; Dolan *et al.*, 1999; Flavin *et al.*, 2009; Jung *et al.*, 2004). Although most of these analyses addressed the role of *TP53*, further study of *TMEM88* may be interesting because the 2 genes between TP53 and TMEM88 are separated by only about 200 kb.

A recent study showed that down regulation of TMEM88 expression is related to non-small cell lung cancer (Jang *et al.*, 2012). They analyzed the mRNA and microRNA (miRNA) expression profiles in matched lung adenocarcinoma and uninvolved lung tissues and found that TMEM88 expression was downregulated by miRNA-708 expression in non-small cell lung cancer. They found that the increased TMEM88 expression appeared to reduce the overall risk of death in lung adenocarcinoma in patients who never smoked. In addition, the TMEM88 mRNA level is directly inhibited by overexpression of miRNA-708 in transduced cells. Given that overexpression of Dvl has been reported in non-small cell lung cancer (Wei *et al.*, 2008; Zhao *et al.*, 2010), it will be fascinating to investigate the role of TMEM88 as a Dvl-binding protein in cancer in more detail.

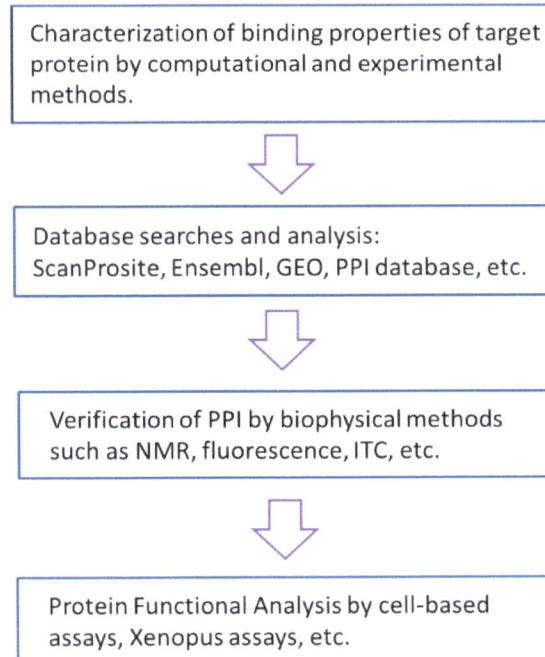

**Figure 2:** An overview of a combinatorial approach to find binding partners for a given protein

# 3   Conclusion

We identified a novel binding partner for a given protein by using a combinatorial approach (Figure 2). We showed that knowledge of the binding motif that is essential to bind a target protein is required to search for the uncharacterized protein. Bioinformatics can be used to search for the protein that contains the binding motif. Meanwhile, PPI databases can be searched to find clues from the literature and predict PPIs. The putative interaction should be confirmed by independent methods to design further studies. Gain- and loss-of-function experiments using cell-based assays and *Xenopus* assays may be performed to uncover the function of PPIs (Lee *et al.*, 2010).

Since most proteins function through interaction with partners, elucidation of PPIs in genome-wide analyses provides valuable insight into understanding molecular biology. In spite of extensive studies of PPIs using advanced tools, researchers need to use caution to curate PPI information from the literature because of high false-positive or -negative results and thus should verify and characterize PPIs using various methods, which is critical to discovering novel functions of a given protein (Lee & Zheng, 2010). However, given that the PPI information from different experimental methods has been deposited in a number of curated databases (Orchard *et al.*, 2012) and the analysis tools to evaluate the PPI information have been developed (Schaefer *et al.*, 2012; Szklarczyk *et al.*, 2011), we expect that integrative *in silico* analysis from several sources can enhance our ability to discover novel PPIs that will help to reveal their biological activity in normal and cancer cells.

# References

Aebersold, R., & Mann, M. (2003). Mass spectrometry-based proteomics. Nature, 422(6928), 198-207.

Angers, S., & Moon, R. T. (2009). Proximal events in Wnt signal transduction. Nat Rev Mol Cell Biol, 10(7), 468-477.

Appleton, B. A., Zhang, Y., Wu, P., Yin, J. P., Hunziker, W., Skelton, N. J., Sidhu, S. S., & Wiesmann, C. (2006). Comparative structural analysis of the Erbin PDZ domain and the first PDZ domain of ZO-1. Insights into determinants of PDZ domain specificity. J Biol Chem, 281(31), 22312-22320.

Beuming, T., Skrabanek, L., Niv, M. Y., Mukherjee, P., & Weinstein, H. (2005). PDZBase: a protein-protein interaction database for PDZ-domains. Bioinformatics, 21(6), 827-828.

Brown, K. R., & Jurisica, I. (2005). Online predicted human interaction database. Bioinformatics, 21(9), 2076-2082.

Ceol, A., Chatr-aryamontri, A., Santonico, E., Sacco, R., Castagnoli, L., & Cesareni, G. (2007). DOMINO: a database of domain-peptide interactions. Nucleic Acids Res, 35(Database issue), D557-560.

Chang, H., Sloan, S., Li, D., & Keith Stewart, A. (2004). Multiple myeloma involving central nervous system: high frequency of chromosome 17p13.1 (p53) deletions. Br J Haematol, 127(3), 280-284.

Cheyette, B. N., Waxman, J. S., Miller, J. R., Takemaru, K., Sheldahl, L. C., Khlebtsova, N., Fox, E. P., Earnest, T., & Moon, R. T. (2002). Dapper, a Dishevelled-associated antagonist of beta-catenin and JNK signaling, is required for notochord formation. Dev Cell, 2(4), 449-461.

Cousin, P., Billotte, J., Chaubert, P., & Shaw, P. (2000). Physical map of 17p13 and the genes adjacent to p53. Genomics, 63(1), 60-68.

de Castro, E., Sigrist, C. J., Gattiker, A., Bulliard, V., Langendijk-Genevaux, P. S., Gasteiger, E., Bairoch, A., & Hulo, N. (2006). ScanProsite: detection of PROSITE signature matches and ProRule-associated functional and structural residues in proteins. Nucleic Acids Res, 34(Web Server issue), W362-365.

Dolan, K., Garde, J., Walker, S. J., Sutton, R., Gosney, J., & Field, J. K. (1999). LOH at the sites of the DCC, APC, and TP53 tumor suppressor genes occurs in Barrett's metaplasia and dysplasia adjacent to adenocarcinoma of the esophagus. Hum Pathol, 30(12), 1508-1514.

Eker, F., Cao, X., Nafie, L., & Schweitzer-Stenner, R. (2002). Tripeptides adopt stable structures in water. A combined polarized visible Raman, FTIR, and VCD spectroscopy study. J Am Chem Soc, 124(48), 14330-14341.

Eker, F., Griebenow, K., Cao, X., Nafie, L. A., & Schweitzer-Stenner, R. (2004a). Preferred peptide backbone conformations in the unfolded state revealed by the structure analysis of alanine-based (AXA) tripeptides in aqueous solution. Proc Natl Acad Sci U S A, 101(27), 10054-10059.

Eker, F., Griebenow, K., Cao, X., Nafie, L. A., & Schweitzer-Stenner, R. (2004b). Tripeptides with ionizable side chains adopt a perturbed polyproline II structure in water. Biochemistry, 43(3), 613-621.

Eker, F., Griebenow, K., & Schweitzer-Stenner, R. (2003). Stable conformations of tripeptides in aqueous solution studied by UV circular dichroism spectroscopy. J Am Chem Soc, 125(27), 8178-8185.

Ernst, A., Gfeller, D., Kan, Z., Seshagiri, S., Kim, P. M., Bader, G. D., & Sidhu, S. S. (2010). Coevolution of PDZ domain-ligand interactions analyzed by high-throughput phage display and deep sequencing. Mol Biosyst, 6(10), 1782-1790.

Fire, A., Xu, S., Montgomery, M. K., Kostas, S. A., Driver, S. E., & Mello, C. C. (1998). Potent and specific genetic interference by double-stranded RNA in Caenorhabditis elegans. Nature, 391(6669), 806-811.

Flavin, R. J., Smyth, P. C., Laios, A., O'Toole, S. A., Barrett, C., Finn, S. P., Russell, S., Ring, M., Denning, K. M., Li, J., Aherne, S. T., Sammarae, D. A., Aziz, N. A., Alhadi, A., Sheppard, B. L., Lao, K., Sheils, O. M., & O'Leary, J. J. (2009). Potentially important microRNA cluster on chromosome 17p13.1 in primary peritoneal carcinoma. Mod Pathol, 22(2), 197-205.

Gao, C., & Chen, Y. G. (2010). Dishevelled: The hub of Wnt signaling. Cell Signal, 22(5), 717-727.

Gfeller, D., Butty, F., Wierzbicka, M., Verschueren, E., Vanhee, P., Huang, H., Ernst, A., Dar, N., Stagljar, I., Serrano, L., Sidhu, S. S., Bader, G. D., & Kim, P. M. (2011). The multiple-specificity landscape of modular peptide recognition domains. Mol Syst Biol, 7, 484.

Grandy, D., Shan, J., Zhang, X., Rao, S., Akunuru, S., Li, H., Zhang, Y., Alpatov, I., Zhang, X. A., Lang, R. A., Shi, D. L., & Zheng, J. J. (2009). Discovery and characterization of a small molecule inhibitor of the PDZ domain of dishevelled. J Biol Chem, 284(24), 16256-16263.

Gray, R. S., Bayly, R. D., Green, S. A., Agarwala, S., Lowe, C. J., & Wallingford, J. B. (2009). Diversification of the expression patterns and developmental functions of the dishevelled gene family during chordate evolution. Dev Dyn, 238(8), 2044-2057.

Hagarman, A., Measey, T., Doddasomayajula, R. S., Dragomir, I., Eker, F., Griebenow, K., & Schweitzer-Stenner, R. (2006). Conformational analysis of XA and AX dipeptides in water by electronic circular dichroism and 1H NMR spectroscopy. J Phys Chem B, 110(13), 6979-6986.

Hawkins, J. C., Zhu, H., Teyra, J., & Pisabarro, M. T. (2012). Reduced False Positives in PDZ Binding Prediction using Sequence and Structural Descriptors. IEEE/ACM Trans Comput Biol Bioinform.

Jang, J., Jeon, H. S., Sun, Z., Aubry, M. C., Tang, H., Park, C. H., Rakhshan, F., Schultz, D. A., Kolbert, C. P., Lupu, R., Park, J. Y., Harris, C. C., Yang, P., & Jin, J. (2012). Increased miR-708 Expression in NSCLC and Its Association with Poor Survival in Lung Adenocarcinoma from Never Smokers. Clin Cancer Res, 18(13), 3658-3667.

Jung, H. L., Wang, K. C., Kim, S. K., Sung, K. W., Koo, H. H., Shin, H. Y., Ahn, H. S., Shin, H. J., & Cho, B. K. (2004). Loss of heterozygosity analysis of chromosome 17p13.1-13.3 and its correlation with clinical outcome in medulloblastomas. J Neurooncol, 67(1-2), 41-46.

Kannengiesser, K., Maaser, C., Heidemann, J., Luegering, A., Ross, M., Brzoska, T., Bohm, M., Luger, T. A., Domschke, W., & Kucharzik, T. (2008). Melanocortin-derived tripeptide KPV has anti-inflammatory potential in murine models of inflammatory bowel disease. Inflamm Bowel Dis, 14(3), 324-331.

Kapushesky, M., Adamusiak, T., Burdett, T., Culhane, A., Farne, A., Filippov, A., Holloway, E., Klebanov, A., Kryvych, N., Kurbatova, N., Kurnosov, P., Malone, J., Melnichuk, O., Petryszak, R., Pultsin, N., Rustici, G., Tikhonov, A., Travillian, R. S., Williams, E., Zorin, A., Parkinson, H., & Brazma, A. (2012). Gene Expression Atlas update--a value-added database of microarray and sequencing-based functional genomics experiments. Nucleic Acids Res, 40(Database issue), D1077-1081.

Kaushansky, A., Allen, J. E., Gordus, A., Stiffler, M. A., Karp, E. S., Chang, B. H., & MacBeath, G. (2010). Quantifying protein-protein interactions in high throughput using protein domain microarrays. Nat Protoc, 5(4), 773-790.

Lee, H. J., Finkelstein, D., Li, X., Wu, D., Shi, D. L., & Zheng, J. J. (2010). Identification of transmembrane protein 88 (TMEM88) as a dishevelled-binding protein. J Biol Chem, 285(53), 41549-41556.

Lee, H. J., Park, H. M., & Lee, K. B. (2007). The beta-turn scaffold of tripeptide containing an azaphenylalanine residue. Biophys Chem, 125(1), 117-126.

Lee, H. J., Wang, N. X., Shao, Y., & Zheng, J. J. (2009a). Identification of tripeptides recognized by the PDZ domain of Dishevelled. Bioorg Med Chem, 17(4), 1701-1708.

Lee, H. J., Wang, N. X., Shi, D. L., & Zheng, J. J. (2009b). Sulindac inhibits canonical Wnt signaling by blocking the PDZ domain of the protein Dishevelled. Angew Chem Int Ed Engl, 48(35), 6448-6452.

Lee, H. J., & Zheng, J. J. (2010). PDZ domains and their binding partners: structure, specificity, and modification. Cell Commun Signal, 8, 8.

Liu, X., Liu, B., Huang, Z., Shi, T., Chen, Y., & Zhang, J. (2012). SPPS: a sequence-based method for predicting probability of protein-protein interaction partners. PLoS One, 7(1), e30938.

McDowall, M. D., Scott, M. S., & Barton, G. J. (2009). PIPs: human protein-protein interaction prediction database. Nucleic Acids Res, 37(Database issue), D651-656.

Orchard, S., Kerrien, S., Abbani, S., Aranda, B., Bhate, J., Bidwell, S., Bridge, A., Briganti, L., Brinkman, F. S., Cesareni, G., Chatr-aryamontri, A., Chautard, E., Chen, C., Dumousseau, M., Goll, J., Hancock, R. E., Hannick, L. I., Jurisica, I., Khadake, J., Lynn, D. J., Mahadevan, U., Perfetto, L., Raghunath, A., Ricard-Blum, S., Roechert, B., Salwinski, L., Stumpflen, V., Tyers, M., Uetz, P., Xenarios, I., & Hermjakob, H. (2012). Protein interaction data curation: the International Molecular Exchange (IMEx) consortium. Nat Methods, 9(4), 345-350.

Pan, W. J., Pang, S. Z., Huang, T., Guo, H. Y., Wu, D., & Li, L. (2004). Characterization of function of three domains in dishevelled-1: DEP domain is responsible for membrane translocation of dishevelled-1. Cell Res, 14(4), 324-330.

Park, T. J., Gray, R. S., Sato, A., Habas, R., & Wallingford, J. B. (2005). Subcellular localization and signaling properties of dishevelled in developing vertebrate embryos. Curr Biol, 15(11), 1039-1044.

Parkinson, H., Sarkans, U., Kolesnikov, N., Abeygunawardena, N., Burdett, T., Dylag, M., Emam, I., Farne, A., Hastings, E., Holloway, E., Kurbatova, N., Lukk, M., Malone, J., Mani, R., Pilicheva, E., Rustici, G., Sharma, A., Williams, E., Adamusiak, T., Brandizi, M., Sklyar, N., & Brazma, A. (2011). ArrayExpress update--an archive of microarray and high-throughput sequencing-based functional genomics experiments. Nucleic Acids Res, 39(Database issue), D1002-1004.

Pawson, T., & Nash, P. (2003). Assembly of cell regulatory systems through protein interaction domains. Science, 300(5618), 445-452.

Pellecchia, M., Sem, D. S., & Wuthrich, K. (2002). NMR in drug discovery. Nat Rev Drug Discov, 1(3), 211-219.

Phizicky, E. M., & Fields, S. (1995). Protein-protein interactions: methods for detection and analysis. Microbiol Rev, 59(1), 94-123.

Rebhan, M., Chalifa-Caspi, V., Prilusky, J., & Lancet, D. (1997). GeneCards: integrating information about genes, proteins and diseases. Trends Genet, 13(4), 163.

Rifai, Y., Elder, A. S., Carati, C. J., Hussey, D. J., Li, X., Woods, C. M., Schloithe, A. C., Thomas, A. C., Mathison, R. D., Davison, J. S., Toouli, J., & Saccone, G. T. (2008). The tripeptide analog feG ameliorates severity of acute pancreatitis in a caerulein mouse model. Am J Physiol Gastrointest Liver Physiol, 294(4), G1094-1099.

Rothbacher, U., Laurent, M. N., Deardorff, M. A., Klein, P. S., Cho, K. W., & Fraser, S. E. (2000). Dishevelled phosphorylation, subcellular localization and multimerization regulate its role in early embryogenesis. EMBO J, 19(5), 1010-1022.

Runyon, S. T., Zhang, Y., Appleton, B. A., Sazinsky, S. L., Wu, P., Pan, B., Wiesmann, C., Skelton, N. J., & Sidhu, S. S. (2007). Structural and functional analysis of the PDZ domains of human HtrA1 and HtrA3. Protein Sci, 16(11), 2454-2471.

Sakurai, M., Aoki, T., Yoshikawa, S., Santschi, L. A., Saito, H., Endo, K., Ishikawa, K., Kimura, K., Ito, K., Thomas, J. B., & Hama, C. (2009). Differentially expressed Drl and Drl-2 play opposing roles in Wnt5 signaling during Drosophila olfactory system development. J Neurosci, 29(15), 4972-4980.

Schaefer, M. H., Fontaine, J. F., Vinayagam, A., Porras, P., Wanker, E. E., & Andrade-Navarro, M. A. (2012). HIPPIE: Integrating protein interaction networks with experiment based quality scores. PLoS One, 7(2), e31826.

Schapira, M., Totrov, M., & Abagyan, R. (1999). Prediction of the binding energy for small molecules, peptides and proteins. J Mol Recognit, 12(3), 177-190.

Schwarz-Romond, T., Fiedler, M., Shibata, N., Butler, P. J., Kikuchi, A., Higuchi, Y., & Bienz, M. (2007a). The DIX domain of Dishevelled confers Wnt signaling by dynamic polymerization. Nat Struct Mol Biol, 14(6), 484-492.

Schwarz-Romond, T., Metcalfe, C., & Bienz, M. (2007b). Dynamic recruitment of axin by Dishevelled protein assemblies. J Cell Sci, 120(Pt 14), 2402-2412.

Schweitzer-Stenner, R., Eker, F., Perez, A., Griebenow, K., Cao, X., & Nafie, L. A. (2003). The structure of tri-proline in water probed by polarized Raman, Fourier transform infrared, vibrational circular dichroism, and electric ultraviolet circular dichroism spectroscopy. Biopolymers, 71(5), 558-568.

Schweitzer-Stenner, R., Measey, T., Hagarman, A., Eker, F., & Griebenow, K. (2006). Salmon calcitonin and amyloid beta: two peptides with amyloidogenic capacity adopt different conformational manifolds in their unfolded states. Biochemistry, 45(9), 2810-2819.

Semenov, M. V., & Snyder, M. (1997). Human dishevelled genes constitute a DHR-containing multigene family. Genomics, 42(2), 302-310.

Shan, J., Shi, D. L., Wang, J., & Zheng, J. (2005). Identification of a specific inhibitor of the dishevelled PDZ domain. Biochemistry, 44(47), 15495-15503.

Simons, M., Gault, W. J., Gotthardt, D., Rohatgi, R., Klein, T. J., Shao, Y., Lee, H. J., Wu, A. L., Fang, Y., Satlin, L. M., Dow, J. T., Chen, J., Zheng, J., Boutros, M., & Mlodzik, M. (2009). Electrochemical cues regulate assembly of the Frizzled/Dishevelled complex at the plasma membrane during planar epithelial polarization. Nat Cell Biol, 11(3), 286-294.

Skelton, N. J., Koehler, M. F., Zobel, K., Wong, W. L., Yeh, S., Pisabarro, M. T., Yin, J. P., Lasky, L. A., & Sidhu, S. S. (2003). Origins of PDZ domain ligand specificity. Structure determination and mutagenesis of the Erbin PDZ domain. J Biol Chem, 278(9), 7645-7654.

Stelzer, G., Dalah, I., Stein, T. I., Satanower, Y., Rosen, N., Nativ, N., Oz-Levi, D., Olender, T., Belinky, F., Bahir, I., Krug, H., Perco, P., Mayer, B., Kolker, E., Safran, M., & Lancet, D. (2011). In-silico human genomics with GeneCards. Hum Genomics, 5(6), 709-717.

Stiffler, M. A., Chen, J. R., Grantcharova, V. P., Lei, Y., Fuchs, D., Allen, J. E., Zaslavskaia, L. A., & MacBeath, G. (2007). PDZ domain binding selectivity is optimized across the mouse proteome. Science, 317(5836), 364-369.

Szklarczyk, D., Franceschini, A., Kuhn, M., Simonovic, M., Roth, A., Minguez, P., Doerks, T., Stark, M., Muller, J., Bork, P., Jensen, L. J., & von Mering, C. (2011). The STRING database in 2011: functional interaction networks of proteins, globally integrated and scored. Nucleic Acids Res, 39(Database issue), D561-568.

Tauriello, D. V., Jordens, I., Kirchner, K., Slootstra, J. W., Kruitwagen, T., Bouwman, B. A., Noutsou, M., Rudiger, S. G., Schwamborn, K., Schambony, A., & Maurice, M. M. (2012). Wnt/beta-catenin signaling requires interaction of the Dishevelled DEP domain and C terminus with a discontinuous motif in Frizzled. Proc Natl Acad Sci U S A, 109(14), E812-820.

Tonikian, R., Zhang, Y., Sazinsky, S. L., Currell, B., Yeh, J. H., Reva, B., Held, H. A., Appleton, B. A., Evangelista, M., Wu, Y., Xin, X., Chan, A. C., Seshagiri, S., Lasky, L. A., Sander, C., Boone, C., Bader, G. D., & Sidhu, S. S. (2008). A specificity map for the PDZ domain family. PLoS Biol, 6(9), e239.

Umbhauer, M., Djiane, A., Goisset, C., Penzo-Mendez, A., Riou, J. F., Boucaut, J. C., & Shi, D. L. (2000). The C-terminal cytoplasmic Lys-thr-X-X-X-Trp motif in frizzled receptors mediates Wnt/beta-catenin signalling. EMBO J, 19(18), 4944-4954.

Wallingford, J. B., & Habas, R. (2005). The developmental biology of Dishevelled: an enigmatic protein governing cell fate and cell polarity. Development, 132(20), 4421-4436.

Wang, N. X., Lee, H. J., & Zheng, J. J. (2008). Therapeutic use of PDZ protein-protein interaction antagonism. Drug News Perspect, 21(3), 137-141.

Wang, W., Donini, O., Reyes, C. M., & Kollman, P. A. (2001). Biomolecular simulations: recent developments in force fields, simulations of enzyme catalysis, protein-ligand, protein-protein, and protein-nucleic acid noncovalent interactions. Annu Rev Biophys Biomol Struct, 30, 211-243.

Wei, Q., Zhao, Y., Yang, Z. Q., Dong, Q. Z., Dong, X. J., Han, Y., Zhao, C., & Wang, E. H. (2008). Dishevelled family proteins are expressed in non-small cell lung cancer and function differentially on tumor progression. Lung Cancer, 62(2), 181-192.

Wharton, K. A., Jr. (2003). Runnin' with the Dvl: proteins that associate with Dsh/Dvl and their significance to Wnt signal transduction. Dev Biol, 253(1), 1-17.

Wong, H. C., Bourdelas, A., Krauss, A., Lee, H. J., Shao, Y., Wu, D., Mlodzik, M., Shi, D. L., & Zheng, J. (2003). Direct binding of the PDZ domain of Dishevelled to a conserved internal sequence in the C-terminal region of Frizzled. Mol Cell, 12(5), 1251-1260.

Wong, H. C., Mao, J., Nguyen, J. T., Srinivas, S., Zhang, W., Liu, B., Li, L., Wu, D., & Zheng, J. (2000). Structural basis of the recognition of the dishevelled DEP domain in the Wnt signaling pathway. Nat Struct Biol, 7(12), 1178-1184.

Yip, K. Y., Utz, L., Sitwell, S., Hu, X., Sidhu, S. S., Turk, B. E., Gerstein, M., & Kim, P. M. (2011). Identification of specificity determining residues in peptide recognition domains using an information theoretic approach applied to large-scale binding maps. BMC Biol, 9, 53.

Yoshikawa, S., McKinnon, R. D., Kokel, M., & Thomas, J. B. (2003). Wnt-mediated axon guidance via the Drosophila Derailed receptor. Nature, 422(6932), 583-588.

Zeng, X., Huang, H., Tamai, K., Zhang, X., Harada, Y., Yokota, C., Almeida, K., Wang, J., Doble, B., Woodgett, J., Wynshaw-Boris, A., Hsieh, J. C., & He, X. (2008). Initiation of Wnt signaling: control of Wnt coreceptor Lrp6 phosphorylation/activation via frizzled, dishevelled and axin functions. Development, 135(2), 367-375.

Zhang, Q. C., Petrey, D., Deng, L., Qiang, L., Shi, Y., Thu, C. A., Bisikirska, B., Lefebvre, C., Accili, D., Hunter, T., Maniatis, T., Califano, A., & Honig, B. (2012). Structure-based prediction of protein-protein interactions on a genome-wide scale. Nature.

Zhao, Y., Yang, Z. Q., Wang, Y., Miao, Y., Liu, Y., Dai, S. D., Han, Y., & Wang, E. H. (2010). Dishevelled-1 and dishevelled-3 affect cell invasion mainly through canonical and noncanonical Wnt pathway, respectively, and associate with poor prognosis in nonsmall cell lung cancer. Mol Carcinog, 49(8), 760-770.

www.ingramcontent.com/pod-product-compliance
Lightning Source LLC
Chambersburg PA
CBHW050837220326
41598CB00006B/388

* 9 7 8 1 9 2 2 2 2 7 4 2 3 *